Veterinary
Immunology

Veterinary Immunology

P. M. OUTTERIDGE

CSIRO
McMaster Laboratory
Glebe, New South Wales
Australia

1985

ACADEMIC PRESS

(Harcourt Brace Jovanovich, Publishers)

London   Orlando   San Diego   New York
Toronto   Montreal   Sydney   Tokyo

ACADEMIC PRESS INC. (LONDON) LTD.
24–28 Oval Road
LONDON NW1 7DX

United States Edition published by
ACADEMIC PRESS, INC.
Orlando, Florida 32887

British Library Cataloguing in Publication Data

Outteridge, P. M.
 Veterinary immunology.
 1. Veterinary immunology
 I. Title
 636.089'6079   SF757.2

Library of Congress Cataloging in Publication Data

Outteridge, P. M.
  Veterinary immunology.

  Includes index.
  1. Veterinary immunology. I. Title
 SF757.2.087 1985   636.089'6079   84–14482
 ISBN 0–12–531130–3 (alk. paper)

PRINTED IN THE UNITED STATES OF AMERICA

85 86 87 88   9 8 7 6 5 4 3 2 1

Contents

3   Immunology of Reproduction

4   Immunoglobulins

5 Local Immunity

6 Immunity to Bacteria

7 Immunity to Viruses

viii Contents

8   Immunity to Internal Parasites

9   Immunity to External Parasites

10   Immunogenetics

Appendix of Methods

Glossary   259

Foreword

This book is the first of its kind, and it will fill a position that has been vacant in the immunological literature. The volume deals with modern immunology as it relates to the physiology and diseases of food-producing vertebrates. These have been topics of traditional responsibility for the veterinary medical profession, and Dr. Outteridge's background in veterinary medicine and science gives him an appropriate perspective for writing such a treatise.

Although restricted to the veterinary field, this book offers much information that will be of interest to all immunologists. Investigators in veterinary immunology have some modifications in approach to their subject which differ from those encountered in more conventional experimental immunology. It is an advantage that experiments are performed on the species of ultimate interest. This is in contrast to the more typical problem of relating work on laboratory animals to human health. However, some factors which slow the progress in veterinary immunology are the high cost of purchasing and maintaining experimental animals, the usual lack of genetic controls due to the necessity for research on outbred animals, and, last, the relatively small number of competent research workers in veterinary immunology. Despite these handicaps Dr. Outteridge's book presents a fascinating array of accomplishments in veterinary immunology that will stimulate ideas and perhaps revise old assumptions.

It is appropriate that this book was written by an Australian. A remarkable number of outstanding contributions to immunology have come from scientists in that country. In addition, applied aspects of veterinary immunology are of great value in Australia, where food animal production is an important part of the national economy. Readers will readily appreciate the scientific breadth of this author, who understands the thrust of the "new immunology" for explaining immune phenomena and the translation of that knowledge to the health of animals and the production of wholesome food products.

The author has organized a prodigious and diverse literature into a readable compendium. The presentation assumes that the reader has already gained an introductory knowledge of immunology. Consequently, when topics such as immunoglobulins, cellular immunology, and local immunity are discussed, it is timely for him to emphasize directly the unique aspects of the subjects as they concern species such as sheep, swine, and cattle.

Dr. Outteridge recognizes that problems associated with infection and immunity will continue to dominate veterinary immunology in the foreseeable future. Valuable chapters are presented on diseases caused by bacteria, viruses, internal parasites, and external parasites. Preventive medicine is stressed through the use of immunization procedures and immunodiagnostic testing. This is appropriate to veterinary medicine, where much has been accomplished to protect human health and diminish the loss of animal life, at minimal cost to society. Readers will, no doubt, be surprised at the large number of immunization procedures now in use and the unique techniques used in some situations. In each chapter Dr. Outteridge offers thoughtful ideas on directions for future advances. The possibilities for the preparation of immunizing antigens from synthetic peptides and the use of recombinant DNA technology are examples of work that is currently under way. Chapters on reproduction and immunogenetics deal in part with novel concepts such as a "fecundity vaccine" to increase the ovulation rate of sheep, and use of the genetic linkage between the major histocompatibility complex with *Ir* genes regulating high and low responders to helminth immunization. An appendix dealing with useful variations of immunological methods will be especially valuable to researchers planning work on species such as cattle, sheep, horses, swine, dogs, and cats.

Dr. Outteridge has done an outstanding job in recognizing trends in basic research and indicating ways that the information might be used for answering new questions in veterinary immunology. This book will appeal to several groups of readers. Immunologists will encounter many aspects of comparative immunology about which they may not have been aware. For advanced students and investigators in veterinary immunology, the book presents a wealth of data and references, in addition to revealing areas that need future research.

John W. Osebold
Department of Veterinary Microbiology
School of Veterinary Medicine
University of California, Davis
Davis, California

Preface

This book on Veterinary Immunology is an attempt to cover the subject in its broadest sense. Among the specialised areas which embrace aspects of immunology are bacteriology, virology, parasitology and veterinary medicine, all of which rely on manifestations of the immune response for vaccination or diagnosis.

If there is a bias towards the animals of economic importance in this book it is because it is the author's opinion that immunology has had the greatest impact and promises the most for the future with the animals which provide meat, milk and animal fibres. As an example, a section has been included on the regulation of hormones such as somatostatin and oestrogens by antibodies, since this is a practical application of immunology in the veterinary field which may well increase production in sheep, both in size and in the birth of twin lambs. The book also places some emphasis on the problems in vaccination and diagnosis of economically important diseases such as tuberculosis and Brucellosis of cattle, which involve skin testing and laboratory serology, respectively, but which also provide a great challenge to the veterinary immunologist to find improved techniques which will lead to the complete eradication of these diseases.

There has also been a conscious attempt in this book to describe aspects of immunology which have been proven to be correct for the domestic animals—if you like, an attempt to describe more than just 'dressed-up mouse immunology'. There is a widespread feeling amongst veterinary immunologists that although the findings in mice may be broadly correct, the details for the domestic species may be quite different. An example is the selective concentration of IgG_1 by the ruminant mammary gland, which is different from other species because of the requirement to transfer antibodies to the neonate by the colostrum, a requirement dictated by the unique syndesmochorial placenta in the ruminant species.

In the last three decades we have seen the definition of the cells involved in antibody production, the lymphocytes and plasma cells; the unravelling of the immunoglobulin molecule and its amino-acid sequence; the genetic code for the synthesis of the heavy and light chains of the immunoglobulin molecule and, finally, present-day research on the genetic basis of antibody variability using the techniques of molecular biology. Most of this work has been carried out in the mouse and human cell systems. However, there will no doubt be attempts to manipulate the immune response in the domestic species to correct immunodeficiencies or to alter the genetic potential of individual animals by insertion of new genetic codes into the genome. The subsequent history of veterinary immunology may well be the slow accumulation of data concerning fitness genes which will allow domestic species of animals to survive in areas of the world in which natural disease now prevents their presence.

For the moment, however, there are many problems remaining to be solved in providing the most effective vaccines and in the accurate diagnosis of disease which need to be investigated by basic research into the mechanisms of the immune response of domestic animals. Therefore, this book attempts to describe the currently-accepted ideas in veterinary immunology as well as certain background details in which veterinary immunology has made contributions to basic immunological concepts, such as the immune tolerance in freemartin twin calves. Some sections are short. This is not necessarily a measure of the importance of the topic but a measure of the space available in a book of this size. Other topics, such as autoimmune diseases, have been omitted in line with the general thrust of the book, which is firstly to present details of economically important aspects of immunology and secondly to discuss clinical conditions which can be prevented by vaccination. Autoimmunity falls into neither of these categories. There is also a section on methods, which is by no means exhaustive but which includes many techniques currently used in veterinary research.

I would like to acknowledge friends, colleagues and members of my family who have all helped in the preparation of this book. Acknowledgements are also given to the authors and publishers who gave permission for the use of their illustrations, and they are mentioned individually in the legends to the figures they provided. The author wishes to acknowledge professional colleagues who provided help and encouragement: Dr. Kevin Fahey, Dr. Hugh Gordon, Dr. Frank Nicholas, Dr. Tony Lepper, Dr. Doug Burrell, Dr. David Stewart, Dr. David Emery, Mr. George Merritt and Dr. Chee-Seong Lee. Thanks are also due to Mr. Ian Roper for the preparation of photographs and to my wife, Adèle, and Miss Sandy Bruch for the preparation of line drawings. I would also like to acknowledge the typists, who have worked hard on the manuscript: Mrs. Helen Brown, Mrs. Patricia Dutt, Mrs. Kerry McKillop and Mrs. Clarita Barnes. Special thanks are given to Miss Jill Franklin for obtaining references for use in the book and to the CSIRO, Division of Animal Health, for allowing me to write this book.

Finally, I would like to thank my wife, Adèle, and my children, without whom this book would not have been completed.

Peter M. Outteridge

Veterinary
Immunology

1
Prologue

The general use of vaccines in the veterinary field effectively started with the discoveries of Louis Pasteur in the 1880s which established that living micro-organisms were the cause of disease. Before this time, vaccines against Smallpox in humans had been developed by empirical means using inoculation with Cowpox virus beginning from the era of Edward Jenner in 1778. However, the success of the interspecies immunisation between cow and human with Cowpox virus led to a prolonged period in which it was attempted to immunise cattle against Cattle Plague (Rinderpest) with Cowpox virus, Cowpox with the material obtained from the lesions of Glanders in horses, and dogs against Canine Distemper with Sheep-Pox virus. None of these attempts to cross-immunise with disease material from one species to another was particularly successful, and there was a slow realisation that each species had distinct disease entities which could not generally be used for cross-immunisation.

The one cattle disease which did appear to respond to vaccination with material from other infected cattle was Contagious Bovine Pleuropneumonia. For inoculation against this disease, serous fluid strained out of the lungs of mildly-infected cattle was introduced into superficial incisions on the tip of the tail. Usually, string which had been soaked in the serous fluid was tied around the tail at the point of incision. It was found that this procedure protected about 60% of cattle while 10% died from Pleuropneumonia. The remaining 30% were protected but suffered the side-effect of gangrene of the tail tip, which had to be amputated, producing large numbers of stumpy-tailed cattle as a result of the inoculation. Despite the risk to cattle of death or deformity after inoculation with

1

virulent Pleuropneumonia organisms, the method was used in vaccination campaigns in England and in North America, where the disease was controlled from about 1852. It was not eradicated from North America until 1892, after a system of compensation of owners, testing, quarantine and slaughter of infected animals had been introduced. A similar eradication of disease in Australia was achieved 76 years later, after a vaccination campaign which switched to test and slaughter in the latter stages, resulting in complete eradication of the disease.

Therefore, the early history of veterinary immunology was closely tied with control and eradication of infectious diseases (Fig. 1.1), as indeed was that of medical immunology. For the veterinary field, it is still true today that the diagnosis of and vaccination against diseases are the most important aspects of veterinary immunology. However, the medical field has taken other directions such as the immunotherapy of cancer, immunodeficiencies and the transplantation of organs. The vaccination of humans against infectious diseases is still a vital part of public health, but active research into infectious diseases in the developed countries is limited to a few project areas such as influenza virus, Rabies vaccines and the Acute Immunodeficiency Syndrome (AIDS), which have a need for active expansion of knowledge before effective vaccines are produced.

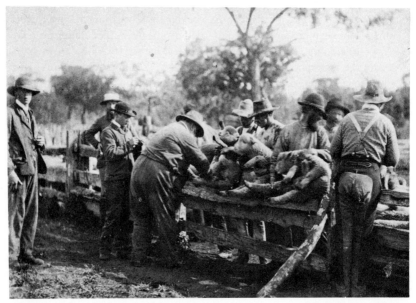

Fig.1.1. The vaccination of lambs against anthrax carried out in Australia in the 1890s. (Reproduced by courtesy of the Department of Agriculture, N.S.W., Australia.)

Although research workers in the veterinary immunology field are still actively working on infectious diseases, these too are often residual problems, in which it had been found too difficult to achieve results using the earlier techniques, which had been effective with the major diseases. For example, the vaccination of sheep against *Cysticercus ovis* (cause of Cysticercosis), *Corynebacterium ovis* (Caseous Lymphadenitis) and *Bacteroides nodosus* (foot-rot) had been attempted for some time, but modern knowledge was required to produce effective vaccines. In the case of *Cysticercus ovis,* the antigens released from tissue culture of the oncospheres from hatched tapeworm eggs were found to be protective if the ewes were inoculated before lambing, so that lambs could be protected by colostral antibodies from the larvae penetrating the gut wall after ingestion of tapeworm eggs on contaminated pastures. The vaccine against *Corynebacterium ovis* required the demonstration of extracellular toxins by the bacteria, important in the pathogenesis of the disease. Toxoids of the extracellular toxins, added to killed bacteria and adjuvant, led to the manufacture of commercial vaccines which now produce good protection in inoculated animals. Finally, the realisation that there were structures radiating from the surface of *Bacteroides nodosus* called pili, which were important in anchoring the bacteria to make them more pathogenic than unattached bacteria, led to vaccines which incorporated pili to stimulate antibodies in the sheep which prevented the acute pathogenic effects of the microorganism.

1.1   CONTRIBUTIONS TO BASIC IMMUNOLOGY

However, some natural phenomena of immunological origin in domestic animals have had a profound influence on the development of theories on the ontogeny of the immune response. A particular case is the freemartin twin calves which were found to share placental blood supply during gestation, and therefore during the pre-natal period, each calf shared red and white blood cells from the other twin. These foreign tissue cells persisted throughout the life of the animal but were not rejected, and the chimaerism, as it was termed, was demonstrated by Owen in 1945 to extend to the prolongation of acceptance of reciprocal skin grafts between the co-twins. This was despite the fact that skin grafts from unrelated donor calves were rapidly rejected.

This finding in cattle lent support to the 'self-marker' hypothesis put forward by Burnet and Fenner (1949), and led to experiments in mice by Billingham, *et al.* (1953), which demonstrated that the injection of allogeneic lymphocytes or any other cells into foetal mice *in utero* led to a tolerance which was expressed in the post-natal period by prolonged acceptance of skin grafts from the donor mice.

It was also incorporated into the clonal selection hypothesis of Burnet, which suggested that clones of lymphocytes which are normally able to recognise incompatible donor graft cells can be made tolerant because they are conditioned to do so during intrauterine life, and that they recognise all antigens present during this time as 'self' antigens. This allowed the body to produce antibodies to foreign antigens after birth without the aberration of autoimmunity, but more importantly, it focussed attention on the development of clones of antibody-forming cells which proliferated in response to antigenic challenge.

It is interesting that the ruminant also provided evidence to refute the original self-marker hypothesis, since skin rafts from unrelated donors were rejected quite normally by lambs which were skin-grafted *in utero*. The work of Schinckel and Ferguson (1953) demonstrated that the skin graft tolerance which could be induced with foetal mice could not be induced in sheep. The reason for the difference between the rodent and the ruminant species was thought to be due to the relative immaturity of the newborn mouse compared with the newborn ruminant. Nevertheless an important principle had been established during this period of experimentation: that clones of cells did proliferate during graft rejection or during specific antibody production, and that this immunological reaction was in the first instance the result of genetic programming of individual antigen-reactive cells.

1.2   LYMPHOCYTE RECIRCULATION

In the early 1960s another phenomenon was demonstrated by Gowans and colleagues, and this was that lymphocytes underwent a process of recirculation from blood to lymph (Gowans and Knight, 1964; Marchesi and Gowans, 1964). This concept of lymphocytes recirculating through lymph nodes and spleen via the post-capillary venules was established by direct observation of sections of the high endothelial cells of the venules using the electron microscope. It was found that large numbers of lymphocytes traversed the high endothelial cells, and some apparently crossed by penetrating the cytoplasm of the cells. Later research by other workers failed to confirm the direct penetration of lymphocytes into endothelial cells, most apparent penetrations being explicable on the basis of the lymphocytes squeezing between cells and only appearing to be within cells in thin sections.

This work in rats was soon confirmed in sheep by Hall and Morris (1965), who cannulated both the afferent and efferent lymphatic ducts of the popliteal lymph node. They then perfused the node with the radioactive DNA precursor [³H]thymidine and found that in the antigenically-stimulated node only about 5% of cells had DNA labelled by the [³H]thymidine. This was very good evidence that in the sheep too, the majority of the unlabelled cells in lymph were recirculating from blood to lymph.

1.3 THEORIES OF ANTIBODY FORMATION

1.3.1 Ehrlich's Side-Chain Hypothesis

The original selection theory of antibody formation was proposed by Paul Ehrlich (1900). He suggested that toxin molecules (antigen) combined with side-chains or antitoxin molecules on the surface of cells and stimulated the cells to produce more side-chains, which appeared in the serum as antitoxin antibody. This original idea is not far removed in concept from the modern ideas on antibody formation, but for many years it was not accepted because of the work of Landsteiner which demonstrated antibody formation against non-biological materials such as dinitrophenyl (DNP) groups. Since it was not thought that side-chains could already exist for the large number of synthetic haptens that were shown to be antigenic, another theory was put forward, which bestowed an instructional role on the antigen.

1.3.2 Pauling–Haurowitz Template Hypothesis (1935–1955)

The template theory proposed that antigen instructed cells to produce specific antibody by moulding non-specific γ-globulin around the antigenic determinant. This was suggested to take place during protein synthesis, but difficulties were encountered in explaining how γ-globulin was instructed by antigens which could not gain access to the interior of the cell, such as bacteria. Various hypotheses were advanced, such as macrophage processing of antigen, to produce small fragments which gained access to lymphocytes. However, further difficulties were encountered when it was appreciated that the primary amino-acid sequence of antibodies determined their protein structure. Moreover, completely-unfolded antibodies could be made to refold in the absence of antigen and regain some of their former antibody activity.

1.3.3 Clonal Selection Theory (1955–Present)

The selective theory of antibody formation was put forward by Jerne (1955). It was proposed that the receptors for antigen were generated on cells in the absence of antigen—in a fashion similar to Ehrlich's side-chain theory. This idea was developed further by Burnet (1957), who suggested that these cells with pre-existing receptors were selectively stimulated by specific antigen to divide and proliferate into a clone of specific antibody-forming cells. This became the clonal selection hypothesis. In modern terminology, it was the receptors on the B-cells which were 'selected' by antigen, and this meant that each B-cell was committed to producing the same antibody that was present in the cell membrane as a receptor. This was the cornerstone of the clonal selection hypothesis, and in practice, many experiments have shown that very few B-cells produce antibody of more than one specificity.

1.4   GENERATION OF DIVERSITY

The two theories put forward to explain the generation of diversity (GOD) were the germ-line theory and the somatic mutation theory. The germ-line theory argued that all immunoglobulin genes were inherited and that antibody diversity arose by selection and mutation during evolution of the species. The somatic mutation theory argued that mutation continued during the lifetime of the individual. The argument has not been settled, but available evidence favours the somatic mutation theory. This is based on amino-acid sequence studies which have examined monoclonal antibodies and found that apparently homogeneous, idiotypic, monoclonal antibodies, positive to the arsenate group, contain a variety of substitutions which are explicable on their being the products of a large number of separate clones which differ from each other by a small number of amino-acid replacements. The simplest explanation for this is that variants have arisen through somatic mutation of genes in the descendants of the hybridoma cell which produced the initial monoclonal antibody.

However, a more balanced theory will probably prevail in which both germ-line and somatic mutation influences are involved in the generation of diversity. Theories which are all-encompassing are out of fashion, but with the evidence from the molecular biology of immunoglobulin genes, it may be possible to map precisely where the generation of diversity is centred and also the frequency with which combinations of genes will arise.

1.5   THE THYMUS AND BURSA OF FABRICIUS

In the decade following the postulation of the clonal selection hypothesis, work was carried out on another aspect of the immune response (the ontogeny of the cells responsible for producing antibodies and of those which developed into the alternative arm): the cell-mediated immune response.

It is interesting that it was not until the period immediately after World War II that the plasma cell was finally demonstrated to be the one responsible for the production of antibody. An association between the increase in plasma cells in the spleen and the secondary immune response in rabbits was found by Fagreaeus (1948), and she suggested that there was a chain of development from a 'transitional cell' to 'immature plasma cell' and finally to the mature plasma cell.

Again, it was not until 1955 that antibody was actually demonstrated within plasma cells. The technique developed by Coons and associates (1955) involved the use of a fluorescent-antibody 'sandwich' method, which demonstrated that antibody against human γ-globulin or ovalbumin could indeed be seen microscopically within the plasma cells of the red pulp of the spleen and in other tissues also.

However, one lymphoid organ remained an enigma and this was the thymus, since very few antibody-forming cells could be demonstrated in the substance of this organ, although it was largely composed of lymphoid cells. The work of Miller and colleagues established that the thymus was vital for the normal immunological development of the neonatal mouse. Removal of the thymus caused an immunodeficiency resulting from lymphopoenia and was accompanied by poor body growth rate and susceptibility to infectious diseases.

It was work in chickens by Warner and Szenberg (1964) which really demonstrated the dichotomy between the two types of lymphocytes: the thymus-derived or T-cells and the bursa-derived or B-cells. Surgical removal of the thymus led to lymphopoenia, but antibody production by the chickens was largely unaffected. On the other hand, removal of the bursa of Fabricius resulted in a profound drop in antibody-producing potential, and it became obvious that the bursa was a primary lymphoid organ in the chicken and that it generated cells which ultimately matured into the antibody-forming cells of the spleen and other lymphoid tissues (Fig. 1.2).

In mammals, the work in mice by Miller and Mitchell (1968) more-or-less established that the bone marrow was the equivalent of the bursa. This was because bone marrow could be used to reconstitute lethally-irradiated recipients which would otherwise have died. The cells which reconstituted the mice contained the normal range of antibody-forming cell precursors but were deficient in cells which mediated other functions such as delayed hypersensitivity and graft rejection. It was also apparent that further reconstitution with thymus-derived cells restored normal antibody levels compared with reconstitution with bone marrow alone and that there was a collaboration between the thymus (T)- and bone marrow (B)-derived cells.

However, there was also some evidence which suggested that the large colon of the rabbit might be more equivalent to the bursa of birds than was the rabbit bone marrow. Surgical removal of the large colon gave variable results, but the idea survived, and more recently attention has been focused on the Peyer's patches of the large intestine as being the most likely equivalent in mammals of the bursa. For example, the Peyer's patches of lambs develop lymphoid follicles in pouches surgically isolated and removed from contact with the normal antigenic stimulation of gut contents, previously thought to be required for their development. The removal of the segment of intestine containing the Peyer's

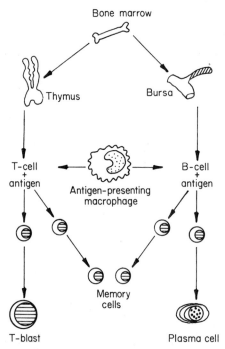

Fig.1.2. Sequence of maturation of the two major lymphocyte populations. These are the thymus-derived or T-cells, and the cells derived from the bone marrow in mammals and the bursa of Fabricius in birds, the B-cells. The presentation of antigen by macrophages is required for further maturation of the two cell lines into T-blasts or plasma cells. These cells are involved in cellular immunity and antibody production, respectively, and in the process of cell division they generate daughter memory cells of both types, which are then available for the secondary immune response.

patches has been demonstrated to lead to depletion of circulating B-cells in newborn lambs (Reynolds *et al.*, 1982), and so the original work in chickens appeared finally to be also applicable to ruminants and possibly other mammals.

1.6   HELPER AND SUPPRESSOR CELLS

The way in which T-cells collaborated with the B-cells to promote antibody production was clarified by the work of Mitchison (1971) and colleagues in mice. They found that the immune response to a hapten consisting of, for example, bovine γ-globulin (BGG) linked to DNP groups, depended on the B-cells recognising the BGG part of the hapten and the T-cells recognising the DNP part of the molecule (Fig. 1.3). Once these events had occurred, a soluble factor from the T-cells appeared to boost the proliferation of the clone of B-cells which produced specific antibody.

Suppression of the response, once antibody production had reached a certain point, was shown in mice by various workers such as Herzenberg *et al.* (1973) and Basten *et al.* (1974), to involve an inhibition of the activities of the collaborating T-cells, or 'helper' (Th) cells, as they became known (Fig. 1.3). The inhibitory cells were called 'suppressor' T-cells (Ts) and were found to be distinguishable from helper cells by their possession of distinctive membrane glycoproteins. These glycoproteins have ultimately been demonstrated in mice using specific monoclonal antibodies which combine with the products encoded by particular genes in the major histocompatibility complex (MHC).

For domestic animals this further subdivision of T-cells into T-helper and T-suppressor cells has not been clear-cut. As in the human, the system of T-cell

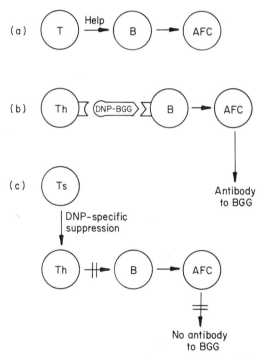

Fig.1.3. (a) Cell collaboration between T- and B-cells is required for thymus-dependent antigens to produce antibody-forming cells (AFC). (b) The cell collaboration may sometimes involve the recognition of different sites on the antigen by T- and B-cells. In this case, the B-cells recognise the bovine γ-globulin (BGG) part of the hapten, and the T-cells recognise the dinitrophenyl (DNP) groups. (c) Suppression of antibody responses appears to involve the inhibition of the helper cells (Th) by suppressor cells (Ts), so that T- and B-cell collaboration is blocked.

markers in domestic animals lagged behind that of the mouse, which had the advantage of the congenic strains bred in the laboratory and which could be used in cross-immunisation experiments to produce antiserum of fine specificity for the lymphocyte membrane glycoproteins. Although it is evident that non-specific suppression can be demonstrated with lymphocytes of domestic animals, specific suppression has yet to be demonstrated in any of the domestic species. Furthermore, there are competing ideas on the mode of help and suppression, which involve either anti-idiotype networks or the soluble factors produced by helper cells, the interleukin molecules, and these ideas must also be considered in any discussion of the regulation of the immune response.

1.7 ANTI-IDIOTYPE ANTIBODIES

The control of the immune response was generally assumed to be regulated by antibody concentration, antigen–antibody complexes or the availability of unbound antigenic determinants. However, Jerne (1974) was not satisfied that this provided a sufficiently selective mechanism, and he suggested that the regulation of the immune response might be mediated through recognition of idiotypic determinants on the surface receptors of the antibody-forming cell progenitors. Each B-cell displays on its membrane a receptor, which represents an accurate sample of the antibody synthesised by its progeny. It has been shown that anti-idiotype, anti-allotype and anti-isotype antibodies given passively to neonatal animals modulate (i.e., may stimulate but usually suppress) the expression of that particular isotype, allotype or idiotype in a subsequent immune response. Based on this, a suggestion was made that during an immune response, the induction and progression of individual clones of antigen-specific antibody-forming cells was regulated by another set of antibody-forming cells, specific for the idiotype of the first set of cells (Fig. 1.4).

A problem with the regulation of T-cells is that they do not produce immunoglobulin. However, it has been suggested that they produce enough of a part of the immunoglobulin molecule, the V_H region (see Chapter 4), to provide a site for regulation by anti-idiotype antibodies. Some of these questions should be amenable to investigation with monoclonal antibodies which show a high degree of specificity for membrane proteins.

Another problem is that for each anti-idiotype antibody, there has to be an anti-anti-idiotype antibody and so on, until a huge network is built up. This is a weakness of the theory, since much of the immune system may be taken up in suppression of idiotypes, rather than in responding to antigen. It also presupposes that the idiotypes do not induce tolerance in the immune response, as do other body proteins. Although the injection of anti-idiotype antibodies modulates the immune response, this is not evidence enough to sustain convincingly a physiological role for anti-idiotype antibodies in the regulation of the immune

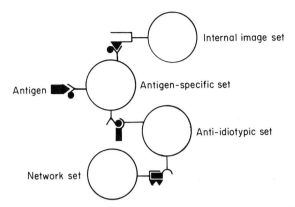

Fig.1.4. The network theory of regulation of the immune response depends on each anti-gen-combining site expressing a set of idiotypic determinants. These are recognised by a set of cells with anti-idiotypic receptors, which in turn are recognised by a network set of cells. Since the combining sites which recognise idiotypes are the same as the combining sites which recognise external antigen, the idiotypes can be regarded as an internal image of foreign antigen. Therefore all immunoglobulin molecules are directed against idiotypes, and their useful function is the recognition of foreign antigen. When antigen induces clonal expansion of the reactive cells, appropriate idiotype-bearing and anti-idiotype sets of cells are stimulated which control the immune response. [Reproduced by kind permission from McConnell *et al.* (1981).]

response. Nevertheless, anti-idiotypic antibodies have been found following immunisation with various antigens; for example, the response of rabbits to streptococcal and staphylococcal antigens is accompanied by the appearance of anti-idiotype antibodies.

Anti-idiotype reactive T-cells (Ts) are suggested to be the effector cells in suppression, and it is thought that they recognise the target idiotype by virtue of receptors on their membranes. They are suggested to regulate both T- and B-cell responses, with the T-cells being either those involved in delayed hypersensitivity (Tdh) or in T-cell help (Th) (Fig. 1.3). The selective removal of idiotype-reactive (i.e., anti-idiotype) B- and T-cells has been shown to augment the humoral immune response. Other experiments have demonstrated that the transfer of idiotype-reactive T-cells from idiotype-suppressed mice resulted in a pronounced suppression of the idiotype expression both in humoral and cell-mediated responses in the recipient mice.

1.8 LYMPHOKINES

The concept of soluble products of stimulated lymphocytes which 'mediated' or modified the response of surrounding lymphocytes grew out of earlier work on lymphocyte 'chalones' postulated in the early 1960s by Bullough (1962). This hypothesis suggested that all the cells in the body released molecules called chalones, which were responsible for limiting the growth of cells. For example, in wound healing, the control of epithelial cell growth in the final stages of wound repair was said to be due to the epithelial cells releasing chalones, which inhibited further proliferation of cells in the area of wound repair once they were packed closely together in the intact epithelium.

For lymphocytes, the idea received serious attention when it was demonstrated by Kamrin (1959) that a fraction of serum containing α-globulins prolonged the time taken for graft rejection. A similar fraction of bovine serum (fraction C) was shown by Mowbray (1963) to have immunosuppressive effects on antibody responses of mice to sheep erythrocytes. It also directly inhibited the *in vitro* proliferative responses of lymphocytes to mitogens, as did a similar fraction containing the α-globulins from human serum. This fraction from human serum was named immunoregulatory α-globulin (IRA) by Cooperband and colleagues (1969). The effects of these fractions of serum were to cause suppression of lymphocyte functions, and in many ways they were similar to suppressive factors, which in the early 1970s, were discovered to be released from lymphocytes proliferating in response to antigens and mitogens in tissue culture. The problem was that many other factors were found to be suppressive, particularly in the conditions of tissue culture. For example, prostaglandins, low pH and even the presence of unlabelled thymidine, reduced the uptake of radioactive [^{3}H]thymidine into the deoxyribonucleic acid (DNA) of the lymphocytes.

At present, the serum factors remain an enigma, since their suppressive actions are non-specific and their importance in control of lymphocyte proliferation *in vivo* has never been adequately explained. In contrast, the factors released by lymphocytes after stimulation continue to be closely examined since 1969 when they were collectively defined by the term 'lymphokines' by Dumonde and colleagues (1969). They were defined as 'cell-free soluble factors which are generated during interaction of sensitized lymphocytes with specific antigen, but which are expressed without immunological activity'.

Several biological activities besides suppression could be demonstrated in the lymphokine preparations. Some such skin-reactive factors were demonstrable *in vivo*, while others such as macrophage migration inhibition factor were demonstrable *in vitro*. The exact chemical nature of these factors, which are defined by their functional effects, has yet to be determined, because it has been difficult to obtain enough material for analysis. In fact it was largely the production of lymphokines by continuously growing lymphoblast lines, which led to the next phase in research on these substances, which were given the name 'interleukins' to replace the older 'lymphocyte-stimulatory factors' which had been found in the culture supernates of antigen-stimulated lymphocytes.

It also began to be appreciated that both lymphocytes and macrophages interacted with each other by means of soluble factors. In particular, the stimulatory effects of interleukin I (IL I) produced by macrophages and interleukin II (IL II) produced by T-cells have been studied for their effects on the immune response of T- and B-cells. This is because it has been found easier to study the stimulatory lymphokines first in that their effect is positive rather than negative. It is for this reason that attention has been transferred from the suppressive to the stimulatory factors which affect the immune response.

1.9   INTERLEUKIN I

Interleukin I has been shown to be derived from macrophages, and its function appears to be the stimulation of T-cells to express receptors for interleukin II. It is also thought that more than one signal is required to do this, and the interaction of antigen with Ia antigens (see Chapter 10) on the surface of the macrophage produces a complex which is recognised by receptors on the T-cell. This event has become known as signal 1 (Fig. 1.5).

The next step is the production of soluble interleukin I by the activated macrophage, and this is called signal 2, since it is thought to stimulate the appearance of receptors for interleukin II on the surface of the T-cell.

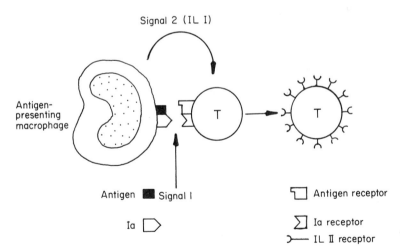

Fig. 1.5.   The involvement of interleukin I (IL I) in the immune response is suggested to arise from the interaction of antigen-presenting macrophages with antigen-reactive T-cells. Both cell determinants (Ia) and antigen are recognised as a complex on the macrophage surface by the T-cell receptors, and the process of recognition causes the production of IL I by the macrophage. The IL I, in turn, stimulates T-cells to express receptors for the other soluble factor interleukin II (IL II).

1.10   INTERLEUKIN II

The expression of receptors for interleukin II makes the activated T-cell receptive to soluble interleukin II, which is itself derived from activated T-cells possessing receptors for interleukin II (Fig. 1.6).

Interleukins I (IL I) and II (IL II) appear to be distinct entities, both being proteins of 12,500 MW for IL I and 15,000 for IL II. The amino-acid sequence of IL II is known, and it has been cloned by recombinant DNA techniques. Both molecules appear to be species-specific, and mouse and human interleukins do not have cross-stimulatory effects on cells from each other.

The work on soluble lymphokines and interleukins has mostly been carried out on human and mouse lymphocytes and macrophages. Work is in progress on the soluble lymphocyte factors of sheep, pigs and cattle, but this has yet to reach a stage where it is of practical importance to veterinary immunology. This research has as its final objective the manipulation of the immune response in animals to adjust the immune response to suit the problem at hand.

1.11   VACCINES

The shift in emphasis to present-day studies on the cells responsible for the immune response was preceded by an era in which the immunoglobulins produced by the immune system were closely studied. This was because many vaccines depend for their protective effects on the production of specific antibodies, and it appeared important to know which immunoglobulin classes were produced and to estimate their likely site of action.

For example, the realisation that IgA was predominantly an immunoglobulin

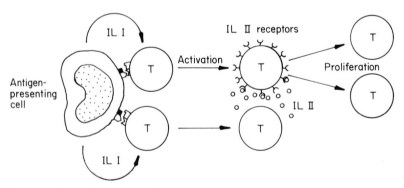

Fig. 1.6.   The stimulation of T-cells by IL I not only causes some to express receptors for IL II but also in turn stimulates other T-cells to produce the IL II which stimulates the IL II receptor-bearing cells to proliferate into T-cell clones.

of mucous membranes led to work on the local immune response to pathogenic microorganisms. In ruminants, the local immune responses of the mammary gland, reproductive tract, respiratory tract and gut have all been studied from the aspect of the immunoglobulins present in secretions and also the immunoglobulin class in which specific antibody is found.

Another major area of activity has been the transmission of immunoglobulins from mother to offspring. In the ruminant, the predominant immunoglobulin class in colostrum is IgG_1, and this is the most important route of transmission of immunoglobulins for this species. This is not so for dogs and cats for which placental transmission of immunoglobulins occurs, although antibodies in colostrum are still important in the protection of the gut mucous membrane in the neonatal animal.

Therefore, much of the research in the 1970s in veterinary immunology was directed towards improving the transmission of colostral immunoglobulins by immunisation of the mother to stimulate antibodies against disease in the neonate. An example is the immunisation of sows against *Escherichia coli* to stimulate serum antibodies which would be concentrated in colostrum, which when ingested by suckling piglets would protect them against this form of neonatal diarrhoea. This area of veterinary immunology is still one of the most important practical areas of research today, particularly with the advent of genetically-engineered vaccines against scours in piglets.

However, it is a reasonable generalisation to say that many of the diseases of economic importance to livestock have vaccines which are commercially available. Furthermore, the length of time the vaccine remains on the market is directly related to the importance of each disease. It also appears to be related to the effectiveness of the vaccine, and partially-effective vaccines against the less common diseases do not generally remain long on the market.

Therefore, efforts are generally directed towards improving the efficacy of vaccines towards the ideal vaccine which provides total protection for the animal. At the same time, an effort is made to increase the shelf-life of the vaccine, so that it can be stored for some time between outbreaks of the disease.

The development of vaccines against diseases which remain persistent problems depends therefore on a variety of factors, which include the efficacy of the vaccine, cost of manufacture, shelf-life and the importance of the disease in the eyes of the client or farmer with whom the veterinarian has to deal. It also seems important that there be an effective acquired resistance to the disease in the field before it is worth close attention into ways of enhancing the immune response against the disease.

Some diseases such as bovine tuberculosis have no effective vaccine, although it seems likely that individual cattle are resistant to challenge infection in the field. Therefore, studies of the immunology of bovine tuberculosis have been directed towards improving diagnosis of the disease using the tuberculin skin test. The disease stimulates a highly-active T-cell response which can be measured in a delayed-hypersensitivity response in the skin of cattle when they are injected intradermally with a purified protein derivative (PPD) from heat-killed *Mycobacterium bovis* culture supernate. Antibodies in tuberculosis are much less apparent and appear to require the prior antigenic stimulus of a tuberculin skin test to stimulate their appearance in the blood.

In contrast, another disease of cattle, Bovine Brucellosis, stimulates high titres of serum antibodies directed towards the bacterial lipopolysaccharide. There are also vaccines against Brucellosis which provide about 80% protection. Campaigns against Brucellosis have usually begun by using vaccination and ended by a test-and-slaughter policy. The intermediate phase of testing cattle in the face of vaccination with living Strain 19 or killed 45/20 vaccines, has led to much research effort into distinguishing vaccinated cattle from actively-infected cattle. It has been found, for example, that the indirect haemolysin test (IHLT) does distinguish vaccinated from infected cattle with much higher reliability than the complement fixation test (CFT). Again the examination of the immunoglobulin classes, in which the antibodies are found, has led to a rational approach to the improvement of serological procedures for diagnosing Brucellosis.

However, the vaccines which have really stood the test of time are those for the clostridial diseases of sheep and cattle. The early vaccines of the 1920s onwards were gradually improved and with continued research, individual toxins were characterised and their importance for vaccines were each assessed. For example, in Pulpy Kidney of lambs caused by *Clostridium welchii* Type D, circulating antitoxin directed towards the ϵ toxin is very effective against experimental enterotoxaemia. Even ileal contents containing between 10,000 and 20,000 mouse minimal lethal doses (MLD) per gram, cannot produce the disease in the face of circulating antitoxin levels of 10 to 20 units/ml in serum (Bullen and Batty, 1957). It is precisely the effectiveness of these vaccines in sheep and cattle which ensures their continued use today in large numbers of animals. Clostridial vaccines are considered one of the standards of veterinary immunology, against which all newer bacterial vaccines must attempt to match, if they are to be considered effective vaccines.

1.12   REMAINING CHALLENGES IN VETERINARY IMMUNOLOGY

Most of the bacterial and viral diseases have effective vaccines, or if they do not, there is a high likelihood that vaccines will be developed. A remaining challenge is the area of parasites—the protozoal parasites and the internal and external parasites of cattle and sheep.

For some parasitic infections such as lungworm of cattle caused by *Dictyocaulus viviparus*, there already is an effective irradiated larvae vaccine. This is true even though effective anthelmintics exist which can control the parasite. The advantage of vaccination is its effectiveness and prolonged action, which makes it unnecessary to drench calves repeatedly with anthelmintics. Similarly, some protozoal diseases such as Babesiosis of cattle also have an effective vaccine. However, generally, the production of vaccines against protozoa and helminths has proved far more difficult than against bacteria and viruses. The complexity of the parasite or its ability to change its surface antigens, particularly in protozoa, have been factors which have made difficult the production of specific vaccines.

The manipulation of the immune response, so that it is directed against some susceptible stage of the parasite life cycle, has proved effective in some parasitic infections. For example, larvae may be prevented from penetrating the gut wall or they may be inhibited from growing past a certain stage of the life cycle of the parasite.

The isolation of antigens from protozoa and parasites has not yet proved particularly useful in formulating vaccines, but the problem has been in identifying those antigens which have the potential to be protective. The use of recombinant DNA techniques to manufacture quantities of these antigens for experimental vaccine trials appears a useful direction for research.

Therefore, the remaining challenges in veterinary immunology seem to be the development of vaccines against protozoa and parasites, many of which are problems of the tropical climates. The helminths of sheep and cattle do, however, extend from the tropics into temperate regions and provide an invisible challenge to the host in terms of production and health. The breeding of sheep and cattle which are resistant to helminths appears feasible and may be the best long-term approach to solving the problem of worm resistance to anthelmintics.

For other vaccines, directed against viruses and bacteria, this approach may also be useful, since partially-effective vaccines may become fully effective when used in a population of animals selected for high immune responsiveness.

1.13 GENETIC ENGINEERING AND GENETIC SELECTION

There is already a vaccine against *Escherichia coli* in pigs which has been genetically engineered to stimulate immunity specifically against the pili of *E. coli,* but it is a non-pathogenic strain of the bacterium. Recombinant DNA techniques also appear to be ideal for the production of virus vaccines, since many irrelevant antigens can be discarded, while concentrating on the peptides from the coat proteins which stimulate protective antibodies. Vaccines against Foot-and-Mouth disease virus of cattle are an example of an area which will benefit from such work. It has even reached the stage where peptide sequences are being chemically synthesised rather than being produced by *E. coli.* Thus it appears likely that highly-protective vaccines against many viruses could soon be produced, which will stimulate the required antibodies with little risk of reversion of living vaccines, or partially-inactivated vaccines, to the virulent virus.

For bacteria, it also appears likely that various recombinant DNA techniques or chemical syntheses will allow economical production of protective antigens, free of irrelevent antigens found in many vaccines today. However, again, economic factors may dictate that for some vaccines, the present style of production is still the more effective, particularly if the recombinant DNA-produced antigens are no better than the older vaccines. This will be the test for commercial success or otherwise of the newer vaccines.

For parasites and protozoa, the problem still remains of identifying the protective antigens. The monoclonal antibodies against parasite antigens have not proved to be as useful as had been hoped, either for diagnosis or in the isolation of protective antigens. The problem appears to be that monoclonal antibodies are too specific, and this results in many important antigens being missed. Research workers are now returning to the conventional polyclonal antibodies to isolate groups of antigens, amongst which there may be some that are protective.

Once isolated, the protective antigens can be analysed for amino-acid sequence and the sequence in turn translated into nucleotide sequences which are synthesised and inserted into the DNA of *E. coli*. The bacteria will then synthesise the required antigen. Such vaccines for parasites and protozoa have yet to be produced, but active research is being undertaken to see if such vaccines can be made. The future of immunisation against parasites may well lie with these vaccines.

The other aspect of immunity to parasites, which may well be useful to explore, is the genetic selection of the host for responsiveness to vaccination against the parasite. This is already possible with intestinal nematode *Trichostrongylus colubriformis* of sheep. In this work an irradiated larvae vaccine induces protection against experimental challenge with normal larvae in 8- to 12-week-old lambs. The selective breeding of two lines of sheep called 'high' and 'low' responders has allowed the analysis of some of the membrane glycoproteins or 'antigens' on lymphocytes from the two lines of sheep. This analysis has revealed that 70% of the high responders have a particular lymphocyte antigen (SY1) and that only 21% of the low responders possess this antigen. Thus it is possible that this will provide a predictive marker for responsiveness to vaccination against the parasite and hopefully for resistance to the parasite in unvaccinated sheep in the field.

Similar lymphocyte antigens are being characterised for the horse, dog, cat, cow, pig and chicken, and if present trends continue, it seems likely that the prediction of the genetic inheritance of disease resistance will play a large role in future developments in veterinary immunology.

Finally, it must be said that it would be difficult, if not impossible, to review all that has happened in immunology in the last few years in this book on veterinary immunology. Rather it is the aim of the author to define those areas in the field of veterinary immunology which appear to be of current relevance to domestic animals, particularly ruminants, and also to describe those techniques which may prove useful in the technical development of diagnostic techniques and research on vaccines against animal diseases.

REFERENCES

Basten, A., Miller, J. F. A. P., Sprent, J. and Cheers, C. (1974). *J. Exp. Med.* **140,** 199–217.
Billingham, R. E., Brent, L. and Medawar, P. B. (1953). *Nature (London)* **172,** 603–606.
Bullen, J. J. and Batty, I. (1957). *J. Pathol. Bacteriol.* **73,** 511–518.
Bullough, W. S. (1962). *Biol. Rev. Cambridge Philos. Soc.* **37,** 307–342.
Burnet, F. M. (1957). *Aust. J. Sci* **20,** 67–69.
Burnet, F. M. and Fenner, F. (1949). 'The Production of Antibodies'. Macmillan, Melbourne.
Coons, A. H., Leduc, E. H. and Connolly, J. M. (1955). *J. Exp. Med.* **102,** 49–60
Cooperband, S. R., Davis, R. C., Schmid, K. and Mannick, J. A. (1969). *Transplant. Proc.* **1,** 516–523.
Dumonde, D. C., Wolstencroft, R. A., Panayi, G. S., Matthew, M., Morley, J. and Howson, W. T. (1969). *Nature (London)* **224,** 38–42.
Ehrlich, P. (1900). *Proc. R. Soc. London* **66,** 424–448.
Fagreaeus, A. (1948). *J. Immunol.* **58,** 1–13.
Gowans, J. L. and Knight, E. J. (1964). *Proc. R. Soc. London, Ser. B.* **159,** 257–282.
Hall, J. G. and Morris, B. (1965). *J. Exp. Med.* **121,** 901–910.
Herzenberg, L. A., Chan, E. L., Ravitch, M. M., Riblet, R. J. and Herzenberg, L. A. (1973). *J. Exp. Med.* **137,** 1311–1324.
Jerne, N. K. (1955). *Proc. Natl. Acad. Sci. U.S.A.* **41,** 849–857.
Jerne, N. K. (1974). *Ann. Immunol. (Paris)* **125C,** 373–389.
Kamrin, B. B. (1959). *Proc. Soc. Exp. Biol. Med.* **100,** 58–61.
McConnell, I., Munro, A. and Waldmann, H. (1981). 'The Immune System: A Course on the Molecular and Cellular Basis of Immunity,' Blackwell Scientific Publications.
Marchesi, V. T. and Gowans, J. L. (1964). *Proc. R. Soc. London, Ser. B* **159,** 283–290
Miller, J. F. A. P. and Mitchell, G. F. (1968). *J. Exp. Med.* **128,** 801–820.
Mitchison, N. A. (1971). *Eur. J. Immunol.* **1,** 10–17.
Mowbray, J. F. (1963). *Immunology* **6,** 217–225.
Owen, R. D. (1945). *Science (Washington, D.C.)* **102,** 400–401.
Reynolds, J. D., Miyasaka, M. and Trnka, Z. (1982). *Annu. Rep. Basel Inst. Immunol.* pp. 74–75.
Schinckel, P. G. and Ferguson, K. A. (1953). *Aust. J. Biol. Sci.* **6,** 533–546.
Warner, N. L. and Szenberg, A. (1964). *Annu. Rev. Microbiol.* **18,** 253–268.

2

Cellular
Immunology

In the veterinary field, the study of cellular immunity was first directed towards the diseases caused by facultative intracellular parasites. These include the bacteria *Mycobacterium bovis* and *Mycobacterium paratuberculosis,* which cause tuberculosis and Johne's disease in cattle, and *Listeria monocytogenes* and *Toxoplasma gondii,* which cause disease in sheep. Historically, the immunity of macrophages to experimental infection was studied first *in vitro* to find out if there were changes induced in the cells after immunisation of the animals from which they were obtained. In particular, evidence was accumulated that live vaccines were necessary for macrophage cellular immunity in domestic animals, where effective vaccination against facultative intracellular parasites was required.

In the late 1960s, a second line of research, on the lymphocyte, showed that in mice at least, this cell was responsible for not only antigen recognition, memory and production of antibodies but also the direction of macrophage responses to bacterial infection. In this last function, it was shown, in mice and guinea pigs, that soluble mediators or 'lymphokines' were released from lymphocytes sensitised to bacteria and that these hastened the conditioning or activation of the macrophages to resist the destructive effects of intracellular infection. The lymphokines themselves were not found to be capable of inhibiting bacterial multiplication, but it was assumed that they had a non-specific effect in causing the macrophages to acquire more lysosomal enzymes and to become physically larger, more phagocytic and more capable of killing intracellular microorganisms than macrophages unstimulated by lymphokines.

Since the lymphocyte was thought to be responsible for the phenomenon of cellular immunity in macrophages, experiments have been carried out to see if particular lymphocyte types were necessary for activation. By analogy with the immunoglobulins, where subclasses such as IgM, IgG and IgA could be recognised, lymphocytes were examined for subpopulations which had specific functions, amongst which were the population of cells activating macrophages.

2.1 THE LYMPHOCYTE

The study of lymphocytes in domestic animals has the considerable background of the work of Morris and his associates in sheep and Kronkite and associates in calves. During the 1950s and 1960s, the prevailing philosophy was the physiological approach to immunity, which was an extension of Florey's work in Oxford. This philosophy, in summary, insisted that studies on immunity or experimental pathology should be undertaken with as little disturbance as possible to the physiology of the experimental animal. In particular, this led to the development of techniques of lymphatic cannulation, which allowed the collection of lymphocytes floating in lymph, on their way back to the blood.

The pioneering work of Hall and Morris (1965) studied the recirculation of lymphocytes in sheep, in which both afferent and efferent lymphatic vessels supplying the popliteal lymph node were cannulated with plastic tubing (Fig. 2.1). The infusion of a radioactive DNA precursor, [^{3}H]thymidine, into the afferent lymphatic vessel, was not accompanied by a large rise in cells with labelled DNA in the efferent lymph of antigenically-stimulated lymph nodes. Rather, there was a surprisingly low proportion of labelled (<5%) cells in efferent lymph. This suggested that most of the cells came from a source outside the node and that this was most likely to be the blood.

The implications of this finding were that the lymph node of the sheep and other species could now be visualised as crossroads of intersecting streams of cells. These were firstly from the tissue spaces via the afferent lymph, secondly from the blood via recirculation through the walls of the microcapillaries or venules and from within the node itself (Fig. 2.2). In the rat and the sheep, the only outlet of lymphocytes from the node appeared to be the efferent lymphatic vessel. Very few cells appeared to leave via the blood. However, this did not appear to be the case in the lymph node of the pig. In this species, it was shown by Binns and Hall (1966) that efferent lymph from the lymph nodes of pigs contained less than 10% of the numbers of cells found in the efferent lymph of sheep. They concluded that lymphocytes recirculated into pig lymph nodes from the blood and then went back out of the node via the blood vessels again. The

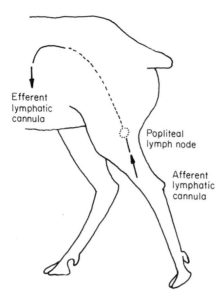

Fig. 2.1. The cannulation of both afferent and efferent popliteal lymphatic vessels in the sheep by Hall and Morris (1965) allowed the perfusion of [³H]thymidine through the afferent cannula and the collection of free-floating cells from the efferent cannula. These experiments showed that during the immune response after antigenic stimulation of the node, most of the cells in efferent lymph were derived from the blood, rather than from within the lymph node itself.

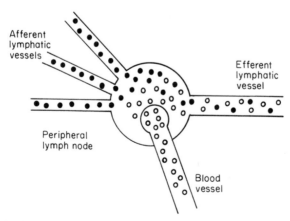

Fig. 2.2. The lymphocytes in efferent lymph from a lymph node are derived from three sources: recirculation from blood and from the afferent lymphatic vessels draining to the node, and from within the lymph node itself.

high circulating blood lymphocyte count in pigs compared with the sheep was supporting evidence that not many lymphocytes went from lymph node to lymph node in the pig via the efferent lymphatics.

The anatomy of the pig lymph node was also known to be different from other species, with an apparent reversal in the normal relationship between the cortex and medulla—the cortical tissue being on the inside and the medullary tissue on the outside of the pig lymph node (Fig. 2.3). However, the principle of mixing of cellular streams was the same as that of sheep, in that specifically-sensitised lymphocytes from many sources came into contact with antigens and micro-organisms which had drained to the regional lymph nodes from peripheral sites, such as the skin. Certainly there is no evidence that pigs are at a disadvantage in their resistance to invading microorganisms. In fact *Mycobacterium bovis* infection in wild pigs in Australia is generally a non-progressive disease, even though lymph nodes under the jaw are infected. The different lymph node anatomy and physiology in the pig most likely stems from changes of the pig lymph node during evolution.

2.2 EXPERIMENTAL USE OF THE ISOLATED LYMPH NODE

A use of the isolated lymph node technique in a practical vaccination problem is illustrated by the work of Burrell (1978) on *Corynebacterium pseudotuber-*

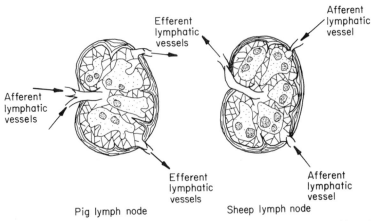

Efferent lymphatic vessels

Afferent lymphatic vessel

Afferent lymphatic vessels

Efferent lymphatic vessels

Afferent lymphatic vessel

Pig lymph node   Sheep lymph node

Fig. 2.3. The pig and sheep lymph nodes are shown with the direction of lymph flow indicated by arrows. In the pig lymph node, the lymph enters via the hilus and leaves via efferent lymphatic vessels from the greater curvature of the node. This arrangement is opposite to that found in most other species in which the lymph enters by several afferent lymphatic vessels on the greater curvature of the node and leaves from the hilus. However, with the reversed cortex and medulla in the pig lymph node, the lymph still traverses the cortex before the medulla, as it does in other species.

culosis (ovis) in sheep. In this bacterial disease, the lymph nodes are invaded by the microorganisms, become swollen and eventually become filled with greenish pus, causing an obvious problem with the mutton industry when the sheep are sent for slaughter.

It is possible to vaccinate against the disease, and during the development of a vaccine, a challenge procedure was used which depended on the infusion of *C. pseudotuberculosis* organisms into the afferent lymphatic vessel of the popliteal lymph nodes of sheep during surgery. If effective vaccination had first been carried out, the lymph node was resistant to challenge. Two weeks after surgery, the node could be excised at postmortem and weighed in comparison with the control popliteal node in the other leg which had not been challenged (Fig. 2.4). Partially-effective vaccination could be objectively assessed by increased weight of the challenged lymph node. This technique allowed the rapid assessment of different procedures using the target organ, the lymph node, to measure the effectiveness of the vaccination.

2.3 CELLS IN LYMPH

In central lymph, such as the thoracic duct of the sheep and cow, a diverse population of lymphocytes can be found after smearing and staining of the cells. The gut microflora provide enough antigenic stimulus for some of the cells to transform and divide. There is a range in size and degree of staining, from small, medium and large lymphocytes, to blast cells and even a few macrophages. In particular, there are large pyroninophilic cells which can be shown to contain RNA but not much antibody. These large pyroninophilic cells from the antigen-stimulated popliteal lymph node have been transferred between identical twin sheep and have been shown to transmit antibody-producing potential from one sheep to the other (Hall *et al.*, 1967). They presumably normally travel via the lymphatic vessels, from lymph node to lymph node, providing for transmission of the immune response around the lymphoid system. In present-day nomen-clature, these cells would most likely be identified as B-cell blasts (Fig. 2.5a), since they possess surface immunoglobulin. Under the electron microscope they can be seen to have a small amount of endoplasmic reticulum in contrast to the well-developed endoplasmic reticulum of the plasma cell (Fig. 2.5b). They are not normally found in the blood in large numbers, and there is good evidence that they home to lymphoid tissues, particularly the gut, where they supplement the gut-associated lymphoid tissue. Although not proven, it is possible that these cells also leave the gut-associated lymphoid tissue and home to the lung and mammary gland, where they produce antibodies in mucus, milk and colostrum, specific for gut microorganisms. These antibodies are thought to be involved in the defence of the neonatal animal against enteric microorganisms.

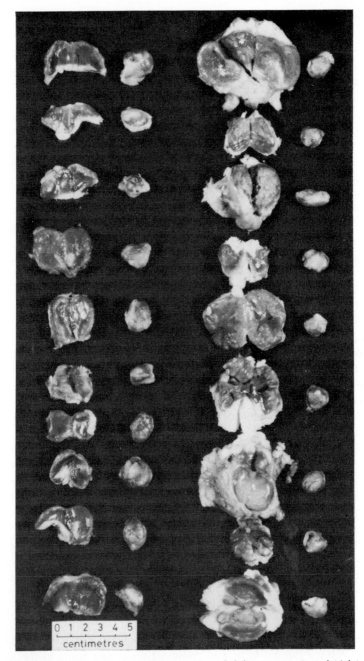

0 1 2 3 4 5
centimetres

Fig. 2.4. The lymph nodes from sheep vaccinated (left) or unvaccinated (right) against *Corynebacterium pseudotuberculosis* (ovis) are shown. Systemic vaccination 1 year previously protected the sheep against experimental challenge with 5×10^6 colony-forming units of virulent bacteria, and this was reflected in the smaller size of nodes excised from the vaccinated

The cellular content of peripheral lymph, in contrast to central lymph, is generally much more uniform. There are mostly unstimulated lymphocytes in the efferent popliteal lymph of sheep. In the afferent popliteal lymph there are larger cells among the unstimulated lymphocytes. In the pig, these cells have been identified as Langerhans cells (Fig. 2.6), and these cells appear to be involved as accessory cells in the transmission of the immune response. Their role would appear to be mainly as antigen-localising cells in the subdermis, and their occurrence in lymph may be coincidental. They certainly do not emerge from the lymph node to which afferent lymph drains, and it must be assumed that they are retained and join the reticulum cells of the node itself.

Another interesting aspect of recirculation of lymphocytes in the sheep is the apparent separation of the cells into two distinct pools (Cahill *et al.*, 1977). From labelling experiments, it is apparent that lymphocytes from the intestine selectively recirculate through the intestinal lymph nodes, while those from peripheral popliteal lymph selectively recirculate through the popliteal lymph node. The significance of this finding may be that at least for the intestine, there is a pool of lymphocytes that are committed to immune responses against gut microflora or pathogens.

2.4 THE THYMUS

The thymus in domestic animals has been the subject of considerable study, following work in the mouse which showed that surgical removal of the thymus in neonatal mice, reduced the capacity of the animal to mount an immune response. In the neonatal mouse, the removal of the thymus has further effects, such as a 'wasting' syndrome which results in poor growth and susceptibility of the 'thymectomised' mice to bacterial infection.

In domestic animals, such as the sheep, this wasting syndrome is not seen, even though in an attempt to duplicate the immaturity of the neonatal mouse, the thymus is removed *in utero* from the foetus (Cole and Morris, 1973). There is, however, a persistent lymphopoenia and a long-term immunodeficiency, which makes animals with their thymus removed, more susceptible to gut infections and infectious virus diseases than the controls. However, in pigs, the removal of the thymus, together with sublethal irradiation, produces a syndrome which closely parallels the wasting syndrome of the mouse (Fig. 2.7). In these experiments performed by Binns *et al.* (1977), the naturally-large litter size of the pig

compared with the unvaccinated sheep. Only one abscess was was found in the vaccinated nodes, while all unvaccinated nodes had abscesses. For both vaccinated and unvaccinated sheep, the contralateral lymph nodes which were not challenged, are also shown to provide a contrast in size within each animal. (Reproduced by kind permission of Dr. D. H. Burrell, CSIRO, McMaster Laboratory, Sydney, Australia.)

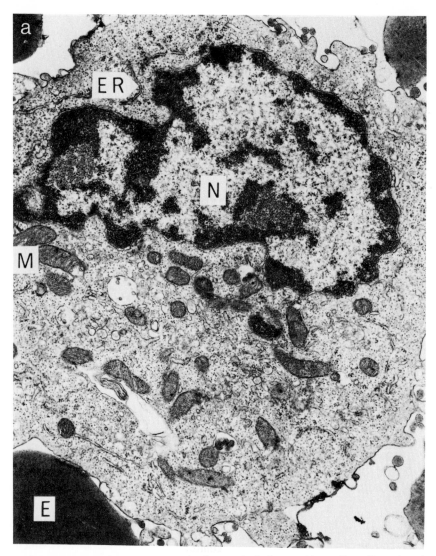

Fig. 2.5. (a) An electron micrograph of an antibody-forming blast cell in efferent lymph from a sheep after antigenic stimulation of the popliteal lymph node with killed *Salmonella muenchen* bacteria. The antigen-coated erythrocytes (E) used to detect the antibody-forming cell can be seen around the cell membrane. The cell has a large nucleus (N) with numerous mitochondria (M) but only sparse endoplasmic reticulum (ER). (Reproduced by kind permission of Dr. J. B. Smith, The John Curtin School of Medical Research, Australian National University, Canberra.) (b) An electron micrograph of a plasma cell from sheep colostrum. The cell has a characteristic 'clock-face' nucleus and numerous cisternae of rough endoplasmic reticulum, some of which are flattened (small arrows) while others are dilated (large arrows). This cell is in marked contrast to the blast cell in (a), which has poorly-developed endoplasmic reticulum. (Reproduced by permission from J. E. Butler, ed. (1981), 'The Ruminant Immune System', Plenum Press.)

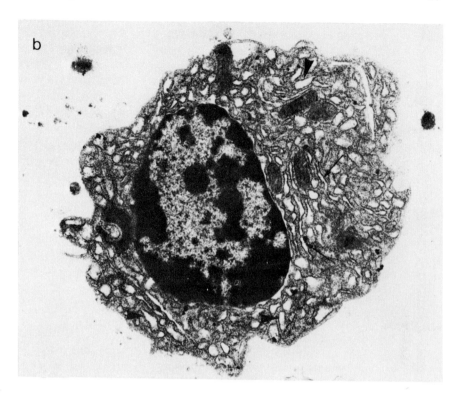

allowed carefully-controlled experiments on litter-mates which were irradiated without removal of the thymus. The syndrome is marked by poor growth rate and lymphopoenia, which persists for a long period accompanied by an apparent deficiency in the remaining circulating T-lymphocytes to mitogens, such as phytohaemagglutinin (PHA) and concanavalin A (Con A). There is also an apparent drop in the numbers of cells which can be identified as neither T- nor B-cells with certainty. These so-called null cells also drop in numbers in the blood of thymectomised sheep and appear to be an immature T-cell in both species. It is interesting that the percentage of mature T-cells does not drop after thymectomy in sheep and pigs. This contrasts with the mouse and rat, in which animals with extremely low T-cell counts can be produced by thymectomy and reconstitution with bone marrow cells after irradiation. In the sheep and pig, the mature T-cells appear to have either migrated before thymectomy or have been produced in sites other than the thymus.

The practical problem of thymus deficiency is rarely encountered as a clinical syndrome in food animals. However there is a trait of Black Pied Danish cattle of Friesian descent which is called 'lethal trait A46'. It is inherited as an autosomal-

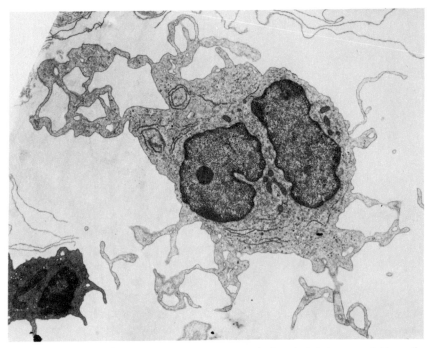

Fig. 2.6. An electron micrograph of a veiled cell in the lymph draining normal skin on the foreleg of a pig. This cell has a large, elongated nucleus with extensive cytoplasm, containing mitochondria and lysosomes. This type of cell has also been identified as a Langerhans-type cell, involved in the presentation of antigen to lymphocytes. (Reproduced by kind permission of Dr. B. Balfour, Clinical Research Centre, Harrow, England.)

recessive trait with a reduced capacity of the calf to absorb zinc in the diet. All the signs point to a progressive immunodeficiency accompanied by skin and gut lesions and atrophy of the thymus, spleen and lymph nodes. There is depletion of lymphocytes in the gut-associated lymphoid tissues and hyperactivity of blood lymphocytes to T-cell mitogens (Brummerstedt *et al.*, 1974; Flagstad, 1976).

Oral treatment of calves with large doses of zinc oxide or zinc sulphate reverses the syndrome and leads to long-term improvement, which, however, depends on the continued treatment with zinc. The mode of action of the zinc is not known, but it is speculated that the zinc is required for metalloenzymes involved in the synthesis of DNA and RNA.

In horses, the thymus deficiency syndrome certainly exists and can be diagnosed as one of several types of immunodeficiency with varying degrees of severity (Chapter 3).

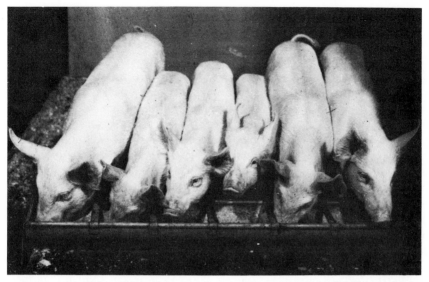

Fig. 2.7. Six piglets which are litter-mates. Three of the piglets have not grown as fast as the others, and the smaller animals have had their thymus removed (Tx) and have received 480 rads of radiation. The other three piglets have had their thymus surgically exposed without removal (STx) and received 480 rads of radiation. The Tx piglets exhibit slow growth, which is a manifestation of induced T-cell deficiency. (Reproduced by kind permission of Dr. R. M. Binns, ARC, Institute for Animal Physiology, Babraham, Cambridge, England.)

2.5 SUBPOPULATIONS OF LYMPHOCYTES

The effects of thymectomy on the lymphocyte subpopulations alerted immunologists to the possibility that lymphocytes with quite similar physical appearance might have different functional properties. This was obviously true of the thymus-derived (T)-cells and the bone marrow-derived (B)-cells in the mouse. The work of Miller and Mitchell (1968) established that removal of the thymus in neonatal mice caused a marked drop in non-antibody-producing functions of the immune response, such as delayed hypersensitivity. There was also a drop in the antibody-producing potential of the remaining B-cells, and the concept of the collaborative 'helper' T-cell was put forward. To balance this idea, evidence of a suppressor T-cell was obtained, and this cell was suggested to control antibody in the induction phase of the immune response.

In humans, the work in mice could not be immediately applied for several reasons. For one, there were no reliable marker systems for T-cells, although B-cells could be identified by their possession of surface immunoglobulin (sIg). For another, there was no way of proving experimentally by thymectomy and irradiation, that the same subpopulations existed in the human that existed in the mouse. A chance finding that sheep erythrocytes bound non-specifically to a large population of human peripheral lymphocytes (Coombs *et al.*, 1970), offered the possibility of a marker, the erythrocyte (E)-'rosette', and this was subsequently proven to define cells which did not bear surface immunoglobulin, that is, the T-cells. Attempts to demonstrate helper and suppressor cells with human lymphocytes have depended mostly on various *in vitro* assays of antibody production after pokeweed mitogen (PWM) stimulation of B-cells or the production of specific antibody by cells in tissue culture. The addition of certain T-cell populations such as cells with receptors for IgG (FcG) was found to suppress the production of immunoglobulin by B-cells, and these cells were thought to be the equivalent of the suppressor cells in the mouse.* Conversely, the IgM receptor-bearing cells (FcM) stimulated immunoglobulin production and were thought to be the equivalent of helper cells. This broad division has not stood up to close scrutiny, although helper and suppressor cells probably possess receptors for immunoglobulin of either type. This idea has been replaced with that of subdivisions of lymphocytes obtained with the use of monoclonal antibodies directed towards lymphocyte membrane glycoproteins. The OKT series of monoclonal antibodies produced by the Ortho Company as well as those produced by Becton-Dickinson and Coulter, for use in their fluorescence-activated cell sorters (FACS), have been suggested to define helper, suppressor and cytotoxic T-cells in human peripheral lymphocyte populations (see Table 4.1 in Chapter 4). At the time of writing, these monoclonal antibodies were still being evaluated from the basic research point of view as well as in clinical immunology. The results of this work are accumulating, but there is yet to be consensus reached on the accuracy of classification of lymphocytes, using these monoclonal antibodies.

2.6   LYMPHOCYTE SUBPOPULATIONS IN ANIMALS

Animal lymphocyte subpopulations can be best described species by species, since there are some variations in the markers used.

2.6.1   Pigs

In the pig, T-cells have been identified with accuracy using the SRBC marker (E-rosette) used with human lymphocytes. In particular, the use of dextran or Ficoll (Pharmacia, Uppsala, Sweden) to enhance the agglutination of the SRBC

*See Chapter 4 for a full explanation of the Fc nomenclature.

(Binns, 1978, 1982), has allowed the identification of most mature pig T-lymphocytes in blood, thymus, lymph nodes and spleen. Another feature of the pig peripheral blood lymphocytes (PBL) is the presence of a population of unmarked or 'null' cells. These cells are depleted after neonatal removal of the thymus in piglets and do not respond in tissue culture to the T-cell mitogens PHA or Con A. They account for up to 40% of PBL in aged pigs. These cells would appear therefore to be present at the time when the thymus makes up a significant amount of the body weight of the pig but not in mature adults, when the thymus has regressed. They would appear, by most criteria of sensitivity to removal of the thymus, density and adhesiveness, to be T-cells, but this population may prove to be more heterogeneous and contain precursors of B-cells and perhaps some immature cells of the erythroid series.

On a percentage differential count, the B-cells of pig PBL appear to be low. However, when the total absolute count of 10,000 to 20,000 PBL is considered, the B-cell count is corrected to absolute counts which are similar to other species, with fewer total PBL, such as the sheep and cow. The reason for the high blood count for PBL in the pig is open to speculation. One possibility is that the return of lymphocytes directly to blood in the lymph nodes, reduces the number of lymphocytes in lymphatic vessels while increasing the number of blood lymphocytes compared with other species. The high blood lymphocyte count in pigs is therefore probably a predictable physiological result of unusual lymphocyte recirculation, and a similar lymph node variation may also be a good reason for the high blood lymphocyte count in chickens and in ducks. In these birds, the lymph node architecture is appreciably different from most mammals. It has been suggested that the thick walls of the post-capillary endothelium prevent migration of lymphocytes directly from blood into lymph, and these cells appear to concentrate in lymphoid follicles distributed through the tissues of birds and in haemolymph nodes, which are a feature of these species.

2.6.2 Sheep

In the sheep, T-lymphocytes have also been detected by a rosette technique using sheep erythrocytes. In fact lymphocytes and erythrocytes from the same sheep can be made to form erythrocyte rosettes. The bond between lymphocyte and erythrocyte is weak, however, unless the strength of the agglutinate is enhanced by the presence of dextran or Ficoll.

As in the pig, there remains a population of unmarked or null cells which, in contrast to pig null cells, respond to phytomitogens such as PHA. This population is larger in lambs than in adult sheep but even in adults, accounts for a high proportion (40%) of PBL (Outteridge et al., 1981). This apparent anomaly is undoubtedly due to the weakness of the bond between erythrocyte and sheep lymphocytes in the rosettes, which makes the E-rosette in the sheep a less comprehensive T-cell marker than in the pig, or even the cow. The anomaly is less evident when fluorescein-labelled peanut agglutinin (PNA) is used as a T-cell marker for the sheep (Fahey, 1980). The null cell population using this technique is only 5–10% in adult sheep, and for most current studies this technique is additionally useful, since the cells can be differentiated using the FACS.

Both E-rosette formation and fluorescent PNA detect the depletion of null T-cells after the removal of the thymus in the foetal lamb. The effect of foetal thymectomy in the lamb persists after birth for up to 1 year. During this period, there is a slow recovery of total lymphocyte count in blood, largely through increase in the null cell population. Also during this period of recovery, lambs are apparently more susceptible to bacterial gut infections and generalised virus infections, than 'sham'-thymectomised control lambs. Growth rate is not generally impaired, although examination of the lambs at post mortem reveals changes in the lymph nodes consistent with depletion of the thymus-dependent cortex.

2.6.3   Cattle

The search for T-cell markers in cattle has probably been the most intensive of any of the domestic species. Cattle lymphocytes form rosettes with sheep erythrocytes, and their numbers have been enhanced by a variety of techniques. These fall into two main categories: enhancement of the spontaneous agglutination and the chemical treatment of the erythrocytes.

In the case of enhancement of E-rosette formation by dextran, Ficoll or foetal calf serum (FCS), these are added separately in various concentrations, to enhance the normal E-rosette formation which occurs in saline alone. These methods have the advantage of not detecting appreciable overlap between T-cells and surface immunoglobulin-positive (sIg^+) B-cells.

In contrast, chemical treatment of sheep erythrocytes with aminoethylammonium bromide (AET) or enzyme treatment with neuraminidase (NA) both enhance E-rosette formation but decrease specificity. In particular, the use of AET or NA in conjunction with dextran enhancement, causes some sIg^+ B-cells to form rosettes with sheep erythrocytes, resulting in inaccurate T-cell counts.

Allowing for the possibility of a small overlap between E-rosette-forming cells and those bearing sIg, this T-cell marker has proved useful for cattle blood lymphocytes. It has been shown, for example, that 89% of calf thymocytes form E-rosettes and that a high proportion (40–80%) of peripheral blood lymphocytes do also. The cells that form E-rosettes appear to be mature cells, since their numbers in blood progressively increase with the age of the foetus and calves are born with blood lymphocytes which form about 40% E-rosettes. As the calves grow, there is a steady increase in the proportion of E-rosette-forming cells, which reaches a plateau of 70 to 80% of total cells at 2 years of age. At the same time, there is a proportional decrease in the B-cells, which reach a plateau of about 20%. Null cells are present in the blood of calves, and they also decrease inversely with the increase of T-cells. In mature cattle, 7 years and older, null cells are present in very low numbers or are absent in blood.

2.7 SUBPOPULATIONS OF T-CELLS

In human blood, the E-rosette-forming cells can be further subdivided on the basis of various other receptors they may possess. As mentioned before, FcM and FcG receptors were at one stage thought to reflect functional helper and suppressor T-cells, respectively. This concept has not stood up to close scrutiny, and it is now thought that the possession of FcM receptors represents a stage in maturation of T-cells towards a cell type which possesses FcG receptors. The function of the Fc receptors is not known, but presumably they are involved somehow in the feedback regulation of the immune response.

Pig, sheep, dog and cattle lymphocytes possess FcM, FcG and complement (C') receptors. There is no convincing evidence to suggest that possession of these receptors is associated with help or suppression of the immune response. None of the domestic species has been studied sufficiently to confirm the findings with the lymphocytes of humans and mice. However, there is no reason to suppose at this stage that they are basically different.

Developments with monoclonal antibodies against human lymphocyte subpopulations, suggest the direction in which research on animal lymphocyte subpopulations may go. The OKT series of monoclonal antibodies identify populations of peripheral human blood lymphocytes, which are thought to be functional helper (OKT4$^+$), suppressor and cytotoxic cells (OKT8$^+$). They have the advantage of being applicable to fluorescent labelling of cells for identification and separation of lymphocytes in the FACS.

Again, considerable work is under way to test these new markers in functional cellular interactions *in vitro*. At the time of writing, it is uncertain whether they are any better than FcM or FcG receptor assays for the identification of helper and suppressor cells. There is some doubt that peripheral blood lymphocyte samples contain all the potential antibody-forming cells of different specificities, as well as the cells which provide control of these specific immune responses. Certainly, lymph nodes and spleen, when available, appear to possess cells which have greater specific antibody-forming potential than those of peripheral blood, and it is possible that many lymphocytes of the controlling series are sessile cells in lymphoid tissues and do not recirculate.

2.8 FUNCTIONAL PROPERTIES
OF LYMPHOCYTE SUBPOPULATIONS

Examination of T-cell markers in the sheep reveals that there are differences in proportion between peripheral blood and efferent popliteal lymph. The E-rosette-forming cells constitute 40% of cells in peripheral blood and 70% of cells in lymph. Conversely, B-cells with sIg constitute 20% of cells in blood but only 11% in lymph. There is also a lack of FcG receptor-bearing cells in lymph, while in sheep blood these cells constitute 40% of cells (Outteridge *et al.*, 1981). The significance of these findings is that there is selection of subpopulations at the level equivalent of the post-capillary venule of the peripheral lymph node. It would appear, as with other species such as the mouse and rat, that T-cells recirculate more rapidly than B-cells. Secondly, there appears to be a barrier to cells with FcG receptors whether they are monocytes or lymphocytes.

Functionally, the E-rosette-forming cells appear to be the subpopulation involved in initial antigen recognition. They are widely distributed through the body and appear to recirculate selectively through lymph nodes as a prerequisite to exposure to antigen. The B-cells also recirculate, but true plasma cells, into which B-cells transform, are mostly sessile cells in sheep lymph nodes and other lymphoid tissue (Fig. 2.5b).

From studies with human blood lymphocytes the connection between FcG receptors and suppression appears tenuous, and there are no studies in domestic animals which prove that these cells suppress the immune response. In cattle it has been demonstrated that blood lymphocytes contain a subpopulation of cells which inhibit transformation of Con A-stimulated cells (Smith *et al.*, 1981). These suppressor cells require an initial pre-stimulation with Con A to make them suppressive. No connection between FcG receptor-bearing cells and suppression has been noted. Also in progressive myelopathy of dogs a suppressor cell appears to be generated during the autoimmune response (Waxman *et al.*, 1980).

Another point which can be made is that a likely reason for exclusion of FcG receptor-bearing cells from lymph, is the known lack of monocytes in lymph. These cells also bear FcG receptors and are often confused with FcG receptor-bearing T-cells in blood lymphocyte suspensions. In certain concentrations (>10%), monocytes are suppressive in tissue culture, and rigorous technique is necessary to exclude the presence of monocytes in suppressor T-cell assays.

From studies on cells in sheep lymph, there appear to be helper T-cells which enhance *in vitro* responses to tuberculin PPD (Outteridge and Fahey, 1981), and enhance the numbers of plaque-forming cells to horse red blood cells or chicken red blood cells (Heron *et al.*, 1982). The FcM receptor-bearing cells have not been proven to be the helper cell subpopulation in domestic species of animals. They account for a considerable proportion of T-cells (30%) in cattle blood, and it seems likely that if helper cells are present in PBL of cattle, some of them would bear FcM receptors. The difficulty is in finding assay systems which will prove that FcM receptor-bearing cells are indeed helper cells. The work with human lymphocytes is still controversial, since FcM receptor-bearing cells appear capable of either enhancing or suppressing *in vitro* antibody responses.

2.9 RESPONSE OF SUBPOPULATIONS TO MITOGENS AND ANTIGENS

One of the accepted criteria of T-cells is that they respond to certain mitogenic substances. These are classically represented by phytohaemagglutinin (PHA) derived from the red kidney bean (*Phaseolus vulgaris*) and concanavalin A (Con A) from the jack bean (*Canavalia ensiformis*). Few immunologists indeed would not have used these lectins at some stage of their careers. The mitogens have become a standard method for studying T-cells in tissue culture in many species, including domestic animals, and yet the way in which they stimulate cells has yet to be clearly explained.

Phytohaemagglutinin is a lectin which binds to glucosyl residues of glycoproteins in the cell membranes of both B- and T-cells. However, it is only the T-cells which respond to the stimulus by undergoing blast cell transformation. The exact mechanism of cell membrane stimulation is not known, but the substance cyclic AMP (adenosine monophosphate) is known to be involved in the initial steps of the blast cell transformation.

In the veterinary field, PHA has been used to stimulate lymphocytes of sheep, cattle, pigs, horses, dogs, cats and chickens. Some information has been obtained on the optimum concentrations of PHA required for stimulation of lymphocytes from all these species. The interpretation of results in animals except those with gross T-cell deficiencies, such as Severe Combined Immunodeficiency (SCID) of horses, is open to question. The PHA stimulation causes a large proportion of T-cells to transform non-specifically, so that this *in vitro* test does not assess T-cell functions for specific immune responses.

In terms of confirming lymphocyte markers, PHA stimulation has been useful in defining T-cells, purified from mixed populations in sheep, cattle, pigs and horses. In this work, the purified T-cells from nylon wool or E-rosette concentration, are found to respond more strongly than the T-cell-depleted population.

Antigens have also been used to stimulate lymphocytes cultured *in vitro*. The use of tuberculin with bovine lymphocytes from tuberculous cattle for *in vitro* assays, has been thoroughly explored. Correlations between delayed hypersensitivity to skin testing with tuberculin in cattle and *in vitro* responsiveness of their blood lymphocytes to tuberculin, have been found. Similar findings for delayed skin hypersensitivity to Johnin and *in vitro* responsiveness of cattle blood lymphocytes to this antigen have been demonstrated. To a lesser extent, correlations exist between Brucallergen delayed skin hypersensitivity and the response *in vitro* to Brucallergen by lymphocytes from cattle infected with *Brucella abortus*. However, the manifestation of delayed hypersensitivity is not the same as that of macrophage cellular immunity, and *in vitro* lymphocyte responsiveness has not been found to correlate with immunity to the diseases just listed. This point is discussed in more detail in Chapter 6 dealing with immunity to bacteria.

It is also possible to stimulate B-cells *in vitro* to produce antibody. For instance, human lymphocytes have been stimulated to produce antibody to influenza virus in tissue culture. This is usually the result of previous immunological stimulus by natural infection with the virus, so that the phenomenon studied is a secondary immune response. It is also possible to stimulate a primary response to some antigens *in vitro*, but the number of cells producing antibody is understandably small. This is because the number of specifically-reactive cells in a small sample of blood lymphocytes is very low.

This technique has been used to measure the quantity of specific antibody in different immunoglobulin classes produced by blood lymphocytes in humans. However, as with PHA stimulation, the method only really demonstrates gross immunological deficiency. It does have the advantage of examining a specific immune response, for instance to influenza virus, diphtheria toxoid or tetanus toxoid. It has not been used at all in the veterinary field.

The stimulation of B-cells non-specifically by two mitogens, pokeweed extract (PWM) and lipopolysaccharide (LPS) has been used to assess B-cell function. Pokeweed mitogen from *Phytolacca americana* has been used to stimulate B-cells non-specifically for suppressor cell assays in humans. The mitogen stimulates a T-cell subpopulation also, but its interest in the laboratory has been its ability to stimulate all B-cells to produce immunoglobulin, detectable by immunofluorescence techniques. In suppressor cell assays, human FcM and FcG cells have been added back to purified B-cell populations, and the degrees of help or suppression of antibody production after PWM stimulation have been measured. This approach has not been explored with domestic animals, although pig lymphocytes have been stimulated and examined for specific immunoglobulin classes after PWM stimulation.

The other mitogen used to stimulate B-cells is the lipopolysaccharide from *Escherichia coli*. Again, LPS has been found to stimulate human B-cells non-specifically to transform into blasts, measurable by [^{3}H]thymidine uptake. It does not work with mouse lymphocytes but does work with pig, sheep and cattle lymphocytes if the donor animals have been previously sensitised naturally or artificially to *E. coli* LPS. Therefore, it appears that the response to LPS in domestic species is a secondary immune response.

Finally, anti-immunoglobulin antibodies have also been used to stimulate pig

B-cells. The effect is similar to LPS, in that only B-cells are stimulated and the response can be measured by [³H]thymidine uptake by the cells.

2.10 HELP AND SUPPRESSION IN DIAGNOSTIC TECHNIQUES INVOLVING LYMPHOCYTES

A practical problem involving the diagnosis of tuberculosis in cattle is thought to be affected by the presence of suppressor cells. This disease is diagnosed by the intradermal injection of tuberculin, followed by the development of a lump at the injection site in tuberculous but not in uninfected cattle.

Various factors affect the development of this delayed-hypersensitivity response to tuberculin. It is known that frequent, repeated skin testing of cattle will lead to desensitisation or even total anergy to further skin testing. Concurrent infection with non-specific soil mycobacteria or the avian strain of mycobacteria, will also produce either desensitisation of positive cattle or non-specific positive reactions in uninfected cattle.

In the case of desensitisation or anergy, the current ideas suggest that this is due to the presence of suppressor T-cells, which specifically suppress tuberculin-reactive lymphocytes. Competing theories include selective removal of reactive lymphocytes by the spleen or lymph nodes, or the presence of circulating antigen–antibody complexes, which block tuberculin receptors on T-cells in cattle.

Suppressor cells have never actually been demonstrated with cattle lymphocytes, reactive to tuberculin, although there is some evidence with human blood lymphocytes, that suppressor T-cells can suppress tuberculin-sensitive lymphocytes *in vitro*. The situation is further complicated by the apparent division of suppressor cells into T-cells and monocytes, the latter being demonstrated to inhibit T-cell responses to tuberculin in tissue culture. This point has been mentioned previously in the section on the functional properties of T-cell subpopulations.

It is known, however, that after desensitisation of cattle, circulating T-cells, responsive to tuberculin, cannot be demonstrated by *in vitro* tests (Corner *et al.*, 1976). Furthermore, work in sheep suggests that specifically-sensitised cells are removed from the circulation via the post-capillary venules in lymph nodes, and if these cells are drained from the animal by lymphatic vessel cannulation, the animals become desensitised to tuberculin (McConnell *et al.*, 1974). It only requires a further step to visualise T-cells failing to recirculate through lymph nodes and instead, becoming trapped in the node where they are suppressed by sessile cells such as macrophages. Specifically-sensitised cells would not reach the blood stream and react to the intradermal injection of tuberculin. This scenario does not require the presence of circulating suppressor T-cells or immune complexes, which have been difficult to demonstrate, but does explain specific desensitisation to tuberculin without any effect on the responses to other antigens.

2.11 LYMPHOKINES

The effects of lymphokines, such as macrophage migration inhibition factor, have been demonstrated with cattle lymphocytes. The interleukins have also been described for cattle (Outteridge and Lepper, 1973), and they can be produced in quantity from bovine lymphocyte cell lines in tissue culture (Baker and Knoblock, 1982a,b). They have also been described for pigs (Gasbarre *et al.,* 1983), and it would seem likely that they are found in all domestic species.

The presence of a suppresive factor in the serum of dogs with Demodectic Mange has has been described (Hirsh *et al.,* 1975), but it appears that accompanying bacterial infection of the skin is also required to stimulate the appearance of this suppressive factor in serum (Barta *et al.,* 1983). Most of the suppressive factors described are not antigen-specific, and in sheep lymph the factor has been found to be prostaglandin E_2 (Hopkins *et al.,* 1981).

At the moment the importance of the interleukins and the immunosuppressive factors in the control of the immune response remains to be determined.

2.12 ANALYSIS OF LYMPHOCYTE SUBPOPULATIONS: THE FLUORESCENCE-ACTIVATED CELL SORTER

The FACS was developed in the early 1970s in California, in the laboratory of the Herzenbergs at Stanford University. The machine directs a stream of cells in single file through a fine nozzle, immediately below which, the beam of an argon laser intersects the stream of cells passing through and excites fluorescein-labelled cells in the population. The stream then breaks into microdroplets and passes between two plates with an electrical potential between them. The light from the laser excitation of the fluorescein tag is collected by an optical system and registered as counts in a photomultiplier tube which in turn, is connected to an oscilloscope display. Cells which appear as dots on the screen, form clusters representing cells with similar fluorescence properties.

The mechanism exists by which clusters can be electronically isolated or 'gated', and by means of a series of pulses, the microdroplets containing the selected fluorescent cells, can be deflected to the left or to the right, between two charged plates, after a suitable deflection delay time. The selected population is then collected in a centrifuge tube, and upon examination, the desired cells are found to be high in purity (>98%).

The FACS has allowed the close analysis of the lymphocyte subpopulations in the mouse and, more recently, with the development of monoclonal antibodies, human lymphocyte subpopulations. The rate of cell sorting is about 3000 cells/ second, but if a particular subpopulation is present in low frequency, large numbers of cells have to be sorted to accumulate the desired subpopulation. This requires an increase in sorting time compared with more numerous cell populations, but even with more common cells the long sorting time of several hours often precludes the use of this machine for producing large numbers of cells for subsequent experiments.

The greatest use for the cell sorter has not been in the physical sorting of lymphocytes but in the analysis of cells. The sorting of selected clusters has allowed each subpopulation to be characterised, but the subsequent purification of large numbers of selected cells (10–100 million) is still carried out with techniques such as density-gradient separation of rosettes or by nylon wool columns. These techniques are described in the Appendix of Methods.

At the moment, cell sorters are being used extensively with cells labelled with monoclonal antibodies, to characterise different lymphocyte subpopulations. The monoclonal antibodies are available from companies such as Becton-Dickinson, Ortho, and Coulter, which also sell the cell-sorting machines. The OKT series of monoclonal antibodies, from the Ortho Company, label lymphocytes which are claimed to be T-cells, thymocytes, monocytes, suppressor and helper cells. They are being used to test lymphocytes in a variety of clinical conditions, such as the various immunodeficiencies and virus infections. They have, for example, proved useful in detecting Acute Immunodeficiency Syndrome (AIDS) in humans.

This type of work has yet to be carried out with lymphocytes of the domestic species. Monoclonal antibodies to bovine lymphocytes have been produced, but there are no published data on the use of the cell sorter to analyse labelled bovine lymphocyte subpopulations. The costliness of the monoclonal antibodies and of the instrument has limited the use of this machine, with lymphocytes from domestic animals, to a few research institutes. At the moment it is difficult to visualise such machines being used outside these institutes for clinical studies on animals.

2.13 ISOLATION TECHNIQUES FOR LYMPHOCYTES

2.13.1 Rosette Techniques

The subdivision of lymphocytes into T- and B-cells, on the basis of spontaneous rosette formation with sheep erythrocytes, has been exploited for initial purification of T-cells. The T-cells which form E-rosettes, assume a density closer to SRBC than lymphocytes and can be separated from non-rosette-forming lymphocytes by separation on Ficoll-Paque (Pharmacia, Uppsala, Sweden). This technique is described in the Appendix of Methods.

The technique allows separation of up to 100 million T-cells in a large centrifuge tube after allowing the formation of the E-rosettes overnight at 4°C. The technique works well for blood lymphocytes from humans and pigs and less well for cattle, sheep and goats. The ruminant species require dextran or Ficoll to enhance E-rosette formation, and this can lead to clumping. These clumps end up in the red-cell pellet, reducing the purity of the E-rosette fraction. A more effective way of initially purifying E-rosette-forming lymphocytes in ruminants, is the nylon wool column technique described in the next subsection.

The concentrated E-rosette-forming cells are mixed with ammonium chloride Tris buffer (ACT) to lyse the red cells (see Appendix); the cells are reconcentrated by centrifugation and, if necessary, layered again over a half-strength Ficoll-Paque gradient for removal of red-cell 'ghosts' by centrifugation. A purity of >90% E-rosette-forming cells has been obtained with pig blood lymphocytes, using this method.

The rosette-forming cells with C', FcM and FcG may also be separated on Ficoll-Paque, so that successive subdivisions of E-rosette-forming cells are obtained. Lymphocytes are subjected to a series of centrifugations on Ficoll-Paque to produce subpopulations of T-cells. Despite the use of the FACS, the rosette-forming cell separations are still commonly used for initial purification of lymphocyte subpopulations for large numbers of cells.

2.13.2 Nylon Wool Columns

This technique, first described by Julius et al. (1973) for human blood lymphocytes, has been widely used to purify T-cells. The mechanism is not precisely known, but it is thought that different membrane properties make T-cells non-adhesive and B-cells adhesive, under the conditions used in the technique.

These conditions require that 10% foetal calf serum (FCS) be added to the tissue culture medium used to soak the nylon wool. No added serum results in all cells adhering to the nylon wool. Undiluted serum results in no cells adhering to the wool. Experiments with varying proportions of serum to medium, generally arrive at about 10% FCS for the required medium (see Appendix).

The technique has been used effectively with sheep, cattle and pig lymphocytes. The non-adherent population usually is depleted of B-cells (<3% sIg[+]) and shows enhanced responsiveness to PHA compared with unseparated cells.

The adherent population can be dislodged from the nylon wool by careful teasing and agitation in a sterile petri dish containing culture medium, or by repeated aspiration of the syringe barrel containing the nylon wool, by sucking up the medium through a needle after insertion of the plunger. Not all adherent cells are recovered, and between 14 and 20% of cells are lost. The adherent cells are enriched for B-cells (up to 50% sIg) but not completely depleted of T-cells, since E-rosette-forming cells still form a high proportion of adherent cells. It appears that in cattle at least, these adherent T-cells possess receptors for FcM and FcG and possibly represent populations of helper and suppressor T-cells.

Nylon wool columns offer a rapid method of purifying T-cells with a resultant population containing few B-cells. Not all T-cells are recovered, and it is possible that some of the regulatory T-cells are depleted in the non-adherent population.

2.13.3 Affinity Plates and Columns

In principle, the use of some affinity separation method, whether by beads in a column or by the flat surface of a petri dish, should provide the best way of purifying lymphocyte subpopulations. For example, lymphocytes with Fc receptors should be retained by surfaces to which immunoglobulin molecules are attached. Or, sIg^+ cells should attach to surfaces coated with anti-immunoglobulin and T-cells should be non-adherent.

In practice, the use of these methods produces variable results. The columns of beads give good depletion of certain populations, but recovery of adherent cells is often poor. The use of spacer molecules between the antibodies and the carrier beads has been carried out, to improve attachment and to allow recovery by elution with medium which breaks the bonds in the spacer molecules. Usually the extra effort required in getting these techniques to work is not justified, when the same purification can be attained using rosette centrifugation techniques. The column method is also quite expensive for reagents such as affinity-purified anti-immunoglobulin, $F(ab')_2$ fragments* and the plastic beads themselves. It also appears that B-cells recovered from $F(ab')_2$ anti-immunoglobulin columns are hyporeactive to B-cell mitogens in tissue culture. Commercially-manufactured affinity beads are available from Bio-Rad Laboratories, Richmond, California, but these are expensive and offer little advantage over the cheaper rosette centrifugation techniques. Petri dishes can also be used with reagents, similar to those used in columns. They have the advantage that the removal of the cells from the plate can be observed by inverted microscope. It is often found that cells have to be centrifuged at low speed in the petri dish to obtain the best attachment possible. This however, often results in non-specific attachment of cells, which then reduces the purity of the specifically-adherent population.

Affinity plates have been used effectively to purify pig lymphocytes by an indirect method of goat anti-rabbit IgG attached to the plate by carbodiimide treatment and rabbit anti-pig IgG coated on the pig B-cells (Symons and Loke,

*See Chapter 4 for a full explanation of the Fab nomenclature.

1975). The attached B-cells can be induced to detach by prolonged incubation of the plates at 37°C, which causes the points of attachment of the anti-immunoglobulin to form caps and eventually come off the cell. There also appears to be some activation to blast transformation in pig B-cells purified by this method, and this may cause problems in later cell culture experiments.

Sheep lymphocytes have been enriched for Fc+ cells using a technique which depends first on attachment of bovine red cells (BRBC) to a petri dish using carbodiimide, followed by rabbit anti-BRBC immunoglobulin. The Fc portion of the rabbit immunoglobulin is then available for the Fc+ cells to attach, and these may be recovered by lysis of the BRBC as described for the rosette centrifugation techniques.

2.14   FLUORESCEIN-LABELLED LYMPHOCYTES

A new technique to allow the tracing of lymphocytes which recirculate, has been developed, which does not require the radioactive tracer method. This involves the direct labelling of whole cells, with fluorescein isothiocyanate, by way of their proteins. The cells survive this procedure and have been shown to live for longer than 21 days after labelling and injection back into the experimental animal (Binns *et al.*, 1981a; Pabst and Binns, 1981).

The technique has been used in pigs in which surgically-exposed spleens have been perfused. The conclusion drawn from these experiments is that the null cell population does not recirculate through the pig spleen whereas the other subpopulations do recirculate Binns *et al.*, 1981b). Experiments with sheep indicate that fluorescein-labelled lymphocytes recirculate through the popliteal lymph node in an apparently normal fashion. It would appear therefore that this technique offers the possibility of tracing the recirculation patterns of different lymphocyte subpopulations.

2.15   CHANGES IN SUBPOPULATIONS IN SEVERE COMBINED
IMMUNODEFICIENCY OF FOALS

In the domestic species, it is only the horse which has been found to exhibit the immuno-deficiency syndrome of human infants. This is the result of genetic faults inherited in the Thoroughbred bloodstock. Foals are born which are deficient in lymphocytes of both T- and B-cell series. They can be kept alive by treatment with antibiotics but eventually succumb to natural infections. Examination of their blood reveals the absence of lymphocytes but the presence of large numbers of polymorphonuclear leucocytes. Much has been written on the clinical manifestations of the syndrome but nothing can be done to correct the condition, and it would appear that the best course of action is to detect carriers of the genetic fault and not breed from them. This condition is discussed in greater detail in Chapter 3 on the immunology of reproduction.

2.16 GENERAL CONCLUSIONS

An important question on cellular immunity in domestic animals is whether it is possible to measure the immune responsiveness of individual animals to vaccines, using the currently-available *in vitro* cell culture techniques. At the moment, the answer to this is that there is no test for cellular immunity *in vitro*, which can be applied to circulating lymphocytes, which measures the effect of vaccination. The lymphocyte stimulation and macrophage migration inhibition tests measure lymphocyte reactivity, but appear to be ill-adapted to detect anything other than delayed hypersensitivity or a gross immunodeficiency.

Current research is moving towards the measurement of leucocyte function with such assays as chemiluminescence of cells, during phagocytosis of bacteria. This measures oxidation products such as superoxide, but it does not give any indication of the degree of intracellular killing of the microorganisms by the phagocytic cells. It still appears necessary to use isolated macrophages or neutrophils, mixed with living microorganisms in tissue culture, to assess the effectiveness of intracellular killing of the pathogenic microorganisms.

The measurement of lymphocyte subpopulations by cell sorter to examine the levels of suppressor or helper cells has yet to be developed to the stage where it provides a measure of potential immune responsiveness in individual animals. At the moment it must be said that the study of cellular immunity has yet to provide a useful practical test for measuring the cellular immune response to specific pathogenic microorganisms.

REFERENCES

Baker, P. E. and Knoblock, K. F. (1982a). *Vet. Immunol. Immunopathol.* **3**, 365–379.
Baker, P. E. and Knoblock, K. F. (1982b). *Vet. Immunol. Immunopathol.* **3**, 381–397.
Barta, O., Waltman, C., Oyekan, P. P., McGrath, R. K. and Hribernik, T. N. (1983). *Comp. Immun. Microbiol. Infect. Dis.* **6**, 9–18.
Binns, R. M. (1978). *J. Immunol. Methods* **21**, 197–210.
Binns, R. M. (1982). *Vet. Immunol. Immunopathol.* **3**, 95–146.
Binns, R. M. and Hall, J. C. (1966). *Br. J. Exp. Pathol.* **47**, 275–280.
Binns, R. M., Pallares, V., Symons, D. B. A. and Sibbons, P. (1977). *Int. Arch. Allergy Appl. Immunol.* **55**, 96–101.
Binns, R. M., Blakeley, D. and Licence, S. T. (1981a). *Int. Arch. Allergy Appl. Immunol.* **66**, 341–349.
Binns, R. M., Pabst, R. and Licence, S. T. (1981b). *Immunology* **44**, 273–279.

Brummerstedt, E., Andresen, E., Basse, A. and Flagstad, T. (1974). *Nord. Veterinaermed.* **26,** 279–293.

Burrell, D. H. (1978). *Res. Vet. Sci.* **24,** 269–276.

Cahill, R. N. P., Poskitt, D. C., Frost, H. and Trnka, Z. (1977). *J. Exp. Med.* **145,** 420–428.

Cole, G. J. and Morris, B. (1973). *Adv. Vet. Sci.* **17,** 225–263.

Coombs, R. R. A., Gurner, B. W., Wilson, A. B., Holm, G. and Lindgren, B. (1970). *Int. Arch. Allergy Appl. Immunol.* **39,** 658–663.

Corner, L. A., Outteridge, P. M., Pearson, C. W. and Lepper, A. W. D. (1976). *Int. Arch. Allergy Appl. Immunol.* **52,** 3–14.

Fahey, K. H. (1980). *Aust. J. Exp. Biol. Med. Sci.* **58,** 557–569.

Flagstad, T. (1976). *Nord. Veterinaermed.* **28,** 160–169.

Gasbarre, L. C., Urban, J. F. and Romanowski, R. D. (1983). *Vet. Immunol. Immunopathol.* **5,** 221–236.

Hall, J. G. and Morris, B. (1965). *J. Exp. Med.* **121,** 901–910.

Hall, J. G., Morris, B., Moreno, G. D. and Bessis, M. C. (1967). *J. Exp. Med.* **125,** 91–109.

Heron, I., Cahill, R. and Trnka, Z. (1982). *Int. Arch. Allergy Appl. Immunol.* **68,** 157–163.

Hirsh, D. C., Baker, B. B., Wiger, N., Yaskulski, S. G. and Osburn, B. I. (1975). *Am. J. Vet. Res.* **36,** 1591–1595.

Hopkins, J., McConnell, I. and Raniwalla, J. (1981). *Immunology* **43,** 205–212.

Julius, M. H., Simpson, E. and Herzenberg, L. A. (1973). *Eur. J. Immunol.* **3,** 645–649.

McConnell, I., Lachmann, P. J. and Hobart, M. J. (1974). *Nature (London)* **250,** 113–116.

Miller, J. F. A. P. and Mitchell, G. F. (1968). *J. Exp. Med.* **128,** 801–820.

Outteridge, P. M. and Fahey, K. J. (1981). *Aust. J. Exp. Biol. Med. Sci.* **59,** 157–165.

Outteridge, P. M. and Lepper, A. W. D. (1973). *Immunology* **25,** 981–994.

Outteridge, P. M., Fahey, K. J. and Lee, C. S. (1981). *Aust. J. Exp. Biol. Med. Sci.* **59,** 143–155.

Pabst, R. and Binns, R. M. (1981). *Immunology* **44,** 321–329.

Smith, W. G., Usinger, W. R. and Splitter, G. A. (1981). *Immunology* **43,** 91–100.

Symons, D. B. A. and Loke, R. K. G. (1975). *J. Immunol. Methods* **7,** 251–254.

Waxman, F. J., Clemmons, R. M. and Hinrichs, D. F. (1980). *J. Immunol.* **124,** 1216–1222.

3

Immunology of
Reproduction

The immunological influences on reproduction extend to a number of aspects, including the immune response of the foetus to antigens and pathogens, the exchange of immunoglobulins between the mother and the newborn animal, the maintenance of pregnancy and faults in embryonic development of the lymphoid system. There are other aspects too, such as chimaeric twin calves, which in some way overcome histocompatibility barriers between non-identical twins. A detailed description of all these subjects is not possible in the space of one chapter, but selected areas of importance are discussed from the point of view of possible practical importance in the management of the neonatal animal.

3.1 FOETAL IMMUNOLOGY

The immunology of the mammalian foetus is of particular interest because it was once thought to be immunologically inert. Burnet and Fenner (1949) put forward the hypothesis that if antigen was administered to the foetus during its development, the foetus would not only fail to react and produce an immune response but would also be unresponsive to the antigen during the post-natal period. This was suggested to be the reason for immunologically mature animals failing to react to so-called self antigens, because these antigens had been present at a stage of foetal development when tolerance could be induced.

It was work in sheep by Schinckel and Ferguson (1953) which showed that the foetal lamb was able effectively to reject allogeneic skin grafts. This was direct evidence against tolerance to antigens administered to the foetus. Subsequent work by Silverstein *et al.* (1963) added further evidence that foetal sheep could indeed react to a variety of antigens. This was in contrast to rodents, which only produced antibody or rejected skin grafts at or after birth. The reason for the difference between the rodent and the ruminant species was thought to be due to the relative immaturity of the newborn mouse compared with the ruminant. This meant that mice became reactive to antigen at, or just after, birth, but the ruminant was reactive to antigen in the last third of pregnancy.

The work in foetal sheep also suggested that there might be a 'hierarchy' of antigens, with the foetus reacting to some antigens much earlier in foetal life than to other antigens. For example, foetal sheep produced antibody to a bacterio-phage antigen ($\phi\chi174$) at 66 days gestation, to ferritin at 80 days gestation and to ovalbumin at 123 days gestation. They failed to respond to diphtheria toxoid, *Salmonella typhosa* or Bacillus Calmette–Guérin (BCG) strain of *Mycobacterium bovis*. It was also found that foetal sheep of 77 to 88 days gestation rejected skin allografts, while animals younger than 67 days gestation did not. Thus it was concluded that the foetal lamb did not develop the capacity to produce antibody to all antigens simultaneously but in a series of maturational steps, each of which allowed stimulation of the immune response by a wider range of antigens than the one before.

The hypothesis was challenged by subsequent work on foetal sheep carried out by Fahey and Morris (1974). They found that the foetal lamb responds to most of the antigens used (e.g., chicken red cells, polymerised bacterial flagellin), and primary antibody responses to seven of eight antigens used were detected between 64 and 82 days gestation. The *Salmonella typhimurium* antigen did not stimulate a primary response but primed the foetuses for a secondary immune response to the antigen injected later in gestation.

The magnitude and duration of the response to most antigens was found to depend on foetal age, and antigenic stimulation, in itself, altered the ability of the foetal lamb to synthesise immunoglobulin. It also appeared that the sensitivity of the assay was important in assessing the immune response, and the apparent hierarchy of antigenic stimulation reported by other workers could have been due to differences in sensitivity amongst the assays for the various antibodies.

The work described so far, was carried out in the sheep, which being a ruminant, has a syndesmochorial form of placentation which prevents maternal immunoglobulin and presumably lymphoid cells from reaching the foetus. In this way, the foetal ruminant is an ideal species for studying the development of the immune response, without the complication of the maternal contribution to cir-culating antibody levels. Indeed, it can be shown quite clearly that the foetal ruminant is usually born with extremely low levels of circulating immunoglobulins. These normal foetal immunoglobulins are low-affinity antibodies of the IgM class, but the foetus can be induced to synthesise IgG, when antigen is given as early as 87 days gestation. However the normal lamb usually is born with only circulating IgM and acquires IgG from the colostrum during the first 48 hours after parturition. It is vital therefore for the neonatal ruminant to ingest colostral IgG during the first 48 hours, to receive its complement of maternal antibodies protective against potential pathogens, such as *Escherichia coli,* which could otherwise cause enteritis.

The infection of the foetus with pathogens is a different matter from that found post-natally in lambs and calves after colostrum ingestion. The ruminant foetus is required to mount an immune response with very little contribution from the mother because of the barrier of the syndesmochorial placenta. In this environment, certain pathogens are able to multiply and cause death or deformation of the foetus before an effective immune response can be mounted. This is dependent on the maturity of the foetus.

In sheep, the experimental infection of pregnant ewes with Akabane virus at 30 to 36 days gestation causes congenital deformities such as hydrancephaly and arthrogryposis. Older foetuses produce antibody to Akabane virus, and generally, the congenital deformities are in much lower incidence than those produced after inoculation at 30 to 36 days, when 80% of foetuses have virus-induced deformities. Similar findings have been made with the injection of Bluetongue virus into foetal sheep, which were able to produce neutralising antibody to the virus at about 122 days gestation.

Pigs show similar features to the sheep, since direct inoculation of porcine parvovirus into the amniotic sac, on or before 55 days gestation, causes the death of the foetal piglets. After 72 days gestation, piglets survive inoculation with the virus and develop high titres of antibody.

In cattle, the longer gestation period, in comparison with sheep and pigs, is reflected in the longer time required for maturation of the immune response than for the other two species. Antibody responses to *Anaplasma marginale, Leptospira* spp., Parainfluenza-3 virus, *Brucella abortus,* Infectious Bovine Rhinotracheitis and Bovine Diarrhoea virus, become apparent between 140 and 212 days gestation. Infection *in utero* with *Campylobacter foetus,* causes foetal death when inoculated before 212 days gestation, but foetuses older than 226 days gestation, produce IgM antibody against the organisms and survive.

3.2 MATURATION OF THE CELLULAR IMMUNE RESPONSE

Attempts have been made to correlate the acquisition of cellular immune responses in the foetus, with the onset of responsiveness to antigens as the foetus matures.

3.2.1   B-Lymphocytes

The best-studied animal of veterinary interest is the chicken. It has long been known that removal of the bursa of Fabricius in chicks (Fig. 3.1) greatly reduces the antibody-producing potential of the remaining lymphoid tissues. Studies on chicken embryos have shown that haemopoietic stem cells migrate from the yolk sac to the epithelial thymus and to the bursa and undergo extensive and rapid proliferation. In the bursa, cells are found which synthesise IgM and this appears not to be due to antigenic stimulation, because the embryo is in an antigenically-protected environment. Furthermore, IgM-synthesising cells are found in equal numbers, in germ-free chicken embryos and in conventionally-reared chicks.

However, direct antigenic stimulation of the bursa can be induced by the introduction of antigen into the cloaca of young chicks. This has been used in the past as a method of inoculating older chickens against Infectious Laryngotracheitis (ILT) virus. Thus it would seem that the bursa has two potential functions: firstly in providing an environment for the development and differentiation of B-cells in the embryo, and secondly for the post-natal contact with antigens via the cloaca, in a fashion analogous to that in the pharyngeal tonsils of mammals.

The model proposed for the function of differentiation and development of B-cells in the bursa is as follows. Stem cells migrate to the bursa where they differentiate and begin to synthesise IgM. In some of the daughter cells from lymphocyte division, a switch occurs from $C\mu$ to $C\gamma$ genes and from $C\mu$ to $C\alpha$ genes. These commit the cells to produce IgG or IgA. It is these cells which migrate to the peripheral lymphoid tissues where they are committed to synthesise IgM, IgG or IgA, respectively.

In the sheep, the equivalent of the bursa of Fabricius has been suggested to be the Peyer's patches (Reynolds *et al.*, 1982). Pre-natal surgical removal of the

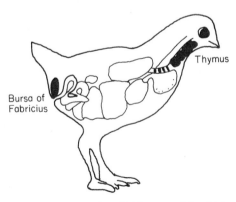

Fig. 3.1.   The figure shows the primary lymphoid organs of the chicken: the thymus and the bursa of Fabricius.

Peyer's patches in foetal lambs is followed by very low B-cell counts in the circulation of these lambs after birth. A bimodal production of B-cells has been observed in the peripheral blood of foetal lambs (Binns and Symons, 1974). Surface immunoglobulin is present on 0.3% of leucocytes at 56 days, on 15% at 78 to 87 days and 2% at 117 days gestation. A slight rise occurs again towards term. The number of peripheral B-cells continues to rise after birth to reach a mean of 22%. The increase in B-cells at 78 to 87 days does not seem to be associated with antigen-binding cells after experimental antigenic stimulation. This rise may therefore be associated with migration of B-cells from the Peyer's patches to the peripheral lymphoid tissues after differentiation and development.

In the pig, surface immunoglobulin-positive cells increase rapidly from 70 to 80 days gestation, from 0.7 to 8.4% of cells. This does not necessarily coincide with the earliest detectable antibody responses, since foetal pigs have been shown to respond to parvovirus as early as 58 days gestation. Although experiments have yet to be performed on this point, it is likely that the 8.4% B-cells found at 70 to 80 days, coincides with the migration of the B-cells from the equivalent of the bursa (e.g., the Peyer's patches) of the foetal pig. The numbers of B-cells are greatly increased by antigenic stimulation of the foetus (17.0–19.1%) compared with controls (8.8%). In this case, it is possible that some cross-stimulation may occur between antigen-stimulated foetuses and non-stimulated foetuses via the placental blood circulation, since the control B-cell counts are also increased.

3.2.2 T-Lymphocytes

As described in Chapter 2 on cellular immunology, the maturation of T-cells was originally studied in mice using neonatal removal of the thymus. This work led to the concept of thymus-derived cells and thymus dependence of immune responses to certain antigens.

Apart from the chicken, this work has not been repeated in domestic animals in exactly the same way that it was carried out in mice. Thymectomy of neonatal ruminants or pigs causes some lymphopoenia but not the wasting disease seen in laboratory rodents. The removal of the thymus from foetal sheep, in the classic experiments of Cole and Morris (1971a,b), again had no effect on the subsequent growth rate of the lambs. In the pig, it was necessary to couple neonatal thymectomy with sublethal irradiation to produce the poor growth rate and susceptibility to infection, comparable with that found with neonatally-thymectomised mice. Even with such severe treatment, piglets recovered rapidly and ultimately reached the same weight as sham-thymectomised litter-mates, albeit at a later time.

The concept of subpopulations of T-cells was also suggested by work in the mouse, where two types of T-cells were found. These were the so-called T1 cells with a high density of thymus θ antigen and T2 cells with a lower density of θ antigen. The T1 cells were found predominantly in the spleen. They were short-lived cells, did not recirculate and were relatively resistant to anti-lymphocyte serum. The T2 cells were found mainly in the blood, thoracic-duct lymph and in lymph nodes. They were long-lived, homed preferentially to lymph nodes, recirculated and were susceptible to anti-lymphocyte serum. Raff and Cantor (1971) suggested that T1 cells were immature T2 cells whose maturation was conditioned by antigen. The T2 cells alone were claimed to be responsible for the T-lymphocyte component of the immune response, while T1 cells became T2 cells in response to antigenic stimulation.

Of the domestic animals, it is the pig which has been most closely studied for changes in these lymphocyte populations during maturation. The work of Binns has shown that there are two main types of T-cells in pigs also. One type does not form E-rosettes and is largely depleted by neonatal thymectomy. Furthermore, while the E-rosette-forming cells react to antigens and mitogens, these 'null' cells appear to be almost totally unreactive, even when macrophages are added to the *in vitro* assay. The null cells have also been shown to remain within the pig spleen and not to recirculate, reinforcing the comparison between these pig lymphocytes and mouse T1 cells.

The maturation of T-cells in the foetus has been followed in two main ways. Firstly, the appearance of E-rosette-forming cells has been measured in the blood of foetuses of different ages. In cattle, it has been found that E-rosette-forming cells are not present in the foetal circulation before 3 months of age. There is a slow increase to a mean of 40% of cells at parturition. After this time, the number of E-rosette-forming cells continues to increase but only reaches a maximum from 7 years of age onwards (Fig. 3.2).

The second method of assaying T-cell maturation is by the use of phytohaemagglutinin (PHA) stimulation. In foetal pigs, this stimulation can be elicited between 72 and 90 days gestation with thymocytes. In sheep, the response can be obtained with liver lymphocytes at 38 days, with thymocytes at about 68 days and with spleen cells at 98 days. In cattle the responses of peripheral blood lymphocytes to PHA can be elicited from 78 to 90 days gestation, and this steadily increases with foetal age. Thus there is a loose association between the acquisition of E-rosette-forming cells and responsiveness to PHA. This is brought into sharper focus in the pig, where it can be demonstrated that it is only the E-rosette-forming cells which are reactive to PHA, with the null cells being completely unresponsive.

Therefore, the ontogeny of T-cell responsiveness in domestic animals would appear to be an initial maturation in the foetal liver, followed by the thymus, spleen and finally the appearance of mature T-cells in peripheral blood. The maturation process then appears to continue after birth, with a steady increase in E-rosette-forming cells and a concomitant decrease in null cells in the peripheral

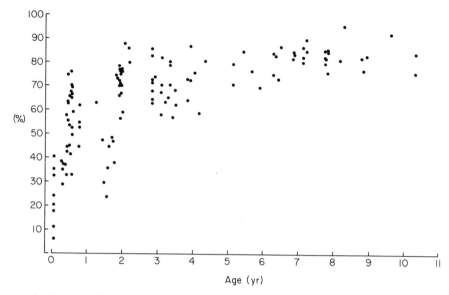

Fig. 3.2. Blood lymphocyte samples from cattle aged from 2 weeks to 10 years were tested for the T-cell marker, sheep erythrocyte (E) rosette formation in the presence of enhancing medium which contained Ficoll 400 (Pharmacia, Uppsala, Sweden). The percentage of T-cells is shown against age in years. (Reproduced by kind permission of the editors of *Res. Vet. Sci.*)

blood. Indeed this post-natal period in calves is characterised by delayed hyper-sensitivity responses to tuberculin which progressively increase in intensity with time after birth, in line with the increase in responsiveness to PHA.

3.3 EXCHANGE OF ANTIBODIES ACROSS THE PLACENTA

The details of experiments on the passive transmission of immunoglobulins from mother to young were the subject of a monograph by Brambell (1970). He reviewed the data for transmission of antibodies or immunoglobulins in birds, rodents, primates, horses, pigs and ruminants. The conclusions from the work summarised in this monograph were that immunoglobulins were transmitted by the uterine blood either across the placenta or across the yolk sac, or by post-natal transmission via the colostrum (Table 3.1).

This work summarised a particular phase of research in immunology in which the relative rates of transmission of immunoglobulins via the placenta were examined in each species using heterologous γ-globulins and compared with the transmission of homologous γ-globulins. In all cases, the selection operated in favour of homologous γ-globulin, and in cases of extreme disparity, the rate of

TABLE 3.1

Transmission of Immunoglobulins from Mother to Neonate[a]

Species	Route	Time of gut closure
Horse	Colostrum	24 hours
Pig	Colostrum	24–36 hours
Ruminant (ox, goat, sheep)	Colostrum	24 hours
Dog and cat	Mostly colostrum	1–2 days
Chicken	Yolk sac	—
Human	Placenta	—

[a] From Brambell (1970).

transmission of heterologous γ-globulin was less than that of the corresponding heterologous albumin.

It is now known that transmission of γ-globulin across the placenta or into colostrum is very much dependent on the Fc piece of the immunoglobulin. This was also appreciated by Brambell, but with subsequent work on amino-acid sequences of immunoglobulins, it appears that the transmission of heterologous γ-globulin must depend on the closeness of the amino-acid sequences to homologous γ-globulin.

Brambell also put forward a hypothesis to explain the transmission of γ-globulin and other proteins through cells into the circulation of the foetus. In this hypothesis, specific receptors on the cell surface (Fc receptors) combined with the γ-globulin, which was then absorbed into pinocytotic vesicles which in turn traversed the cell to secrete their contents on the other side. In Brambell's hypothesis, the pinocytotic vesicle fused with lysosomes in the cell, and a certain amount was digested by the enzymes in the phagolysosomes before the remaining γ-globulin was secreted at the other end of the cell. Subsequent work suggests that appreciable digestion of γ-globulin by the cell is unlikely (Brandon *et al.*, 1971) and that most of the γ-globulin is transmitted intact across the cell (Fig. 3.3). The addition of a 'secretory piece' to IgA has been demonstrated in epithelial cells of mucous membranes and in liver cells, but the necessity of this additional protein for the transmission of IgG has not been shown. It appears that the secretory piece of IgA must provide some protective function against digestion by the enzymes in external secretions such as intestinal fluid.

3.4 INTESTINAL ABSORPTION OF IMMUNOGLOBULIN

In the absorption of γ-globulin by the neonate, a large degree of non-specificity exists in the transmission of macromolecules. Thus although the major protein

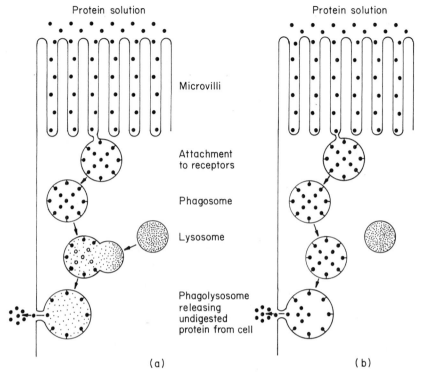

Fig. 3.3. In Brambell's original hypothesis (a) it was suggested that γ-globulin was transmitted across cells by attaching to receptors, which in some way protected some of the γ-globulin from being degraded in the phagolysosome by proteolytic enzymes. This was the mechanism by which the amount of γ-globulin released from the cell after transport, remained constant irrespective of concentration at the apical surface. Later work has suggested that (b) appreciable degradation of the γ-globulin does *not* occur within the cell and that some other mechanism is responsible for regulating the rate of transmission of globulin across the cell. (Adapted from Brambell (1970), 'The Transmission of Passive Immunity from Mother to Young', by permission of North-Holland Publishing Co., Amsterdam and London.)

absorbed is γ-globulin, serum albumin can be absorbed but at a much lower rate. Indeed β-lactoglobulin of whey has been shown to be absorbed by the neonatal calf and then, because of its low molecular weight, re-excreted in the urine, where it appears to cause no untoward clinical effects.

The epithelial cells of the jejunum absorb the immunoglobulin from colostrum, but intact immunoglobulins are not absorbed by epithelial cells in the ileum; they are digested. Receptors for immunoglobulin on epithelial cells of the jejunum have not been demonstrated, presumably because the absorption of immunoglobulin is non-specific and competitive inhibition between immunoglobulin classes cannot be demonstrated.

The 'closure' of the gut of the neonate to immunoglobulin absorption shows considerable variation. In ruminants, horses, pigs, cats and dogs, cessation of intestinal absorption of antibodies occurs at about 24 to 36 hours after birth, while in mice and rats, it is delayed until 16 and 21 days of age, respectively. Experiments have been carried out to determine the basis of 'closure' using the intestinal absorption of polyvinyl pyrrolidone (PVP)(an inert molecule of approximately the same size as γ-globulin) in rats. It was found that cortisone acetate treatment caused precocious closure of the intestine. Experiments with ruminants and pigs suggest that exogenous corticosteroids can reduce the transmission of colostral immunoglobulin but not cause it to cease. It has been concluded from these and other experiments, that the endogenous glucocorticoids are not the physiological inducers of closure. At the moment, it is not known what induces closure of the gut to immunoglobulins.

The immunological responsiveness of neonates is affected by absorption of colostrum. Specific primary antibody responses to *Brucella abortus* vaccines are depressed in colostrum-fed calves compared with colostrum-deprived calves (Husband and Lascelles, 1975). Thus the antibodies from colostrum inhibit the response of the calf to antigenic stimulation during the immediate post-natal period. Therefore, it can be concluded that it is not the immaturity of the calf which prevents a normal immune response but the presence of serum antibodies to *Brucella abortus* vaccine, absorbed with maternal colostrum.

In all cases of transmission of antibodies via placenta, yolk sac or colostrum, the primary purpose is to protect the young against infectious disease. Interruption of this transmission is a well-recognised cause of disease and death in neonates. The immunisation of mothers is often used as a means of providing protection for the newborn animal, as is discussed in more detail in Chapter 5 on local immunity.

3.5 THE MAINTENANCE OF PREGNANCY

The way in which the maternal–foetal barrier is maintained has long intrigued biologists in the field of reproduction. The foetus differs by one haplotype from the mother, due to the father's contribution in the fertilisation of the ovum, and this is accompanied by differences in histocompatibility type between mother and foetus. Normally, the presence of foreign histocompatibility antigens leads to the generation of an immune response with ultimate rejection of the graft.

If the foetus can be regarded as a homograft on the mother's uterine wall, it must be that the placenta provides a barrier to the passage of cells and antibodies from mother to foetus and from foetus to mother. But we know that, except in syndesmochorial placentas, there is exchange of immunoglobulins between mother and foetus and if these antibodies were directed towards the paternal haplotype, they could damage the foetus.

Antibodies are formed against foetal histocompatibility antigens but are usually present in low titre and do not apparently cause any damage to the foetus, even after multiple pregnancies when titres are higher. The presence of these antibodies indicates that cells must pass from the foetus or foetal placenta to the mother, even in ruminants, and also that presumably cells pass from the mother to the foetus. These cells apparently do not set up a graft-versus-host reaction in the recipient, and there must therefore be a controlling mechanism which prevents this.

Several mechanisms have been suggested for the control of immune rejection of the foetus. It was first thought that the epithelial cells of the maternal placenta provided a physical barrier to the passage of foetal antigens by possession of an immunologically inert surface. Indeed, it has been shown that the cells of the amnion grown in culture, do not possess histocompatibility antigens and are immunologically inert to the mother. But it is known that cells and antibodies pass from mother to foetus, and therefore, the inert barrier only provides service in the maintenance of the placenta. Then it was suggested that placental hormones, such as human chorionic gonadotropin and placental lactogen, dampened the immune responsiveness of the lymphocytes in the placenta. Again, this could only be a local placental effect, since antibodies to the foetal histocompatibility antigens are present in the maternal circulation. Next, it was suggested that a 'pregnancy zone' protein was produced by the mother which dampened the transformation of maternal lymphocytes responding to foetal histocompatibility antigens. Indeed, a pregnancy test in sheep has been based on the appearance of this glycoprotein. However, the specificity of this suppression was not necessarily directed towards the immune response to foetal antigens, and it was thought that pregnancy zone protein may only be a contributing factor in dampening maternal–foetal immunity.

The presence of α-foetoprotein, as a result of the developing foetal liver, was also thought to protect the foetus from maternal lymphocytes which could be potentially harmful to the foetus. α-Foetoprotein has been isolated from ovine and bovine serum. Indeed the protein has been demonstrated on the surface of human cord blood lymphocytes, presumably dampening their immune responsiveness. It has been suggested that the placenta acts as a paternal haplotype antigen immunoabsorbent, but again it is obvious that sufficient antigen gets through to cause a maternal immune response.

Studies with transformation of lymphocytes *in vitro* have suggested that the foetal lymphocytes could contain a population of suppressor cells which inhibit mitosis of the maternal lymphocytes. Factors from maternal serum have been shown to inhibit the mixed-lymphocyte reaction (MLR) and responsiveness to mitogens such as PHA. An α-macroglobulin has been suggested to be a cause of the inhibition, since like α-foetoprotein, it can be demonstrated on the surface of peripheral blood lymphocytes. Perhaps a combination of serum glycoproteins and placental hormones is responsible for the dampening of the immune response in the placenta, with specific suppressor cells controlling specific immune responses which may lead to a graft-versus-host reaction.

In cattle, there is evidence that responsiveness of maternal lymphocytes to mitogens, such as PHA, is reduced near full-term gestation and in the immediate post-parturient period. These studies, however, can be criticised on the basis of possible seasonal effects if the animals at different stages of pregnancy are not all sampled at the same time of year. It is known that conglutinin levels in bovine serum fluctuate with season, and the relatively small drop in PHA responsiveness could be a variation due to a seasonal effect. Nevertheless, it is well-known that plasma corticosteroids increase in the circulation of cows close to parturition, and this could have an inhibitory effect on lymphocyte stimulation, particularly if the test is carried out in the presence of autologous serum.

It is also known from field experience that cows at or around the time of parturition may give false-negative tuberculin skin test responses, and this is a factor which must be assessed in the timing of tuberculin skin tests. For the rest of the pregnancy period, however, immune suppression is certainly not obvious and titres of antibodies to *Brucella abortus* actually increase towards parturition, probably as a result of replacement of serum antibodies during colostrum formation in the last month of pregnancy.

3.6   EXCHANGE OF CELLS ACROSS THE PLACENTA

3.6.1   Freemartins

Although not the result of an exchange of cells across the placenta between mother and offspring, the occurrence of freemartins opens intriguing questions on tolerance to foreign lymphocytes and the possibility of bone marrow grafts in the foetal calf.

It was reported by Owen (1945) that two antigenically-distinct types of red blood cells could coexist in the blood circulation of a high proportion of non-identical (di-zygotic) twins (Fig. 3.4). This was given the term 'erythrocyte mosaicism or chimaerism'. The explanation put forward was that vascular anastomoses of foetal blood vessels in the placenta allowed free exchange of developing haemopoietic tissue at a certain stage of development in the foetus. This allowed incompatible cells to be accepted by each twin and by some mechanism, allowed them to persist throughout the life of the individual.

At the same time, lymphoid cell precursors were exchanged, and the lympho-

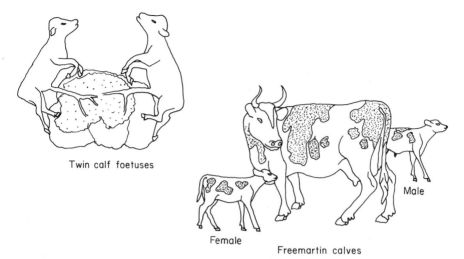

Twin calf foetuses

Female

Male

Freemartin calves

Fig. 3.4. The anastomosis of blood vessels in the placenta of cattle twins *in utero* allows the exchange of haemopoietic tissues. The effect of the pre-natal mixing of blood cells is to produce chimaerism of both erythrocytes and leucocytes which persists in the calves after birth. This tolerance allows the survival of reciprocal skin grafts between the twin calves for a much longer period than grafts from sibling donor calves.

cyte typing of cattle has revealed two antigenically-distinct types of lymphoid cells in the circulation of the twins. Furthermore, reciprocal skin grafts between twins are generally accepted. This naturally-occurring phenomenon in cattle stimulated the classic work on the induction of acquired tolerance by Billingham *et al.* (1953). They showed that if inbred mice were injected with cells from an unrelated strain of mouse during the embryonic period, they would accept skin grafts from the unrelated mouse strain in the post-natal period. As mentioned earlier, this type of result was limited to the laboratory rodent and could not be demonstrated in sheep by Schinckel and Ferguson (1953), who found that foetal lambs rejected allogeneic skin grafts.

Nevertheless, the findings of Owen in freemartin cattle and of Billingham, Brent and Medawar in mice, provided support for the 'self-marker' concept which was proposed by Burnet and Fenner (1949). This was basically a hypothesis to explain why the immune response distinguished 'self' from 'non-self'. It meant that contact with antigens on somatic cells during the foetal period, made the immune system of the embryo tolerant to those same antigens during adult life.

Although this idea has not been found to be true for bacterial and chemical antigens with sheep and cattle foetuses, there remains the evidence of the mixed bone marrow cell types in freemartin calves. Closer examination of the acceptance of reciprocal skin grafts in di-zygotic cattle twins revealed that most of the grafts were rejected ultimately on average 250 days after transplantation (Stone et al., 1965). Therefore, the twins were not completely tolerant to each other's skin. However in a small proportion of cattle twins, the grafts survived indefinitely, even though the reciprocal graft in the other twin was rejected.

A distinction was drawn by Emery and McCullagh (1980a), between survival of skin grafts from two different sites on the calves. The skin grafts from the withers survived for a shorter time than those from the ear, and some of the ear skin grafts survived indefinitely. This is of obvious importance in the assessment of tolerance to reciprocal skin grafts between these twins. It is interesting that even though the mixed-lymphocyte reactions (MLR) between the twins were negative, transplantation rejections still occurred (Emery and McCullagh, 1980b), demonstrating that the MLR is a far less-sensitive test than skin transplantation for histocompatibility between twins.

The study of lymphocyte antigens in domestic animals is still at an early stage of development. However it would be interesting to see if compatibility of skin grafts between freemartin calves was associated with closeness in major histocompatibility complex (MHC) type between them. This is found with human kidney transplants, which are much less likely to be rejected if the donor has some antigens in common with the recipient. In this way, tolerance to a low level of MHC incompatibility can be induced even in adults. In cattle, a special property of the pre-natal environment, which has not been analysed, still appears to operate with regard to somatic cells of di-zygotic twins and between mother and foetus during gestation.

3.6.2   Haemolytic Diseases of the Newborn

Differences in blood groups between mother and foetus may produce a haemolytic syndrome, if antibodies are produced by the mother and reach the foetal circulation via the placenta or after ingestion and absorption of colostrum.

The most important syndrome in the veterinary field is that found in foals which have ingested colostrum containing antibodies to their erythrocytes. The use of foster mothers is an effective treatment for the condition, if it is recognised in time. It is thought that some minor damage to the placenta during pregnancy allows the foetal erythrocytes to pass into the maternal circulation. If the blood group of these foetal erythrocytes is incompatible with that of the mother, antibodies are produced which are transmitted post-natally via the colostrum to the foal.

Haemolytic diseases of the newborn can be induced by the injection of incompatible erythrocytes into the mother during pregnancy. In pigs and dogs, there is sufficient permeability of the placental barrier to allow transmission of antibodies in small amounts to the foetus, but the bulk of the antibodies are transmitted via the colostrum. In this case, the pregnant dam is immunised with erythrocytes from the sire.

In contrast, the immunisation of ruminants such as cattle or sheep with erythrocytes from the sire, has failed to produce haemolytic disease of the newborn after ingestion of colostrum. It has been postulated that anti-erythrocyte antibodies in colostrum are absorbed or neutralised in some way during their passage through the gut. It is not known what this mechanism entails, nor is it known why it does not operate for other species such as the horse. One can only speculate that ruminant IgG_1, which is the predominant immunoglobulin of ruminant colostrum, is not the class of immunoglobulin that contains the haemolytic antibodies.

3.7   MATERNAL ANTIBODIES TO THE MHC ANTIGENS

The appearance of antibodies to the paternal *MHC* haplotype antigens on lymphocytes has been known for some time. These antibodies are usually of low titre but increase with successive pregnancies. They have been found in maternal serum of mares, sows, dogs, cattle and ewes, and their occurrence seems to be independent of the number of layers in the placenta which separate mother from foetus. The mechanism by which they are stimulated is unknown, but presumably they are the result of migration of lymphoid or monocytoid cells from foetus to mother during pregnancy. It is interesting that peak titres in cattle are often achieved up to 3 months after birth, suggesting that resorption of remnants of the foetal placenta by the uterus after birth provides a continuing stimulus. These maternal antibodies have been used as a source of lymphocyte-typing reagents, and this application is discussed in Chapter 10.

At this stage, there is no evidence that these antibodies to the foetal MHC are a cause of infertility or premature birth in animals. Colostrum does contain antibodies to lymphocyte MHC antigens, but their ingestion by the newborn animal does not appear to have the detrimental effects that are found with haemolytic disease of the newborn. One can only assume that the titres are low enough for the antibodies to be absorbed by the tissues during passage into the blood, so that only very low titres appear in the circulation.

The suggestion that certain blood group incompatibilities are involved in reduced fertility has been put forward for many years. At various times, transferrin-, haemoglobin- and serum phosphatase-type incompatibilities have been suggested to be associated with lowered fertility in cattle, sheep and humans, respectively. An obvious example is the erythrocyte Rh and ABO blood group incompatibilities in the human, which are strong candidates for a cause of miscarriages in humans.

At the moment, there is no evidence in domestic animals for a link between poor foetal survival and large histocompatibility differences between mother and foetus. Evidence from mice suggests that haplotype variation may account for 14% of variation in foetal loss and 20% of variation in foetal weight. However, there are no similar studies in domestic animals, due to the lack of typing reagents for histocompatibility antigens in these species. The studies with congenic mice, in which significant associations have been found between genes at or near the *H-2* complex and foetal loss or foetal weight, are difficult to apply to outbred species such as cattle and sheep. At the moment, it remains an open question whether MHC-type incompatibilities in domestic animals are a source of reproductive loss.

It has also been suggested that incompatibility operates at the fertilisation level with antibodies directed towards spermatozoa. Furthermore, seminal plasma in turn may contain antibodies which may be directed towards the ovum. In many of the earlier studies it was found that immunoglobulins reacted with spermatozoa. However, it was not appreciated that spermatozoa can possess Fc receptors and that fluorescent immunoglobulin can combine non-specifically with spermatozoa. It was then suggested that spermatozoa possess MHC antigens themselves, and therefore, antibodies to the incompatible MHC antigens, present in uterine secretions, would inhibit fertilisation. However, the presence of MHC antigens, in particular HLA-D on spermatozoa, has not been confirmed in recent studies. Again it must be concluded that the case has yet to be proven for MHC incompatibilities being a cause of poor fertilisation of ova and subsequent infertility. Possibly antibodies may be present in uterine secretions which are directed towards seminal plasma proteins. If this occurs, it seems likely that spermatozoa could be trapped in an agglutinate of seminal plasma.

3.8 FAULTS IN THE DEVELOPMENT OF THE FOETAL IMMUNE SYSTEM

In the early 1970s investigations into the death of Arabian foals led to the discovery of Severe Combined Immunodeficiency (SCID) by McGuire and associates (reviewed in McGuire and Perryman, 1981). These were the first well-documented series of reports on a congenital immunodeficiency in a domestic species of animal, which could be compared with a similar condition in human beings.

The foals presented clinically as cases of chronic viral or bacterial infections of the lung which eventually led to death before 5 months of age. The most significant finding on haematological examination is a very severe lymphopoenia of <1000 lymphocytes/mm^3 compared with a mean of 4119 lymphocytes/mm^3 for normal foals.

Examination of immunoglobulins in serum before the foals are allowed the suckle, revealed that while normal foals possess IgM, the foals with Severe Combined Immunodeficiency had no IgM, nor did they have any other immunoglobulin. After suckling and ingestion of colostrum, the serum immunoglobulin pattern for the immunodeficient foals was the same as that for normal foals.

Therefore, the foal with immunodeficiency survives on maternally-transferred antibody but by about 1 month of age has metabolised most of its IgM and later its IgA and IgG (T).* However no foals live long enough to metabolise all their maternal IgG.

Thus, there is no synthesis of any class of immunoglobulin by the foals, although free secretory component is present in external secretions. Examination of peripheral blood or lymphoid tissues reveals no surface immunoglobulin (sIg)-bearing cells. Furthermore, immunodeficient foals produce no antibody in response to primary immunisation with sheep erythrocytes (SRBC) or keyhole limpet haemocyanin (KLH) in Freund's incomplete adjuvant.

In general, the mononuclear cells from the blood of immunodeficient foals do not respond to phytohaemagglutinin, pokeweed mitogen, concanavalin A or lipopolysaccharide. However, two cases were found in which 10–40% reactivity of normal foals developed at 3 weeks of age. No response can be obtained to allogeneic lymphocytes, but their own mononuclear cells can act as stimulators in a one-way mixed-lymphocyte reaction. Delayed-hypersensitivity skin tests to phytohaemagglutinin, which causes a reaction in normal foals, are negative in immunodeficient foals. Functional tests reveal that complement levels, neutrophil function and monocyte function are not reduced in immunodeficient foals.

Histologically, there is an absence of lymphoid structure in the spleen and lymph nodes. A feature which distinguishes immunodeficient foals from the condition of partial depletion due to other causes, is the total absence of B-cell-dependent areas in the lymphoid tissues of immunodeficient foals. Periarteriolar cuffs are also absent. These features are usually enough to distinguish immunodeficient foals, but lymph nodes from foals with generalised bacterial infection can also exhibit lymphoid depletion which may be difficult to distinguish from that caused by immunodeficiency.

The thymus of immunodeficient foals shows extreme hypoplasia. The outer capsule is present, but distinct cortex and medulla is lacking. Lymphoid islands may be found, and an epithelial component with Hassal's corpuscles is usually present. Generally there is extreme morphological heterogeneity of thymuses from immunodeficient foals. It is suggested by McGuire that morphology should only be used with caution as a criterion of immunodeficiency.

*See Chapter 4 for a description of the T-globulin of horses.

Severe Combined Immunodeficiency is inherited as an autosomal-recessive gene. No differences in MHC antigen frequency have been detected in MHC type of immunodeficient foals compared with normal foals. Therefore, the genes do not yet appear to be within the MHC. The immunodeficient foals do not exhibit the adenosine deaminase enzyme deficiency seen with a similar condition in humans.

Reconstitution has been attempted using foetal thymus and liver cells. This has generally been unsuccessful except in one case which survived for 11½ months. The major problem is a graft-versus-host reaction due to transplantation of incompatible lymphoid cells. The hope for the future is lymphocyte typing of donors, so that donor and recipient can be matched for MHC antigens and so avoid the graft-versus-host reaction.

Other immunodeficiencies have been found to occur in horses (Perryman, 1982), but these are usually very much less severe than Combined Immunodeficiency. These other conditions include failure or partial failure of colostral immunoglobulin transfer from mare to foal, selective IgM deficiency, agammaglobulinaemia, transient hypogammaglobulinaemia and lymphosarcoma. By far the greatest problem is failure of immunoglobulin transfer, and this can be ameliorated by good management and feeding of colostrum.

3.9 HORMONE REGULATION BY ANTIBODIES

Sheep have been immunised against oestrogen and androgen steroid hormones to alter the endocrine balance and cause increased ovulation (Scaramuzzi et al., 1977). A highly specific anti-steroid response may be obtained by linking the steroids to human serum albumin as a carrier and injecting this into ewes with added adjuvant. The effect of this vaccination is to increase the ovulation rate by about 0.4 ovulations per sheep, and this increases the lambing rate. A commercial 'fecundity vaccine' is being investigated using this technique, and this has just been placed on the market in Australia.

Monoclonal antibodies to progesterone have been found to block pregnancy in mice. The circulating progesterone levels are rapidly reduced by 95%, and this prevents the normal preparation of the endometrium for implantation. This approach has been attempted before with polyclonal antibodies, but the concentration of specific antibody in blood cannot be maintained for long enough to produce the blocking effect. The advantages of monoclonal antibodies in mice are that they are not foreign proteins and they have a relatively low contamination with other proteins, so that high levels of antibody can be maintained in the serum. This approach has not been used with domestic animals because increase in fertility rather than decrease is required. The use of monoclonal antibodies to oestrogen or androgen to increase ovulation may not work, because the mouse immunoglobulin would be treated as a foreign protein by sheep and rapidly cleared from the circulating blood.

The injection of somatostatin (a peptide hormone) linked to human serum α-globulin into sheep, causes the production of antibodies to this growth-regulating hormone. This partially removes the inhibitory effects of the somatostatin, so that the sheep put on weight at twice the rate of controls (Spencer and Williamson, 1981). Because of the current concern over the use of chemical growth promoters, this autoimmunisation method may prove to be more acceptable for controlling growth than the use of artificial hormones.

3.10 GENERAL CONCLUSIONS

The areas included in immunology of reproduction in domestic animals generally involve the control of infectious disease. Infections of the foetus which cause abortion because of the immunological immaturity of the foetus are of concern to the veterinarian. The failure of the neonatal foal or ruminant to absorb colostrum is of prime importance in neonatal infections. The effects of pregnancy on the diagnosis of tuberculosis by the tuberculin skin test should also be taken into account when testing cattle which are close to parturition. The absorption of antibodies to *Brucella abortus* from the colostrum by newborn calves can interfere with both vaccination and diagnosis of the disease in calves.

In general, it is these areas which are of concern to the veterinarian, although specific immunodeficiencies such as SCID of foals can pose a particular problem. Also the preoccupation of the medical world in controlling fertility is not shared by the veterinary clinician, since increased fertility is the goal, possibly by means of a 'fecundity vaccine'. Finally, the question of erythrocyte and MHC incompatibilities as causes of infertility do not really arise in the veterinary field, since herd fertility is assessed as a whole rather than on an individual animal basis.

REFERENCES

Billingham, R. E., Brent, L. and Medawar, P. B. (1953). *Nature (London)* **172,**603–606.

Binns, R. M. and Symons, D. B. A. (1974). *Res. Vet. Sci.* **16,** 260–262.

Brambell, F. W. R. (1970). 'The Transmission of Passive Immunity from Mother to Young' (A. Neuberger, E. L. Tatum and E. J. Holborow, ser. eds.), Frontiers of Biology, Vol. 18. North-Holland Publishing Co., Amsterdam and London.

Brandon, M. R., Watson, D. L. and Lascelles, A. K. (1971). *Aust. J. Exp. Biol. Med. Sci.* **49,** 613–623.

Burnet, F. M. and Fenner, F. (1949). 'The Production of Antibodies'. Macmillan, Melbourne.

Cole, G. J. and Morris, B. (1971a). *Aust. J. Exp. Biol. Med. Sci.* **49,** 33–53.

Cole, G. J. and Morris, B. (1971b). *Aust. J. Exp. Biol. Med. Sci.* **49** 55–73.

Emery, D. and McCullagh, P. (1980a). *Transplantation* **29**, 4–9.

Emery, D. and McCullagh, P. (1980b). *Transplantation* **29**, 17–22.

Fahey, K. J. and Morris, B. (1974). *Ser. Haematol.* **7**, 548–567.

Husband, A. J. and Lascelles, A. K. (1975). *Res. Vet. Sci.* **18**, 201–207.

McGuire, T. C. and Perryman, L. E. (1981). Combined immunodeficiency of arabian foals. *In* 'Immunologic Defects in Laboratory Animals' (M. E. Gershwin and B. Merchant, eds.), Vol. 2, pp. 185–203. Plenum Press, New York.

Owen, R. D. (1945). *Science (Washington, D.C.)* **102**,400–401.

Perryman, L. E. (1982). *J. Am. Vet. Med. Assoc.* **181**, 1097–1101.

Raff, M. D. and Cantor, H. (1971). Subpopulations of Thymus Cells and Thymus-derived Cells. In 'Progress in Immunology' (B. Amos, ed.), Vol. 1, pp. 83–93. Academic Press, New York and London.

Reynolds, J. D., Miyasaka, M. and Trnka, Z. (1982). *Annu. Rep. Basel Inst. Immunol.* pp. 74–75.

Scaramuzzi, R. J., Davidson, W. G. and Van Look, P. F. A. (1977). *Nature (London)* **269**, 817–818.

Schinckel, P. G. and Ferguson, K. A. (1953). *Aust. J. Biol. Sci.* **6**, 533–546.

Silverstein, A. M., Uhr, J. W., Kraner, K. L. and Lukes, R. J. (1963). *J. Exp. Med.* **117**, 799–812.

Spencer, G. S. G. and Williamson, E. D. (1981). *Anim. Prod.* **32**, 376.

Stone, W. H., Cragle, R. G., Swanson, E. W. and Brown, D. G. (1965). *Science (Washington, D.C.)* **148**, 1335–1336.

4

Immunoglobulins

The classification of γ-globulin into the major immunoglobulins of sheep, cattle, pig and horse serum was first achieved when the technique of immunoelectrophoresis was developed. Previous to this time, antibodies were known to be present in the γ-globulin fraction rather than in the α- and β-globulin fractions separated by moving-boundary electrophoresis in a U tube. This arbitrary classification persisted until international agreements were reached on the nomenclature for the serum proteins, so that much of the earlier literature on the immunoglobulins in domestic animals refers to the same immunoglobulins by several names. An example was the naming of the macroglobulin with antibody activity as β2M or γ-M with final nomenclature being IgM. One can see the transition from the older classification of electrophoretic mobility in the α, β, and γ regions of the electrophoresis pattern to the newer, more functional nomenclature, which unified all the immunoglobulins with the prefix Ig to give IgA, IgG, IgM, IgD and IgE, the names by which we know them today.

The first clear description of bovine immunoglobulins was that of Pierce and Feinstein (1965) in Cambridge, England, and Murphy, Osebold and Aalund (1965) in Davis, California. Both groups showed a heterogeneity in the immunoelectrophoretic patterns of cattle serum and by the use, at that time, of the newly-developed cross-linked dextran gels (Sephadex: Pharmacia, Uppsala, Sweden) and ion-exchange chromatography, they were able to divide the major immunoglobulins of cattle serum into IgM, IgG_1 and IgG_2. In the technique of immunoelectrophoresis, the serum proteins are subjected to electrophoresis from wells cut in the gel, and then a trough is cut longitudinally through the gel, into

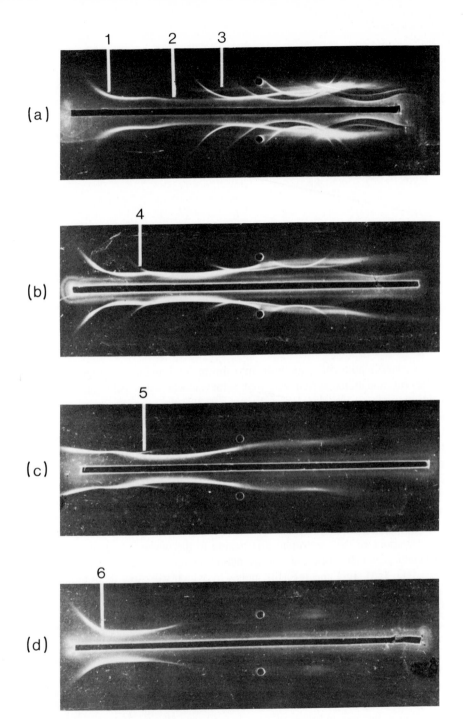

Fig. 4.1. (a) An immunoelectrophoresis pattern of ovine serum, with the serum in the wells and rabbit anti-ovine serum in the trough. The typical 'gull-wing' pattern of ovine IgG is visible.

which are placed rabbit antibodies to cattle serum proteins. The rabbit antibodies diffuse through the gel and precipitate the cattle serum proteins in arcs which reflect the relative mobility and concentration of the cattle proteins, as well as the titres of the rabbit antibodies to each serum protein.

Similar studies were carried out on sheep serum (Fig. 4.1), and the conclusion was reached that the immunoglobulins of both sheep and cattle were unique, in that a particular IgG class, IgG_1, was selectively transferred into mammary secretion during colostrum formation. This finding differed from that in humans, pigs and rodents in which another class of immunoglobulin, IgA, was selectively concentrated in mammary secretion. The difference between ruminants and the other species was attributed to the different types of placentation, which either allowed transfer of immunoglobulins before birth (human, pig, rodent), or required that they be transferred after birth (ruminants). The effect of this work on ruminants was to concentrate attention on the subclasses of immunoglobulins and their possible functions. However, although subclasses of IgG have been demonstrated in humans and rodents, there has been no example of a highly-specific function for these subclasses comparable to the selection of IgG_1 by the mammary gland of the ruminant.

Due to the dependence of these earlier workers on immunoelectrophoretic patterns to identify immunoglobulins, considerable controversy was generated on which line of precipitate represented each immunoglobulin. The gradual improvement in separation techniques eventually led to immunoglobulins which were pure enough to be used as standards against which specific antisera could be checked. These standards have been in use for some time with human immunoglobulins and are in the process of being collected for cattle and sheep immunoglobulins. In particular, the reliable identification of the IgA arc proved to be elusive because of the difficulty in purifying the protein from ruminant serum, where it is present in very low concentrations. The IgA immunoglobulin has been purified from external secretions such as saliva and colostrum in various laboratories around the world but not yet in sufficient quantity to provide an international standard.

Because there were few cases of myeloma tumours found in domestic animals, the study of the serum paraproteins produced by these tumours was not carried out with these species in the detail that it was with the human myeloma proteins.

The lines point to (1) IgG_2, (2) IgG_1 and (3) IgM. (b) An immunoelectrophoresis pattern developed with another rabbit anti-ovine serum. The line (4) points to the spurring of IgG_1 over IgG_2, indicating non-identity of the H chains of these two subclasses. (c) An immunoelectrophoresis pattern of rabbit anti-ovine IgG developed with ovine serum. The line (5) points to the spurring of IgG_2 over IgG_1, again indicating non-identity of the H chains of the two subclasses. (d) A single line developing from the immunoelectrophoresis of anti-ovine IgG_2 against ovine serum (6). In this case the antiserum is specific only for the H chains of IgG_2. (Reproduced by permission from Outteridge, Mackenzie and Lascelles (1968), *Arch. Biochem. Biophys.* **126,** 105–110.)

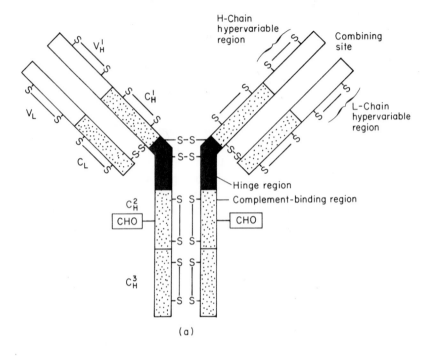

(a)

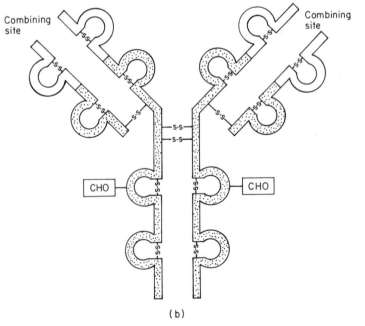

(b)

The advantage of working with myeloma paraproteins is that they are generally-homogeneous proteins which are much easier to analyse than the mixture of immunoglobulin antibodies found in normal serum. An exception has been the dog, in which naturally-occurring myelomas have been studied. These were of the IgM, IgG and IgA classes. Heavy chains (see Fig. 4.2 for IgG structure) of each of these classes were subjected to amino-acid sequence analysis, and it was found that the sequences were, in the main, very similar to those of human heavy chains (Kehoe, 1982). However, there were certain substitutions in individual positions which were comparable to those found with another species, the cat. This is thought to have phylogenetic significance, since the same substitutions were found to occur in pooled normal canine IgG.

The variable region of the heavy chains of IgM and IgA (see Figs. 4.3 and 4.4 for IgM and IgA structure) from canine myelomas has also been examined for amino-acid sequence, and although the data are limited, the canine myeloma heavy chains showed 78% homology with the variable regions of human heavy chains. The constant region of IgM heavy (μ) chain was also examined, and again, there was 81% homology between canine and human constant regions of the IgM heavy chain.

Other homologous amino-acid sequences were found in the secretory pieces from bovine, canine and human origin, and it has been concluded that the basic structure of immunoglobulins is similar both for domestic species and for humans.

4.1 THE STRUCTURE OF IMMUNOGLOBULINS

The structure of immunoglobulins was determined in the 1960s with chemical and electrophoretic studies as well as electron micrographs of purified immunoglobulins. It is interesting that amongst the first immunoglobulins examined by electron microscope were sheep antibodies to the flagellae of *Salmonella* bacteria, described by Feinstein and Munn (1969). These were observed as two classes, IgG and IgM, attached by their combining sites to the surface of the

---

Fig. 4.2. Two models of the IgG molecule: (a) 'stick model' and (b) 'domain model'. Interchain disulphide bonds hold the light (L) and heavy (H) chains together, and intrachain disulphide bonds, which determine the tertiary folding of the L and H chains, are represented as loops in the domain model. The molecule has two major functional regions: firstly, the hyper-variable regions, which combine with antigen, and secondly, the constant regions, which include the Fc piece which combines with receptors on cell membranes and with serum complement. The number and sites of the interchain disulphide bonds vary among immunoglobulin subclasses within species as well as between species. For domestic animals, the arrangement of the chains is thought to be broadly the same, but for some species the details are not known.

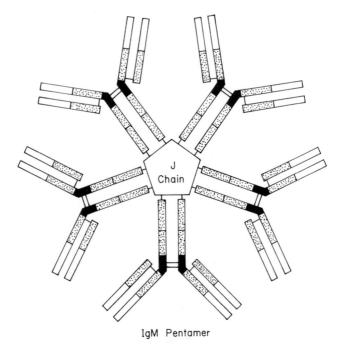

IgM Pentamer

Fig. 4.3. Diagram of the IgM molecule, which is composed of five subunits, each consisting of two L chains and two H chains, joined together by disulphide bonds. The subunits are linked to each other by a J (joining) chain via disulphide bonds. A total of 10 combining sites are available for combination with antigen.

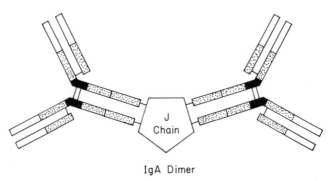

IgA Dimer

Fig. 4.4. Diagram of an IgA molecule, which in this case is represented as a dimer, although other multimeric forms of IgA have been shown to exist. As in the IgM molecule, a J chain joins the subunits of the dimer.

flagellae. The IgG molecules were seen to be predominantly Y-shaped with the two combining sites on the arms of the Y. The IgM molecules were seen as flat pentameric molecules, with the combining sites on the end of the 'fingers' of each IgM molecule.

However, the essential structure of IgG is that of two heavy (H) chains (MW 45,000) and two light (L) chains (MW 22,500). Subsequent work on both ruminant and other immunoglobulins has defined the light and heavy chains of the IgG molecule, folded into a series of globular regions called 'domains'. The combining site for the molecule consists of two 'variable' regions, one on the heavy chain and one on the light chain for each arm of the Y (Fig. 4.2). The genetic control of the variable part of the immunoglobulin molecule is under intense investigation at the moment, but it is assumed to be the result of rearrangement of the DNA molecules in the chromatin of lymphocytes (Fig. 4.7). The light chains and heavy chains are assembled separately within the cell and secreted as complete immunoglobulin molecules. The molecules of the other classes of immunoglobulins, such as IgM and IgA, are also made up of light and heavy chains, and in fact the light chains of all classes of immunoglobulins cross-react in immunodiffusion tests. The immunoglobulin classes differ in their heavy chains, and this is the basis for their distinctive precipitates in immunoelectrophoretic patterns. The IgM molecules have five sets of light and heavy chains joined at the opposite end to their combining sites, into a pentamer, by a 'J' or 'joining' chain (Fig. 4.3). The IgA molecules have two sets of light and heavy chains and are also joined at the opposite end to their combining sites by a J chain (Fig. 4.4). In secreted IgA, there is also a 'secretory piece' attached, which is thought to protect the molecule from disruption by proteolytic enzymes at sites such as the lumen of the gut. This additional secretory piece is found as a glycoprotein attached to the J-chain region of the molecule and is antigenically distinct from the rest of the IgA molecule. Amino-acid sequence studies have shown that there is close homology between the secretory pieces of canine, bovine and human origin. The secretory piece is not limited to IgA, since secreted IgM has also been shown to have a secretory piece.

The point of divergence of the two arms of the IgG molecule is referred to as the 'hinge' region. It has significance in that the combination of antibody with antigen (antigen-antibody complexes) appears to expose previously-hidden sites in the hinge region for interaction with lymphocyte surface receptors. In this case, immunoglobulin can combine via the end opposite to the combining sites, the Fc part of the molecule, with receptors on the plasma membrane surface of mononuclear cells.

Proteolytic enzymes have been used in the laboratory to prepare different pieces of the immunoglobulin molecule. The nomenclature for these different pieces of the IgG molecule is derived from earlier studies with the proteolytic enzymes. When intact IgG molecules are incubated with the enzyme papain, in the presence of sulphhydryl compounds in low concentration, the peptide bonds in the hinge region are split, releasing three fragments. These were originally named fragments a, b and c, until it was realized that fragments a and b were identical but fragment c was quite different. Thus the two arms of the Y-shaped IgG molecule are known as Fab fragments, and the remaining protein, the Fc fragment.

The Fab fragments of the IgG molecules consist of the light chain and the variable region (V_H) and constant ($C_H{}^1$) domains of the heavy chain. They are univalent because each fragment contains a single antibody-combining site, consisting of the variable domains (V_H and V_L) regions of the heavy and light chains. The Fab fragments of antibodies are very often labelled with fluorescein isothiocyanate, so that they can be used to identify the glycoproteins in the surface membranes of lymphocytes. The use of Fab fragments prevents combination of antibodies via their Fc piece to the Fc receptors on the cells. It also prevents cross-linking of the antigen on the cell surfaces, which leads to 'patching' and 'capping' of the antigen–antibody complexes, which eventually detach from the cell.

The IgG molecule may also be digested with the enzyme pepsin. This removes a large part of the Fc end of the molecule but leaves enough of the hinge region to allow the two Fab ends to remain attached to each other. This is usually described as the $F(ab')_2$ molecule and is also used for fluorescent labelling of antibodies directed towards the surface membrane glycoproteins of lymphocytes. Since the two combining sites are still joined, it can still provide cross-linking between different areas in the membrane, with patching and capping of the antigen–antibody complexes.

After preparation of Fab and Fc fragments by papain digestion, the fragments can be detected using immunoelectrophoresis of the digest. Since the Fab and Fc portions do not share antigenic determinants, they appear as two arcs of precipitation which cross each other in a reaction of non-identity, while whole IgG produces a single arc of precipitation.

There are differences between animal species, with the Fc fragments of rabbit IgG being more basic than the Fab fragments, while those of the goat, sheep, horse, pig, cow, chicken, human, mouse, rat and guinea pig are more acidic than their Fab fragments. Generally, Fab fragments can be purified by DEAE ion-exchange chromatography, to produce fractions enriched for Fab and Fc fragments, respectively; an exception is the rabbit, which requires CM ion-exchange chromatography (Mage, 1980). However, the Fab fraction may still have some undigested or partially-digested molecules of IgG which can be detected by double diffusion in gel against antiserum to IgG. These may be removed by affinity chromatography with anti-Fc antibody attached to a cyanogen bromide (CNBr)-activated Sepharose column. However, when the IgG is of a subclass or from an animal species whose immunoglobulin Fc fragment binds to *Sta-*

phylococcus aureus protein A, an affinity column of protein A Sepharose can be used to remove the Fc-containing fragments. The relative binding properties of protein A for the immunoglobulins of different animal species is shown in Table 6.3 (Chapter 6). Unfortunately the ruminant species (cow, sheep and goat) have variable binding affinity between their Fc molecules and protein A, and although some Fab purification may be achieved using protein A columns, it is not a reliable method in these species.

4.1.1 Bence–Jones Proteins

An interesting clinical syndrome associated with multiple myeloma in humans is the appearance of protein in the urine. This is not due to normal serum proteins, which are usually retained by the glomerulus of the kidney, but to low molecular weight proteins which are the breakdown products of the myeloma paraprotein. In particular, light chains with molecular weight of 22,500 are able to pass into the urine. These light chains are either κ or λ allotypes, which are the two genetic variants of light chains. Here they can cause an upset in the normal filtration of urine by the kidney, leading to renal failure. These light chains are known as Bence–Jones proteins and have been used in the laboratory as an enriched source of paraprotein light chains for amino-acid sequence studies in both humans and mice. Bence–Jones proteins have been reported from the urine of cattle with myelomatous disease (Rockley and Kimmell, 1972). These proteins show strong identity with isolated bovine serum light chains on immunodiffusion in gel. Their sedimentation constant (estimated by analytical ultracentrifugation), is 2.75 S, which is close to the sedimentation constant for monomeric human Bence–Jones proteins.

Multiple myeloma has been observed in the cat, dog, pig, horse and rabbit, but Bence–Jones proteins have only been carefully examined in the cow. A clinical test may be used as an indicator of Bence–Jones proteins. Urine is mixed with 2 *M* acetate buffer (pH 4.9) and heated at 56°C for 15 minutes, when marked turbidity of urine appears when compared with control urine. If the tube is then heated to 100°C in a boiling-water bath, the turbidity should disappear, unless other proteins are present which cause some of the turbidity to remain after this treatment.

4.2 THE FUNCTION OF IMMUNOGLOBULINS

4.2.1 IgG

One of the interesting aspects of ruminant IgG, the division into IgG$_1$ and IgG$_2$, has been the subject of many investigations into the functional basis for subclasses of immunoglobulins. These subclasses are characteristically seen as a 'gull-wing' line of precipitate in immunoelectrophoretic patterns (Fig. 4.1). With carefully absorbed antisera, there is a line of non-identity between the two subclasses due to antigenic differences between them. Initially, it was thought that differences in the amino-acid sequences between the H chains of IgG_1 and IgG_2 were the basis of their antigenic differences on immunoelectrophoresis. However, it has been shown that differences in amino-acid sequence between the H chains of IgG_1 and IgG_2 are very minor in cattle and non-existent in sheep (Conde *et al.*, 1975). Therefore, the antigenic differences between these subclasses are due to their Fc fragments.

This has been supported by studies which showed that the Fc end of the immunoglobulin has a function in the selective transfer of IgG_1 immunoglobulin into the colostrum of ruminants. Isolated mammary cells have been shown to possess both IgG_1 and IgG_2 receptors on their surfaces. These receptors are specific for the Fc piece of the immunoglobulin molecules, and experiments have demonstrated that the uptake of either IgG_1 or IgG_2 by each specific receptor is not blocked by the other subclass.

The ratio of receptors for IgG_1 to IgG_2 is about 2:1, but in the week before parturition, a new set of high-affinity receptors appears on the surface of the cells, and this changes the ratio of IgG_1 receptors to IgG_2 receptors to 7:1. After parturition, the normal ratio is restored, and throughout lactation the receptors for IgG_1 continue to outnumber those for IgG_2 in the ratio of 2:1.

Earlier studies on the net electrostatic charge on antigens suggested that, with immunisation of rabbits, the charge on the antigen could affect the predominant immunoglobulin subclass produced. Thus highly positively-charged antigens stimulated antibody of the γ_1 class and negatively charged antigens, antibody of the γ_2 class. Because of the clear delineation between IgG_1 and IgG_2 in their serum, this has also been studied in ruminants. The initial experiments suggested that there were differences in the predominant subclass of immunoglobulin produced by antigens of different charge. These results were not confirmed in subsequent experiments, which showed that both IgG_1 and IgG_2 subclasses contained specific antibody molecules which were produced at the same rate in the primary immune response and at slightly different rates in the secondary immune response. Results in cattle and sheep are conflicting, both within each species and between them. However, at this stage it can only be said that the concept of antigen directing the production of subclasses of IgG has yet to be proven.

Current attention has therefore been directed towards the Fc fragments of IgG_1 and IgG_2, and it is here that functional differences can be demonstrated. As mentioned earlier, the Fc fragment of IgG_1 is responsible for its selective uptake by the epithelial cells of the ruminant mammary gland during the week before parturition. In contrast, the Fc fragment of IgG_2 is responsible for its uptake by receptors on the polymorphs of sheep and cattle. This so-called cytophilic antibody is thought to be involved in the opsonisation of bacteria and adsorption to the polymorphs for subsequent phagocytosis. It is not known why the IgG_2 Fc receptors predominate on polymorphs when the IgG_1 subclass is in higher concentration in serum than IgG_2. As with the absence of IgM Fc receptors on ruminant macrophages, the predominance of IgG_2 receptors on polymorphs has yet to be explained.

The significance of the subclasses of IgG in species other than ruminants has not been determined. There are usually not enough physicochemical differences among the molecules of IgG in many species to warrant clear divisions into subclasses. More often, they appear to form part of a heterogeneous population in which components differ from each other by electrostatic charge, presumably as a result of differences in amino-acid sequence of their Fc fragments. An exception is the horse, in which another immunoglobulin, the so-called T-globulin, is found. This was once thought to represent another major immunoglobulin, closely related to IgA, because of its high carbohydrate content. However, amino-acid sequence studies have shown that the T-globulin of horses is closer to IgG. The reason for its high carbohydrate content is not certain, but it may have some connection with its presence, in company with IgA, at mucous epithelial surfaces.

4.2.2 IgA

The IgA immunoglobulin is the predominant class found in intestinal secretions, and this is thought to be due to its resistance to digestion by the proteolytic enzymes of the gut. It is a poor opsonin, and its bactericidal activity against *Escherichia coli,* in the presence of complement, is much lower than IgG or IgM. It seems likely that specific IgA antibody can prevent the attachment of viruses to epithelial cells causing interference with the Sabin vaccine used against poliomyelitis in humans. In chickens, an IgA is also found which is antigenically distinct from all mammalian IgA immunoglobulins. However, *Eimeria tenella* sporozoites are partially inhibited from penetrating chicken kidney cells *in vitro,* by caecal extracts rich in IgA.

Other functions suggested for IgA include immune elimination of circulating antigens via the bile and enhanced antibody responses to antigens. It has also been suggested that IgA helps to exclude antigens which would otherwise enter the body from the gut. The increased incidence of allergic disease in humans with IgA deficiency has been put forward as evidence that allergens can penetrate the gut and sensitise the immunodeficient patient. However, it has also been shown that there is a compensatory increase in IgM in secretions, and this may provide the means of excluding allergens from the body.

4.2.3   IgM

The IgM macroglobulin is an intriguing immunoglobulin because most of its functions could be taken over by IgG. Phylogenetically IgM appears before the development of IgG, with primitive vertebrates having IgM but not IgG. Ontogenically, IgM is the first immunoglobulin manufactured by the developing foetus. Also in the immune responses of adults, IgM appears before IgG as specific antibody. Monomeric IgM is found in the membrane of B-cells and is thought to be the antigen receptor. In T-cells, the receptor has not been defined, but one suggestion is that it is composed only of the variable region of IgM. Evidence suggests, however, that it is a glycoprotein related to the lymphocyte MHC antigens.

During the early stages of an immune response, the IgM antibody is produced first, and it has been suggested that this is because of the multiple binding sites on the immunoglobulin. These allow the efficient agglutination of large numbers of bacteria in bacteraemic disease and the opsonisation of these organisms for phagocytosis. However, in immunised animals this function is probably taken over by IgG, which has fewer combining sites but is in much higher concentration than IgM. The early production of specific IgM antibodies is followed by a switch to either IgG or IgA antibodies. The genetic basis for this switch is being closely examined by molecular biologists at the present time.

The membrane IgM is anchored by a unique Fc piece which differs in amino-acid sequence from monomers prepared from circulating IgM. However, it does appear that the antibody specificity of the membrane IgM variable chain is the same as that on the IgM which is subsequently produced by the cells following specific antigenic stimulation. Both IgM and another immunoglobulin, IgD, have been demonstrated in the membranes of B-cells. Although the IgM functions as a receptor, the function of IgD remains an enigma. The IgD appears earlier in ontogeny than IgM, but seems to possess no specificity for antigen. It has yet to be isolated from the lymphocytes of domestic animals.

As mentioned earlier, IgM can combine with free secretory piece, and it seems likely that it can be transported across membranes. It has been found as an important component of specific antibodies in milk after local immunisation of the sheep mammary gland. It has also been found in pulmonary and intestinal secretions of sheep and cattle. However, it would appear that the major role is played by IgA in the defence of external mucous membranes and that IgM plays a supporting role.

4.2.4   IgE

The remaining immunoglobulin of importance to be discussed is IgE. This was first described in humans by Ishizaka in 1966 and was shown to be the immunoglobulin involved in Type I immediate hypersensitivity reactions, such as urticaria and anaphylaxis. The IgE immunoglobulin is found in very low concentrations in adult human serum (0.25 μg/ml), but there is a wide range of concentrations (0.066–1.83 μg/ml). This low concentration in humans and other species meant that IgE had to be measured indirectly in animals by the passive cutaneous anaphylaxis (PCA) test. In this test, the serum containing the specific IgE is injected subcutaneously into the skin of a recipient of the same species. After 48 to 72 hours the recipient is injected intravenously with specific antigen (also called reagin) mixed with Evans Blue dye. During the 48–72 hours after the initial injection of the test serum, the IgE becomes attached to the mast cells in the subcutaneous site, and on contact with the intravenously-injected reagin, the mast cells degranulate and release histamine, which causes increased capillary permeability at the site. The function of the Evans Blue is then to provide a coloured marker for the area of increased capillary permeability, and this can be measured by direct observation of the shaved skin. The sites of choice are the non-pigmented areas of the skin of calves, but this is not usually a consideration with sheep and goats. The extent of the subcutaneous blue-coloured areas can then be examined and calibrated against the dose of sensitising serum.

The sensitising or 'homocytotropic' characteristics of IgE are considered so specific that cross-reactivity between species is thought to indicate common evolutionary origins. Thus rats, rabbits, guinea pigs, pigs and dogs fail to develop ovalbumin hypersensitivity after passive transfer of bovine serum containing specific anti-ovalbumin IgE. On the other hand, sheep and goats can develop hypersensitivity, although it has to be tested within 48 hours after bovine serum has been injected, and not all sheep and goats tested exhibit the PCA reaction (Gershwin, 1981). The PCA test has been used to demonstrate reaginic antibodies in cattle to ovalbumin, *Micropolyspora faeni* antigen, human serum albumin, rabbit serum albumin and *Fasciola hepatica*. The IgE immunoglobulin has been isolated from bovine serum using DEAE-cellulose and Sephadex G200 chromatography. The IgE, specific for rabbit serum albumin, has been shown to persist in the skin of calves for at least 8 weeks and still be capable of causing a positive PCA test. There is also strong cross-reactivity between bovine and human IgE in ^{125}I-radiolabelled immunosorbent tests (RIST), but this test has not been used much for the measurement of IgE in bovine serum because of its cost.

Because of the difficulty in isolating useful amounts of IgE from normal serum, most of the structural features of IgE have been deduced from the paraproteins found in a few human IgE myeloma cases. The molecular weight of human IgE is higher than that of IgG (190,000 versus 180,000), and it is thought that the increased molecular weight is due to an Fc piece which is larger in the IgE than the IgG molecule. This unique Fc piece confers on IgE its property of binding to specific receptors on mast cell or basophil plasma membranes, where it remains unreactive until cross-linked by reagin. Then the mast cells are stimulated to degranulate, release histamine and set off a hypersensitivity reaction. In the intestinal wall of the sheep, these degranulated mast cells are known as 'globule leucocytes', and they appear to be associated with the 'self-cure' phenomenon in helminthiasis. Heating of bovine or human IgE for 1 hour at 50°C causes a conformational change in the Fc piece of IgE, rendering it incapable of sensitising mast cells. Removal of the Fc piece of IgE with pepsin also renders it incapable of passively blocking reaginic reactions because the $F(ab')_2$ fragment lacks the combining site for attachment to the mast cell receptor. The bovine IgE molecule is not affected by treatment with 2-mercaptoethanol and iodoacetamide, a treatment which effectively depolymerises IgM.

The IgE in bovine colostral whey is capable of producing the PCA reaction, and calves passively acquire IgE from colostrum (Hammer *et al.*, 1971). Therefore calves can be sensitised passively against antigens to which the cow has been sensitised. As mentioned before, levels of human IgE are measured by the radioimmunosorbent test, which can also be used to measure IgE levels in bovine and canine serum. Bovine serum has also been demonstrated to degranulate rat mast cells *in vitro*, and this is surprising, considering the species specificity of IgE. The IgE immunoglobulin is of great importance in the various skin allergies of dogs, in sensitisation of cattle to inhalation of the spores of the fungus *Micropolysporum faeni* and in the sensitisation of sheep and cattle to nematodes and trematodes. Its precise function in immunity is not certain, but it is thought to play a role in the rejection of intestinal parasites and blood-sucking ectoparasites by virtue of the immediate hypersensitivity reaction at the site of contact or attachment of the parasites.

4.3 COMPLEMENT

Complement (C′) is a collective term for a group of proteins in serum which combine with antibody in antigen–antibody reactions and cause direct lysis of invading microorganisms such as protozoa and some bacteria. Complement may also be utilised in test systems which depend on the prevention of lysis of sheep erythrocytes, such as the complement fixation test.

The combination of complement and immunoglobulin is the initial step in which the first component of complement combines with a region of the Fc piece of IgG or IgM. The activation process is then accomplished by the cleavage of each component of complement in turn into fragments, some of which combine to have enzymatic properties. The system is held in check by the instability of the complexes formed as well as by inhibitors or inactivators present in normal serum. However, not only antigen–antibody complexes activate complement, but also anions such as DNA, RNA, polyinosinic acid, enzymes such as trypsin, plasmin and bacterial components such as endotoxin, will all activate complement, in what is known as the classical pathway.

4.3.1 The Classical Pathway

This pathway consists of three units which are defined by their function. Firstly, there is the unit of recognition of antigen–antibody complexes by C1q, and this component from human complement has been examined in the electron microscope. It has an unusual structure which consists of six peripheral subunits connected by fibrillar strands to a central core, which give it the appearance of a 'pot of flowers' (Fig. 4.5). The heads of the 'flowers' bind to the Fc pieces of immunoglobulin, presumably to sites which are only exposed by conformational changes resulting from combination with antigen.

The second unit is the activation of C2, C3 and C4, and this follows the initial activation of C1q, C1r and C1s (Fig. 4.5 and 4.6). This leads to the cleavage of C4 into two fragments, one of which (C4b) attaches to the target cell membrane. The C1s also cleaves C2 into two fragments, one of which (C2a) attaches to the cell membrane and combines with C4b. Together they form the enzyme convertase, which is directed against C3. The C3 is in turn cleaved into two molecules,

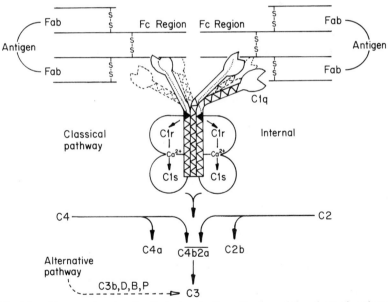

Fig. 4.5. Diagram showing the first steps in the activation of the classical pathway of human complement by combination of C1 with the immunoglobulin Fc piece during antigen–antibody complex formation. The C1 molecule has been observed in the electron microscope to have the 'pot of flowers' appearance represented in the diagram. [Reprinted with permission from *Mol. Immunol.* **19**, Loos, The functions of endogenous C1q, a subcomponent of the first component of complement, as a receptor on the membrane of macrophages. Copyright (1982), Pergamon Press Ltd.]

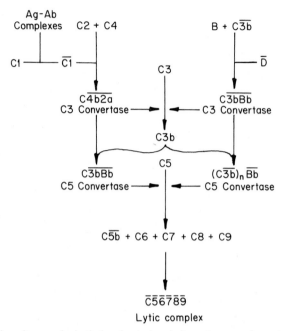

Fig. 4.6. Flow diagram for both the classical and alternative complement-activation pathways. Ag, antigen; Ab, antibody. From Reid and Porter (1981) (Reproduced, with permission, from *Annu. Rev. Biochem.* Volume **50,** © 1981 by Annual Reviews, Inc.)

with C3b combining with C4b and C2a to form another convertase directed towards C5. The C3a which is released into the tissue fluid is a mediator of anaphylaxis.

The third unit of complement activation is the one which mediates the attack on the target cell membrane. The C5 is cleaved by the C5 convertase, and C5b combines with C6 and C7 to form a membrane-bound complex. The final lytic complex requires the combination of C8 and C9 (C5 6 7 8 9), but this is not a proteolytic step as it is with the first five components.

4.3.2 The Alternative Pathway

The alternative pathway was discovered when it was realized that the 'properdin' protein component of human serum could activate complement by a pathway different from the classical pathway. This alternative pathway activated complement from C3 onwards and was also found to be initiated by a variety of other factors such as aggregated IgG and yeast cell walls (zymosan), and by immunoglobulins such as IgA which do not activate complement via the classical pathway. The alternative pathway can also be activated by $F(ab')_2$–antigen complexes, since the combination of the C1q with the Fc piece of immunoglobulin is not required.

The alternative pathway is important because certain strains of *E. coli,* trypanosomes and virus-infected cells can all activate the alternative pathway without the intervention of antibody. The alternative pathway also works with IgA, which then can be seen to have antimicrobial potential in addition to its more obvious role as an agglutinin in external secretions.

There is a component in normal serum which is called factor B, a serine protease demonstrated in bovine serum (Pang and Ashton, 1978), which combines with C3b. This, in turn, is acted on by factor D, a serine proteinase in serum, which leads to the formation of C3bBb, which is a C3 convertase. This then forms a C5 convertase, and the alternative pathway joins the classical pathway to form the lytic complex (Fig. 4.6).

It has been suggested by Lachmann and colleagues that C3b formation takes place continuously *in vivo* at a low level (the 'tick-over' mechanism), and that activators of the alternative pathway either accelerate C3b formation or slow its breakdown.

4.4 PURIFICATION OF COMPLEMENT COMPONENTS

The components of human complement have been purified, particularly the third component (C3), which is a β protein with a molecular weight of 198,000. This protein is composed of two polypeptide chains, a larger α chain (MW 12,600) and a smaller β chain (MW 7200) held together by disulphide bonds. Both canine and feline C3 have been studied by Gorman *et al.* (1981) and found to consist of α and β chains with molecular weights very similar to human α and β chains.

For the other domestic animals, much of the early literature is confusing because detection systems were used which depended on the mixing of complement components from different species. Thus an apparent absence of haemolytic complement activity in bovine serum was found because sheep erythrocytes coated with rabbit antibody were used to assay the bovine complement. Although this system works well with human and guinea pig complement, it does not work with bovine complement, and the absence of haemolytic complement activity was attributed to a lack of bovine C2 or both C2 and C4 components. The ability to interchange complement components from different species is however limited, and earlier reports of the absence of some complement components in animal serum should be accepted with caution.

An example of this confusion is demonstrated by the finding that bovine IgG_1 but not IgG_2 will fix guinea pig complement. When this was examined using homologous bovine complement (McGuire *et al.*, 1979), it was found that both IgG_1 and IgG_2 could fix complement but IgG_1 was generally more efficient than IgG_2 in the fixation process.

The methods for purifying complement from bovine serum have been described by Barta *et al.* (1976). They purified six components (C1, C5, C6, C7, C8 and C9) of bovine complement but could not detect C2, C3 or C4 of bovine origin, because they had to use intermediates formed by sheep erythrocytes, rabbit haemolysin and guinea pig complement to detect the isolated components.

A tentative identification of C2 in sheep serum has been reported by Jonas *et al.* (1982), but this work and that of others in the identification of complement components in domestic animals needs to be pursued vigorously to see if there are in fact differences in the complement system between domestic animals and other species.

4.5 SYNTHESIS OF COMPLEMENT COMPONENTS BY MACROPHAGES

Many of the complement components are synthesised in the liver, but it is of interest that many of them are also synthesised by macrophages. An intriguing possibility has been put forward (Loos, 1982), which is that the receptor for the Fc piece of IgG in macrophage cell membranes is in fact the C1q component of complement. The macrophage may, however, produce complement components for another reason, which is the stimulation of increased vascular permeability at a site of microbial invasion and as a chemotactic factor.

4.6 CONGLUTININ

Conglutinins are present in the serum of all species, but they have been studied most closely in the serum of cattle. The history of conglutinin and its properties have been ably reviewed by Ingram (1982).

Bovine serum contains a protein which will aggregate immune complexes with complement bound to them. This serum component is conglutinin and has a molecular weight of 750,000, consisting of eight polypeptide chains held together by a combination of disulphide and weak intermolecular bonds. It appears to require the activation of complement via the classical pathway, with C1, C4, C2 and C3 all being needed for the reaction with conglutinin. The C3b adsorbed to the target cell membranes is acted upon by a conglutinin-activating factor (KAF), which is an enzyme that splits C3c and C3d from C3, which then acquires the ability to react with conglutinin.

Conglutinin can be purified from heated serum (56°C for 30 minutes) by adsorption to zymosan (Ingram, 1982). It can be found in foetal calf serum and in some colostrum and milk whey samples. The serum levels of conglutinin show marked seasonal fluctuations, and there is a marked fall in levels in cows at calving. Severe infections cause a drop in serum conglutinin titres, and it has been suggested that this indicates a role for conglutinin in the resistance of animals to infectious diseases.

Another type of conglutination is found with bovine serum, and this has been called immunoconglutination. This is due to antibodies of the IgG, IgM or IgA class which appear to be directed towards hidden antigenic determinants on complement proteins exposed during the activation of complement. The immunoconglutinins are produced in response to infection, and they enhance complement fixation and bactericidal activity of serum as well as the phagocytosis of foreign particles by leucocytes. It would seem therefore that the immunoconglutinins amplify the systems which deal with resistance to infectious diseases.

A conglutinating complement absorption test has been developed as a serological test for a variety of infectious agents, but the method is not often used nowadays, despite its ability to react with autologous, isologous or heterologous components of complement.

4.7   IMMUNOGLOBULIN GENES

The primary question about the genes controlling immunoglobulin production has been the mechanism by which the variable regions of the H and L chains for each specific antibody molecule are controlled. The constant regions of the immunoglobulin molecule, in contrast to the variable regions, have been shown to have a small number of alternative amino-acid sequences. From genetic work in rabbits, it has been shown that both variable and constant regions of H chains are controlled by DNA sequences, some distance apart, on the same chromosome. Using human–mouse hybrids, it has been found that heavy-chain genes are on chromosome 14 in humans and on chromosome 12 in mice. The κ light-chain genes are on chromosome 6 in mice. There are no published reports which assign immunoglobulin genes to chromosome number in domestic animals.

The mechanism of generation of diversity for variable regions of the H and L chains has been approached by comparing embryonic with adult genes. The evidence suggests that between embryonic and adult nuclear DNA, there is rearrangement of the DNA nucleotide sequence within the chromosome. There is a shortening of the distance between variable and constant regions on the DNA sequences in embryonic DNA as it becomes adult DNA, with transposition of variable-region genes to any of the J (joining)-segment genes (Fig. 4.7). This has the effect of increasing the diversity of the V regions. While some variability in the variable region is thought to result from this shortening process, it is not clear

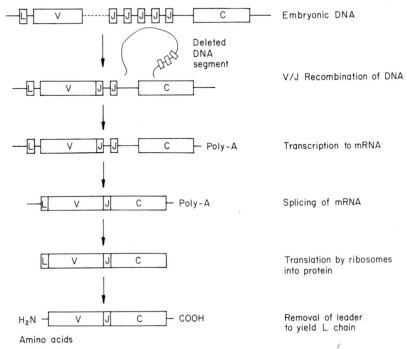

Fig. 4.7. The sequence of steps in L-chain synthesis in the mouse is shown diagrammatically, starting with the organization of the L-chain gene segments in embryonic DNA. There is an initial rearrangement of the variable-region (V) and joining-region (J) genes to bring the V region closer to the constant region (C). This involves the deletion of the intervening segment of DNA. This results in one V sequence, together with a short leader (L) sequence being combined with one of the J sequences and one C sequence to form the κ or λ gene. This entire gene is transcribed into primary RNA, which is in turn transcribed into messenger RNA (mRNA) with removal of the intervening sequences. This is translated by the ribosomes into peptides; the hydrophobic leader sequence is removed and the completed L chain is formed.

whether somatic mutation, specifically within the *V*-region gene, can contribute significantly to antibody variability. This shortening may occur by the formation of loops which are not read into the final messenger RNA (mRNA). Thus the mRNA lacks the intervening sequences found between variable and *J* segments in the adult DNA and only includes nucleotides which correspond exactly to the amino-acid sequences of the light chains.

As B-cells mature, they produce firstly μ chains and then κ or λ chains, but it is not known if this is a regulated process or if it involves the relative rates of DNA rearrangement. A switch between H-chain classes from μ chain to α chain or γ chain also occurs, presumably by some form of recombination between sequences for variable and constant regions for the other types of H chains (Fig. 4.8). Animals heterozygous for immunoglobulin allotypes, inherited from their

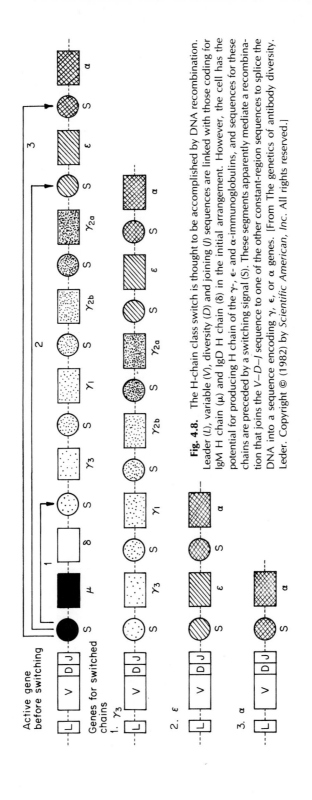

Fig. 4.8. The H-chain class switch is thought to be accomplished by DNA recombination. Leader (L), variable (V), diversity (D) and joining (J) sequences are linked with those coding for IgM H chain (μ) and IgD H chain (δ) in the initial arrangement. However, the cell has the potential for producing H chain of the γ-, ε- and α-immunoglobulins, and sequences for these chains are preceded by a switching signal (S). These segments apparently mediate a recombination that joins the V–D–J sequence to one of the other constant-region sequences to splice the DNA into a sequence encoding γ, ε, or α genes. [From The genetics of antibody diversity. Leder. Copyright © (1982) by *Scientific American, Inc.* All rights reserved.]

parents, make only one of the two allelic forms potentially available. This is known as 'allelic exclusion'. At present, efforts are also being made to determine if this is due to errors in the rearrangement process or whether there is another switch mechanism operating.

The final mRNA for heavy and light chains is translated separately by the ribosomes which synthesise the peptides of the heavy and light chains, which are then assembled in the endoplasmic reticulum of the plasma cell to form complete immunoglobulin molecules. This combination of H and L chains is non-covalent, with disulphide bridges forming between the two types of molecules to produce H_2L_2. Carbohydrate residues are attached within the lumen of the endo-plasmic reticulum of the cell, and with IgM and IgA immunoglobulins, a further J chain (distinct from the J segment of DNA) is attached to form the polymers of H and L chains which make up these classes of immunoglobulins.

4.8 MONOCLONAL ANTIBODIES

A discussion of immunoglobulins would be incomplete without a description of the production of monoclonal antibodies. This technique arose from work carried out at Oxford and Cambridge Universities on cell fusion techniques. It was found that the plasma membranes of cells could be made to fuse using viruses or polyethylene glycol and that during this fusion, often the nuclei of the cells also fused. Some cells with fused nuclei continued to grow with double the number of chromosomes, although during subculture, some of the chromosomes were lost. It was also found possible to produce mouse and human cell hybrids which were to prove valuable in genetic studies on the major histocompatibility complex (MHC) in humans. By this method it was possible to localise chromo-some 6 as the one bearing the DNA sequences for the MHC antigens, since the expression of these MHC antigens on the hybrid cell surface disappeared when chromosome 6 was lost from the cell hybrid nucleus.

The technique of cell fusion was also exploited by Köhler and Milstein (1975), who had the idea of fusing mouse spleen antibody-forming cells with mouse myeloma cells. This elegant idea was translated into practical reality when they demonstrated that mouse spleen cells producing antibodies to sheep erythrocytes could be fused with myeloma cells to produce clones of hybrid cells or 'hybrido-mas', which proliferated in cell culture to produce monoclonal antibodies (Fig. 4.9). These monoclonal antibodies were easily demonstrated because in the presence of complement, they formed haemolytic plaques around hybridoma cells placed on sheep blood agar. It was also possible to distinguish the hybridoma cells from unfused myeloma cells or spleen cells by the use of selective tissue culture medium. The myeloma cells could not grow in medium containing aminopterin and supplemented with hypoxanthine and thymidine

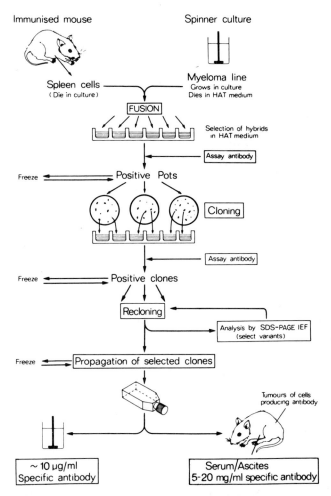

Fig. 4.9. Flow diagram showing the method for cell fusion, cloning and preparation of monoclonal antibodies. (Reproduced by kind permission from Milstein and Lennox (1980), *Curr. Top. Dev. Biol.* **14**, 1–32, Academic Press.)

(HAT medium), because they were unable to utilise the salvage pathway. Hybrids between such cells could be selectively grown because these were the only cells able to multiply in the HAT selective medium. Therefore, the unfused myeloma cells died out, while the unfused spleen cells failed to proliferate because there was nothing in the medium which would stimulate them to divide.

The hybridoma cells proliferated and could be purified by limiting dilution technique in plastic Microtiter trays, which in the case of Köhler and Milstein's original work, could be measured by adding sheep erythrocytes and complement to the wells containing the proliferating anti-sheep erythrocyte hybridomas.

The assay of the products of hybridomas at the screening stage then moved to the use of radioimmunoassays and enzyme-linked immunosorbent assay (ELISA) techniques. Hybridoma monoclonal antibodies have been taken up commercially, and there are inventories of monoclonal antibodies to human and mouse lymphocyte-differentiation antigens, to immunoglobulin fragments and to mouse MHC antigens. The monoclonal antibodies to the human MHC antigens were not, however, as forthcoming as had been originally hoped. It appeared that the mouse spleen cells, immunised with human cells, recognised major differentiation antigens more often than they recognised MHC antigens. Among the large number of human MHC alleles, only nine have been recognised with monoclonal antibodies using mouse spleen cells fused with mouse myeloma cells. Therefore attention has been turned towards the use of human myelomas with human antibody-forming cells to produce hybridomas. Although this has been achieved in the laboratory, it has yet to be taken up commercially. Some work has also been attempted with mixed human and mouse hybridomas, but the instability of the hybrid cells has been a problem in the continued production of monoclonal antibodies.

Monoclonal antibodies are being used therapeutically in human cancer patients. In some work, toxic molecules or drugs are linked to the tumour-specific antibodies, so that when they attach to the tumour, the tumour cells are killed. This work is being carried out with mouse monoclonal antibodies, which are a foreign protein. Repeated treatments carry the risk of Type III hypersensitivity reactions (see Chapter 9 for classification of hypersensitivities), and the treatment is not in common use. In the veterinary field, there are no published reports of the use of hybridoma antibodies in the therapy of disease. The progress towards this will, no doubt, depend on the success of efforts in the therapy of human disease with monoclonal antibodies produced from human hybridomas. At the moment, the likely candidate for similar work is the dog, which has myeloma cell lines available, as well as the need to control neoplastic conditions by therapy.

A major research use for monoclonal antibodies has been in the identification and enumeration of lymphocytes in the fluorescence-activated cell sorter (FACS). As mentioned in Chapter 2 on cellular immunology, these antibodies are available from the Ortho, Becton-Dickinson and Coulter companies, which also sell the machines. A list of the major human lymphocyte-differentiation antigens and subpopulations recognised by these monoclonal antibodies is shown in Table 4.1. Unfortunately there are no comparable monoclonal antibodies for animal lymphocytes, available from commercial sources. Some laboratories have produced their own hybridoma antibodies to bovine and ovine lymphocytes, and these have recognised MHC antigens as well as differentiation anti-

TABLE 4.1

Monoclonal Antibodies Available for Human Lymphocyte Subsets

Cell type	Ortho	Coulter	Beckton-Dickinson
T-cells	OKT3		Anti-leu-4
Suppressor/cytotoxic T-cells	OKT8	T8	Anti-leu-2a+2b
Helper/Inducer T-cells	OKT4	T4	Anti-leu-3a+3b
E-rosette receptor	OKT11	T11	Anti-leu-5
Thymocytes	OKT6	T6	
Activated lymphocytes	OKT9		Anti-HLA-DR
Early stem cells	OKT10		
Monocytes and macrophages	OKM1	M02	Anti-leu-M1
'Ia-like' antigens	OKIa1	HLA D/DR	Anti-HLA-DR
B-cells	OKIa1	B1	Anti-HLA-DR

gens on the lymphocytes. Interestingly, monoclonal antibodies to bovine B-cell membrane IgM heavy chains are also commonly found (Pinder *et al.*, 1980). The study of monoclonal antibodies to animal lymphocytes is still at an early stage of development, but if the need for them arises for typing MHC in animals, they will undoubtedly be developed commercially. One technical problem that may arise is that the monoclonal antibodies cannot always be used in microcytotoxicity tests because they fix complement poorly.

Another major research use for monoclonal antibodies has been in the study of virus structure and in the subdivision of viruses into strains. For example, the haemagglutinin protein of influenza virus has been extensively studied with monoclonal antibodies in attempts to determine important antigenic sites. Strain differences are usually the result of a few amino-acid sequence differences, but these are enough to cause antigenic shifts in the virus coat protein against which a new immune response has to be mounted by susceptible individuals. Monoclonal antibodies recognise antigenic sequences of peptides which make up the influenza virus haemagglutinin molecule, but antibodies to these peptides are not protective by themselves, since it is the tertiary protein structure which determines the antigenic specificity. Therefore the monoclonal antibodies to virus haemagglutinins may not be as protective as natural antibodies of broad specificity.

Another use for virus-specific monoclonal antibodies has been in the recognition of two strains of Rabies virus. The second strain was suspected from the poor efficacy of some vaccine strains against wild Rabies virus. The proof was finally provided by the high specificity of monoclonal antibodies for amino-acid sequences unique for each strain of Rabies virus. The importance of this was that the preparation of vaccines could then be carried out with the confidence that both Rabies virus antigenic types were included.

4.9 GENERAL CONCLUSIONS

Animal immunoglobulins have been studied and found to be different from those of the human and mouse. For example, there is a functional difference in the IgG_1 and IgG_2 subclasses of ruminant IgG, in which the IgG_1 is preferentially concentrated by the mammary gland epithelium, to be transferred to the newborn ruminant after ingestion of colostrum.

The amino-acid sequences of immunoglobulins have been studied in some domestic species, particularly the dog, but in general, these immunoglobulins are not as well-characterised as those of the human and mouse. There are some data which suggest that the amino-acid sequence in the Fc piece of bovine and ovine IgG immunoglobulins determines the electrophoretic mobility of the subclasses and also their combination with specific Fc receptors on the surface membranes of cells.

The equivalent of the human Bence–Jones proteins has been described for bovine urine, and multiple myelomata, reported for the cat, dog, pig and horse. The normal IgG, IgM and IgA immunoglobulins have been found to have much the same specialised functions that they have for other species. The IgM macroglobulin appears before IgG during the immune response, and IgA is present in external secretions of all domestic species so far examined. The IgE immunoglobulin, which mediates immediate (Type I) hypersensitivity, has been found in bovine colostrum and is capable of passively transmitting hypersensitivity after ingestion of colostrum.

Serum complement components have been poorly characterised for most domestic species except perhaps the dog and cow. It is possible that studies on the genetics of complement components would lead to a better understanding of the causes of variation of individuals in resistance to infectious diseases. Bovine serum contains a unique conglutinin which binds to aggregated immune complexes which have fixed complement.

The immunoglobulin genes of the mouse and human are the subject of close scrutiny in current basic immunological research. Comparable studies have not been reported for any of the domestic species.

The production of monoclonal antibodies in mice to bovine lymphocyte membrane components has been reported. It would seem that a myeloma cell line is necessary for each species, to produce monoclonal antibodies adapted for each species. As yet none have been produced for domestic animals, although the dog would be a logical choice, since myeloma tumours have been frequently found. However, the future of the monoclonal antibodies in the animal field appears to lie in the characterisation of strains of infectious viruses, to improve the formulation of vaccines.

REFERENCES

Barta, O., Nelson, R. A. and Kuo, C. Y. (1976). *Immunol. Commun.* **5**, 75–86.
Conde, F. P., Deverson, E. V. and Milstein, C. P. (1975). *Eur. J. Immunol.* **5**, 291–293.
Feinstein, A. and Munn, E. A. (1969). *Nature (London)* **224**, 1307–1309.
Gershwin, L. J. (1981). *Am. J. Vet. Res.* **42**, 1184–1187.
Gorman, N. T., McConnell, I. and Lachmann, P. J. (1981). *Vet. Immunol. Immunopathol.* **2**, 309–320.
Hammer, D. K., Kickhöfen, B. and Schmid, T. (1971). *Eur. J. Immunol.* **1**, 249–258.
Ingram, D. G. (1982). Comparative aspects of conglutinin and immunoconglutinin. *In* 'Animal Models of Immunological Processes' (J. B. Hay, ed.), pp. 221–253. Academic Press, New York.
Ishizaka, K., Ishizaka, T. and Hornbrook, M. M. (1966). *J. Immunol.* **97**, 840–853.
Jonas, W., Stankiewicz, M. and Pulford, H. (1982). *N.Z. Vet. J.* **30**, 85–87.
Kehoe, J. M. (1982). Selected aspects of the canine immune response. *In* 'Animal Models of Immunological Processes' (J. B. Hay, ed.), pp. 1–23. Academic Press, New York.
Köhler, G. and Milstein, C. (1975). *Nature (London)* **256**, 495–497.
Leder, P. (1982). *Sci. Am.* **246**, 72–83.
Loos, M. (1982). *Mol Immunol.* **19**, 1229–1238.
McGuire, T. C., Musoke, A. J. and Kurtti, T. (1979). *Immunology* **38**, 249–256.
Mage, M. G. (1980). Preparation of Fab fragments from IgGs of different animal species. *In* 'Immunological Techniques' (H. Van Vunakis and J. J. Langone, eds.), Methods in Enzymology, Vol. 70, pp. 142–150. Academic Press, New York.
Milstein, C. and Lennox, E. S. (1980). *Curr. Top. Dev. Biol.* **14**, 1–32.
Murphy, F. A., Osebold, J. W. and Aalund, O. (1965). *Arch. Biochem. Biophys.* **112**, 126–136.
Outteridge, P. M., Mackenzie, D. D. S. and Lascelles, A. K. (1968). *Arch. Biochem. Biophys.* **126**, 105–110.
Pang, A. S. D. and Ashton, W. P. (1978). *Immunochemistry* **15**, 529–534.
Pierce, A. E. and Feinstein, A. (1965). *Immunology* **8**, 106–123.
Pinder, M., Pearson, T. W., and Roelants, G. E. (1980). *Vet. Immunol. Immunopathol.* **1**, 303–316.
Reid, K. B. M. and Porter, R. R. (1981). *Annu. Rev. Biochem.* **50**, 433–464.
Rockley, L. S. and Kimmell, A. T. (1972). *Immunochemistry* **9**, 23–28.

5

Local Immunity

The possibility of local immunisation of mucous membranes, separately from parental immunisation of the rest of the animal, has stimulated considerable activity in the veterinary field. Infections of the mammary gland, reproductive tract, gut and lungs, figure large in the day-to-day work of most veterinarians. Vaccines administered parenterally stimulate serum antibodies in high titre, but often the titres of specific antibody are greatly reduced in secretions. Thus the concentration of IgG in bovine milk can be $\frac{1}{20}$ that found in the blood, due to the normal filtration from blood to interstitial tissue fluid and from tissue fluid into milk. If the titre were the only factor, it would seem reasonable to boost titres in serum so that enough antibody crossed mucous membranes to provide protection.

Other factors influence the efficacy of parenteral boosting of titres and subsequent protection at a mucous membrane. One of these is the multiplicity of antigens which are presented to the host by the invading microorganisms or parasites. Some of these antigens, such as the staphylococcal toxins, never stimulate high titres, even when administered parenterally. Therefore, the final titres in secretions, against important antigens, can often be undetectable and consequently non-protective during challenge.

A way around this problem is to provide local stimulation of the immune response by direct immunisation of cells of the mucous membrane. The aim is to cause local plasma cells adjacent to the epithelium, to produce antibody specific to the vaccine. The titres in the secretions are consequently augmented by highly-specific antibody which is always present at the site of challenge. This may be all that is needed for protection; the oral Sabin vaccine against poliomyelitis in humans stimulates a local immune response in the gut, which prevents the virus from infecting the host through its normal point of entry. In this case, the attenuated living vaccine stimulates plasma cells in the gut submucosa to produce specific antibodies which are secreted in two directions, directly into the gut mucus and in the other direction into the intestinal lymph and ultimately into the blood.

Such clear-cut effective vaccines for local immunisation of a mucous membrane are rare in both the human and veterinary fields. However, an apparent parallel to the Sabin poliomyelitis vaccine is found with chickens, where living attenuated-virus vaccines to Avian Encephalomyelitis, Infectious Bronchitis, Infectious Laryngotracheitis (ILT) and Newcastle disease are administered via the drinking water. However, with the possible exception of Avian Encephalomyelitis, immunity appears to depend on the establishment of the viruses in the gut where they stimulate antibodies and antibody-producing cells which have their effect at another site, such as the respiratory system. In this case, it would appear that the introduction of the virus by a relatively abnormal route, stimulates protection, but equally-good protection can be obtained from administration by eye-drop or aerosol spray.

5.1   THE DEMONSTRATION OF LOCAL IMMUNITY

The essential problem in demonstrating local immunity has been to distinguish antibodies in secretions, which are there because of plasma cell concentrations near epithelia, from those antibodies which have diffused from serum, or have been selectively concentrated by epithelial cells.

For example, it was contended by Campbell *et al.* (1950), that in the mammary gland of the cow all the antibodies in colostrum were locally synthesised by plasma cells in the mammary gland interstitial tissues. This was disproved by Pierce (1955), and Larson and Kendall (1957), who found that there was a pronounced drop in serum immunoglobulin levels coincident with a rise in mammary secretion immunoglobulins. Direct labelling of serum immunoglobulins with radioactive iodine (^{131}I) demonstrated that the mammary gland concentrated the protein-bound radioactivity in colostrum as much as 13 times that in serum (Dixon *et al.*, 1961).

Nevertheless, plasma cells do exist in the mammary gland tissue, and their contribution to the immunoglobulin in milk becomes evident once the colostral immunoglobulin transport has declined. In the case of the ruminant, the locally-synthesised immunoglobulin was found to be IgA, which distinguished it from the IgG_1 which was selectively transported by the epithelial cells.

There are several ways of estimating the local synthesis of immunoglobulins.

The most obvious is to compare titres of specific antibody in the secretion with those in serum. If the titre in the secretion is persistently higher than that in serum, the evidence is favourable for local antibody synthesis. This is because there is no evidence to suggest that transport of specific antibody across epithelial surfaces occurs to the exclusion of other molecules of the same immunoglobulin class.

Another method of looking at local synthesis of an immunoglobulin class is to label it with radioactive ^{131}I and inject it back into the animal. This was carried out with the two classes of IgG in ruminants—the IgG_1 being labelled with ^{131}I and IgG_2 class with ^{125}I. If a large amount of IgG_1, for example, is locally synthesised, the amount of labelled serum IgG_1 in secretions will decrease. In this case, the ^{125}I-labelled IgG_2 acts as a control for passive diffusion from serum, because little of this immunoglobulin is synthesised locally. The two immunoglobulins can be counted simultaneously in the γ spectrometer by the use of two different window settings which cover the spectra of ^{131}I and ^{125}I respectively.

Thirdly, the distribution of antibody-containing cells in the subepithelial regions of mucous membranes can be examined in frozen sections using fluorescent anti-immunoglobulin reagents. A concentration of specific antibody-containing cells close to the epithelial surface is strong but not unequivocal evidence for contribution of local synthesis to antibody in secretions. This is because much of the antibody may end up in regional lymph and pass back into the blood stream via the thoracic duct. The high IgA content of intestinal lymph is a good example where immunoglobulin is synthesised by cells in the submucosa and regional lymph nodes to be returned to the blood via the lymphatics and ultimately to be concentrated in bile and returned to the intestinal secretions. Some caution with fluorescent-antibody techniques is also required with phagocytes, since these may take up free immunoglobulin, for example from colostrum, and give the appearance of being antibody-forming cells.

5.2 LOCAL ANTIGENIC STIMULATION
OF THE MAMMARY GLAND

The mammary gland of the cow is subject to mastitis, particularly that caused by *Staphylococcus aureus*. Vaccines administered parenterally have been found to provide some protection, but it was demonstrated in sheep injected intravenously with radiolabelled IgG that immunoglobulin could only cross from serum to milk during acute inflammation. This meant that specific antibody crossed from serum to milk in high titre only after the mastitis was well-established. Therefore, the mammary gland offered great potential for local immunisation to provide protective antibody in milk.

Several other factors, however, can affect the course of the mastitis. It is known that IgG$_1$ is concentrated in preference to IgG$_2$ in the ruminant mammary gland during the period just before calving or lambing. This concentrating function continues for the first week after parturition but then drops to a low background level which persists throughout lactation. It is paradoxical that, at a time of maximum immunoglobulin concentration in mammary gland secretion, the gland is highly susceptible to mastitis. Obviously, not all the IgG$_1$ is specific for bacteria such as staphylococci, but measurable titres against α-haemolysin in colostrum are six times higher than in serum and higher than at any other time during the lactational cycle. It appears that the natural flushing action of milk secretion and removal by calf suckling, is important in the physical removal of staphylococci before they reach numbers which can damage the mammary gland epithelium.

The toxins produced by the staphylococci, such as α- and δ-haemolysin, can also produce severe inflammation when injected on their own, without the bacteria. The neutralisation of the toxins by specific antitoxin, as well as their dilution in milk, appears to be crucial to the outcome of the infection. If the staphylococcal growth is not checked early in the infection, the acute form of the disease ensues, with rapid loss of milk production and, in severe cases, can even lead to gangrenous mastitis. However, more commonly, the acute phase rapidly passes and the chronic form of mastitis persists. This low-grade inflammation is not dangerous to the animal but is a cause of economic loss, through a lower milk production compared with that which could be expected from the uninfected mammary gland. Furthermore, such chronically-infected cattle are a source of infection for the rest of the herd, via the cups of the milking machine.

The mammary gland can be locally immunised with staphylococcal antigens, but this must be carried out during the *non-lactating* or involution phase of the cycle. At the end of lactation, secretion of milk decreases and eventually ceases, if no further milking stimulus is applied. The integrity of the glandular epithelium breaks down and the gland itself becomes smaller, as large areas of glandular tissue are resorbed. There are large numbers of lymphoid cells and macrophages which invade the interstitial tissues between the islands of epithelium which remain. The function of these lymphoid cells is thought to be mainly in the defence of the mammary gland, to prevent bacterial opportunism at a time of breakdown of the integrity of the epithelium. The macrophages also have a function in the removal of fat from the gland and resorption of cell debris. The introduction of vaccines into the gland at this time allows a long-term stimulus to the lymphoid cells there. These cells persist in the gland and mature into plasma cells which produce specific antibody throughout the subsequent lactation.

A particularly good example of local immunity is, in fact, found with the sheep mammary gland (Lascelles and McDowell, 1974). The infusion, 1 month before lambing, of killed *Salmonella* organisms into one side of the mammary gland, simultaneously with the infusion of killed *Brucella* organisms into the other side, provided a well-controlled experiment which demonstrated local production of antibody. The whey from the *Salmonella*-infused side contained antibodies to *Salmonella* in higher titre than in plasma and in higher titre than in whey from the *Brucella*-infused side. The converse was true for the other side, in which antibodies to *Brucella* exceeded those of plasma and those in whey from the *Salmonella*-infused side. The titres of specific antibody in milk remained higher than the titres of specific antibody in serum or in efferent mammary lymph, if the lymphatic duct was cannulated at this time (Fig. 5.1). This is excellent evidence for local antibody production but is further supported by the demonstration of specific antibody-containing cells in histological sections of

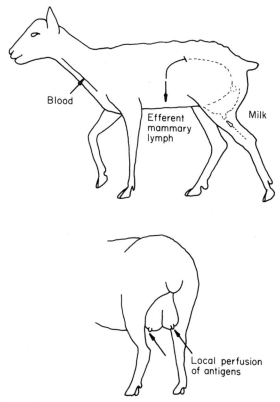

Fig. 5.1. The antibody levels in blood, milk whey and mammary lymph can all be measured after local antigenic stimulation of the mammary gland during the non-lactating period. The titres of specific antibodies in milk remain higher than those in the blood or in efferent mammary lymph during lactation, and this is excellent evidence for local antibody synthesis by the mammary gland of the ewe.

mammary gland. The cells demonstrable in the interstitial spaces produce specific antibody of the IgA, IgM or IgG_1 class.

The specific antibody responses in the secretions of the mammary gland are predominantly of the IgA and IgM subclasses of immunoglobulin. Some antibody of the IgG_1 class is present in milk, but it seems likely that much of this results from the persistence, at a low level, of the selective concentration mechanism of colostrum formation from serum, and that specific antibody is passively transported from blood through the mammary gland epithelial cells as a component of this IgG_1 immunoglobulin. This contrasts with the human mammary gland where the predominant immunoglobulin in milk is IgA, both in colostrum and in milk after local antigenic stimulation. In the sheep, and most likely in other ruminants, the production of specific IgA antibody is nascent, until the stimulus of local immunisation.

The effectiveness of local immunisation against staphylococcal mastitis has been extensively tested in the sheep mammary gland (Watson, 1980). The infusion of killed bacteria with added toxoids of α-haemolysin, δ-haemolysin, leucocidin and coagulase, results in the appearance of specific agglutinins and antitoxins in colostrum and in milk. Again the vaccine must be administered during the non-lactating phase of the mammary gland cycle. Antibody can only be detected in very low levels during full lactation, but experimental challenge with virulent staphylococci causes it to reappear in measurable titres in milk. The protection afforded by these antibodies, is mainly against acute mastitis. The organisms can persist in the gland and cause low-grade chronic mastitis apparently because the small numbers of organisms which remain either do not stimulate the immune response or there is an immune tolerance induced to the staphylococci.

Local immunisation with staphylococcal vaccines infused into the mammary gland has been attempted in cattle. Many of the experiments have attempted immunisation during the lactating phase of the mammary gland cycle. This has proved unsuccessful, presumably because the vaccine did not remain long enough in the gland to stimulate an effective local immune response. There is also some anxiety among owners of dairy cattle that the local infusion of vaccines into the mammary glands of dairy cattle could have an effect of reducing milk production. Certainly anything that causes inflammation in the lactating mammary gland, causes a drop in milk production, and the use of oil or alum adjuvants is contraindicated in the mammary gland. However, vaccines without adjuvant have been infused into the non-lactating mammary gland of dairy cattle and found to induce the production of local antibody. The problem of experimental challenge of valuable cattle, to see if the vaccination has been achieved, has usually prevented critical evaluation of the protection afforded to the animals. Instead, reliance has been placed on natural infection and monitoring of the infection rate in vaccinated mammary glands compared with non-immunised mammary glands. The results of the experiments with herds of dairy cattle have been inconclusive, because of the variable challenge each animal has received. The overall conclusion from such work is that since the vaccine is not highly protective, the expense and effort required in local vaccination is not justified. Therefore, efforts should be logically directed towards improving the efficacy of staphylococcal vaccines experimentally, and once this has been achieved, then the question of local vaccination of the mammary gland should be examined again.

5.2.1 Cells in Milk

Cellular immunity in the mammary gland has been suggested as a possible avenue for research. Certainly the infusion of sterile water into the bovine mammary gland causes a leucocytosis in milk consisting mostly of polymorphs, and these cells are very effective against challenge with *Escherichia coli* or *Pseudomonas* organisms. However, this is, in effect, inducing mastitis to fight mastitis, an approach which may be detrimental to milk production. Furthermore, it does not prevent the colonisation of the mammary gland with staphylococcal organisms, which appear to be capable of surviving within polymorphonuclear leucocytes.

Paape and colleagues (1981) have developed an intramammary device which works on this principle. A polystyrene plastic coil is inserted into the milk cistern of the mammary gland of dairy cattle, and this is left to provide a low-grade irritation, which stimulates the migration of polymorphs into milk. The critical number appears to be 900,000 cells/ml of stripping milk. This protects the gland against experimental challenge with *E. coli* organisms. The intramammary device (IMD) is being tested in field trials to see if the incidence of mastitis is reduced, without a penalty in milk production.

This kind of cellular immunity is only immunologically directed to the extent that local antibody opsonises invading bacteria and causes more rapid mobilisation of polymorphs in immunised rather than in non-immunised glands. There is a Type III hypersensitivity reaction which causes inflammation in locally-immunised mammary glands 4 hours after challenge. It is not known if this is helpful or injurious to the defence of the gland against staphylococcal infections.

The predominant lymphocyte in bovine mammary secretions appears to be the mature T-cell (Schore *et al.*, 1981). In sheep, fluorescein-labelled colostral lymphocytes cross the intestinal epithelium of neonatal lambs but only appear in small numbers in the blood of lambs (Schnorr and Pearson, 1984). Therefore, milk lymphocytes have two potential functions, the defence of the mammary gland and the transmission of immunity from mother to offspring.

Delayed hypersensitivity to staphylococcal antigens has been demonstrated in experimental rabbits and in humans. It is not known if macrophage cellular immunity is important in the long-term control of staphylococcal infection. The

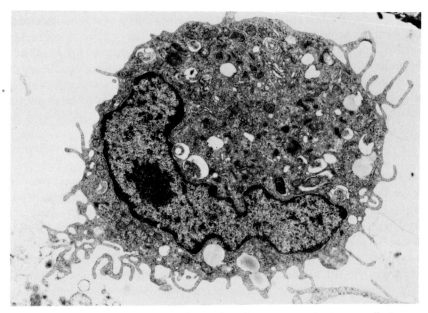

Fig. 5.2. A sheep macrophage from the non-lactating mammary gland, an excellent source of these cells not only in the ewe but also in the cow and the mare. These cells apparently have a defensive function at a time in the lactational cycle when the integrity of the mammary epithelium is incomplete. (Reproduced by kind permission of Dr. C. S. Lee, School of Veterinary Science, University of Melbourne, Australia.)

non-lactating mammary gland contains many macrophages (Fig. 5.2) and has been used as a source of these cells in sheep, cattle and horses (see Appendix). However, staphylococci can persist in the non-lactating mammary gland, and antibiotics are often infused in 'dry udder' therapy. It would seem that if lymphocytes within the gland produce delayed hypersensitivity or macrophage cellular immunity, it is not very effective in the elimination of the bacteria. However, the extent to which staphylococci can wall themselves off in small abscesses is probably a significant factor in their survival in the non-lactating mammary gland.

5.3   LOCAL ANTIGENIC STIMULATION OF THE GASTRO-INTESTINAL TRACT

By its very nature, the gut is a site of constant antigenic stimulation, as a result of the microorganisms and complex antigens present in the gut contents. In the chicken, it has long been known that the removal of the bursa of Fabricius in young birds, leads to an immunodeficiency of B-cells. Until recently, this had not been proven for mammals such as laboratory rodents or the domestic animals. It had been assumed that the mammalian equivalent of the bursa of Fabricius would be some organ such as the large colon in the rabbit, but removal of this piece of gut by surgery did not lead to an immunodeficiency.

It is now known that concentrations of lymphoid cells in the large intestine, the Peyer's patches, are the equivalent of the bursa of Fabricius in the chicken. The removal of the Peyer's patches from the gut of newborn lambs, leads to a long-term deficiency in circulating B-cells. This is one arm of the immune response which is apparently under the control of the Peyer's patches, which must now be regarded as a primary lymphoid organ; that is, one in which the stem cells of the B-cell series originate. This area of the gut is anatomically in close apposition to the gut contents but apparently is not stimulated only by the antigens there. The Peyer's patches develop germinal centres even when surgically isolated in loops which no longer communicate with the lumen of the intestine. Instead, they appear to serve the function in the foetus of supplying pre-B-cells, which are the daughter cells of dividing stem cells within the Peyer's patches.

However, along the length of the rest of the gut there are concentrations of lymphoid cells which are most certainly there solely as a result of antigenic stimulation. For example, in the sheep the proportion of immunoglobulin-containing cells varies along the length of the gut (Table 5.1). The plasma cells demonstrable in tissue sections using fluorescent-antibody techniques, are thought to migrate there as circulating B-cells from the blood stream and mature in the submucosa of the gut to produce specific antibody. It is known that, in sheep at least, blast cells from efferent intestinal lymph preferentially recirculate via the lymphatics of the intestine and settle in the submucosal tissues. There is also evidence that a two-way traffic exists between the gut and other mucous membranes of the body. This has been suggested as a reason for the high content of IgA antibodies in the colostrum of humans which are specific for gut bacteria.

TABLE 5.1

Immunoglobulin-Containing Cells along the Gut of Parasite-Free Sheep[a,b]

Immuno-globulin subclass	Lymph nodes			Abomasum		Small intestine	
	Pre-scapular	Mesen-teric	Abo-masal	Fundic	Pyloric	Jejunum	Ileum
IgA	3.7	7.9	3.6	0	0	43.1	33.8
IgG$_1$	37.9	42.3	35.3	3.7	1.1	29.7	8.6
IgG$_2$	26.1	29.8	18.7	0	0	5.6	2.6

[a] From Curtain and Anderson (1971).

[b] Figures represent mean counts of each cell type for 100 microscope fields at ×100.

In ruminants, however, the IgA system is relatively dormant unless local antigenic stimulation occurs. The predominant immunoglobulin in colostrum is IgG_1, and this contains a heterogeneous collection of specific antibodies which are non-specifically transported across the mammary epithelium into the milk cistern. Another way in which ruminants differ from other species is in the transport of IgA into bile and thence into the gut. In species such as the laboratory rat, it appears that IgA which originates in the submucosa of the gut, is transported to the blood stream via the intestinal lymphatics. A concentrating mechanism occurs in the epithelial cells of the liver, and the IgA is selectively transported from blood into the bile and from there into the gut, where it presumably has an effect in preventing attachment of enteric pathogenic microorganisms.

In ruminants, the results are less clear-cut than in rats. There is IgG_1 in bile and some IgA. At one time it appeared that IgA was not concentrated by the liver of ruminants as it is for other species. More recent evidence (Scicchitano et al., 1984), however, suggests that IgA is returned to the gut via the bile duct in sheep and cattle, as it is for other species (Fig. 5.3). In general, however, it appears that in ruminants there are two instances, the mammary gland and the gut, in which IgA secretory antibody can be at low levels without any detrimental effects on the resistance of the calf or lamb to infection in the gut. Thus a generally-accepted tenet of mucosal immunity, that IgA is vital for immunity,

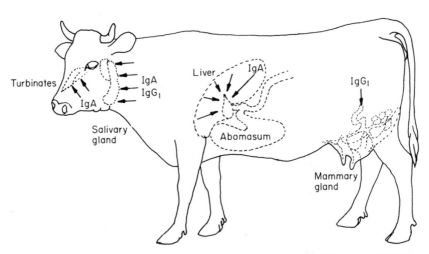

Fig. 5.3. The various external secretory organs of the ruminant which concentrate immunoglobulins. Selective concentration of IgG_1 occurs in the mammary gland and to some extent the salivary gland. The salivary gland also concentrates IgA, and recent evidence suggests that the liver can concentrate IgA in bile, which is the route by which this immunoglobulin can return to the gut lumen via the bile duct.

does not appear to hold true for the ruminant. Admittedly, IgA-containing cells are present in the ruminant gut submucosa, particularly the small intestine, but it is not the major immunoglobulin in the ruminant that it is in the gut of other species such as the rat, pig, rabbit and human.

The IgA system has also been activated in ruminants by injection of antigens into the peritoneal cavity of the sheep. In these experiments, complete Freund's adjuvant was used to provide long-lasting stimulation of the serosal surface of the gut (Husband *et al.*, 1979). In rats, injection of antigen by this route causes increased production of IgA in the gut secretions and in intestinal lymph. In sheep also there is an increase in the IgA-containing cells in intestinal lymph, but the greatest number of specific antibody-containing cells are those with IgG immunoglobulin (Beh *et al.*, 1979).

5.4 LOCAL VACCINATION AGAINST MICROORGANISMS IN THE GUT

Local vaccination of the gut has been demonstrated with piglets fed a heat-killed suspension of *E. coli* mixed in with their feed (Porter *et al.*, 1973; Newby *et al.*, 1977). The commercial vaccine, called Intagen, consists of several different strains of *E. coli* and has been effective in reducing the incidence and severity of scours in piglets which is caused by these organisms. Although the immune response appears to be mainly against the somatic antigens such as the K88 antigen of the heat-killed organisms, there is evidence for production of antibodies against the heat-labile enterotoxin of the enteric pathogen. Specific IgG and IgA antibodies are both present after feeding the Intagen vaccine, but IgM is also found as a prominent immunoglobulin and has specificity for antigens, as it has after vaccination of the mammary gland of the ewe.

However, the most common approach in vaccination against *E. coli* scours in calves and piglets, has been the vaccination of the dam before colostrum formation by the mammary gland. This concentrates specific antibodies in the colostrum, and some of these are directed towards the *E. coli* antigens contained in the vaccine used with the dam. These antibodies are protective to the calf and piglet during the critical 2 months after parturition. It is interesting that the IgA immunoglobulins appear to behave differently in the two species. In calves, IgA is absorbed from the gut with the IgG$_1$, during the first 48 hours after parturition, and then rapidly secreted again by selective concentration by the epithelia of the salivary gland, lachrymal gland, gut and possibly liver. The evidence for this is mostly based on the very short half-life for IgA (48 hours) when injected into cattle. Levels of circulating IgA are low in adults and also return to low levels in calves 48 hours after ingestion of colostrum.

In contrast, the young piglet does not appear to absorb much IgA from the ingested colostrum. Instead, this immunoglobulin remains within the lumen of the gut, where it prevents attachment of *E. coli*. It has been assumed that attachment of the organisms by their pili to the mucosal epithelium is prevented by a coating of specific IgA antibody in piglets and of IgG$_1$ antibody in calves. A most important antigen on the pili is the K88 antigen for pig strains and the K99 antigen for the bovine strains. However, the neutralisation of the enterotoxin from *E. coli*, by antibodies of the IgA or IgG$_1$ class, is undoubtedly important in the prevention of the pathogenic effects of the microorganisms. Vaccines which stimulate antibodies against both the somatic K antigens and the enterotoxin are thought to be the best for preventing scours.

In balance, it appears that local vaccination can have an effect on *E. coli* infections in piglets, leading to improved growth rate and lower incidence and severity of infection compared with unvaccinated piglets. However, the colostral antibodies are also vitally important and probably present a cheaper and easier way of immunisation via the colostrum of the dam. Critical to any vaccine is the inclusion of particular *E. coli* strains which are present in the environment of the animals at risk. It is also becoming apparent that both the heat-stable and heat-labile enterotoxins vary in composition with each strain of *E. coli*, and the characterisation of these enterotoxins is the subject of current research on vaccines against these organisms.

5.4.1 Oral Immunisation against Rabies

The oral route of immunisation has been put to practical use in the vaccination of wild foxes with an attenuated strain of Rabies virus. Swiss veterinarians have used chicken-head baits, with a plastic sachet inserted to contain the virus. It has been found that 63% of baits are taken within 48 hours, mostly by foxes, and this form of vaccination has been found to be very promising as a method for controlling Rabies outbreaks in the Swiss mountain valleys.

Careful laboratory studies have shown that rats, mice and cats are fully protected by oral vaccination with the attenuated vaccine from experimental challenge with wild Rabies virus strains. However, authorities in countries other than Switzerland, have been reluctant to release the attenuated strain of Rabies virus in baits to foxes in case the virus reverts to the wild strain. Therefore, considerable work is being carried out experimentally to measure the reversion of the vaccine strains of virus to the wild virulent strains after oral vaccination.

If the virus proves stable and safe for release in wild foxes, it may be the best way of halting the Rabies epidemic which has been progressing slowly across Europe during the last decade. The mode of action of the vaccine has not been worked out, but it would seem likely that IgA and IgG immunoglobulins and immunoglobulin-forming cells, specific for the Rabies virus, are stimulated in the gut mucosa by slow replication of the virus in the gut.

5.4.2 Immunity to *Cysticercus* Infections in Sheep and Cattle

It has been found that the implantation of diffusion chambers containing the oncospheres of *Cysticercus ovis* into the peritoneal cavity of ewes, leads to the development of antibodies which are concentrated in the colostrum, and when ingested by the lamb, the antibodies provide protection against experimental challenge with *Cysticercus* eggs (see Fig. 8.1, Chapter 8).

It has also been found that the diffusion chambers containing the oncospheres can be replaced with culture filtrates of oncospheres which contain antigens which stimulate protective antibodies. This works for calves challenged with *Taenia solium* and *Taenia saginata* eggs under conditions where cattle graze on pastures which are part of a sewage farm. In both cattle and sheep, the protection is provided against the oncospheres which burrow through the gut wall after hatching from the cestode eggs. The barrier is not complete, since a small proportion of the larvae become established and form cysts after experimental challenge. The larvae which escape the colostral antibody may do so by becoming coated with antibody, so that they are not recognised by the host. At this later stage, the predominant immune response is cell-mediated, and old cysts eventually are destroyed by invading mononuclear cells and resorbed.

Thus, as with *E. coli* scours in pigs, the strategic immunisation of ewes or cows with cestode antigens can provide protection against larvae at the gut surface by means of colostral antibody.

5.5 LOCAL ANTIGENIC STIMULATION OF THE LUNG

The lung is a rather unusual organ in its immune response to invading microorganisms. There is a constant flow of mucus outwards from the alveoli, bronchioles, bronchi and trachea to remove particles and organisms which have been inhaled. Within this mucus are both antibodies and cells which are thought to play a role in the defence of the lung against microorganisms.

The predominant immunoglobulins in bronchial mucus are IgA, IgG and IgM. In the ruminant, there is evidence of IgG_1 transport across the alveolar epithelium, in a fashion similar to that in the mammary gland. The ratio of IgA : IgG varies, with IgA predominating in nasal secretions and IgG predominating in bronchoalveolar secretions (Fig. 5.4). However, the immunoglobulin content of the respiratory tract secretions is not only influenced by their production in mucosal plasma cells. In lambs which have been deprived of colostrum, there is no detectable immunoglobulin in nasal secretions, while colostrum-fed lambs, calves and piglets have immunoglobulin in nasal secretions from the time of feeding. It is interesting that after colostrum ingestion the predominant immunoglobulin in nasal secretions of piglets is IgA while that in the nasal secretion of

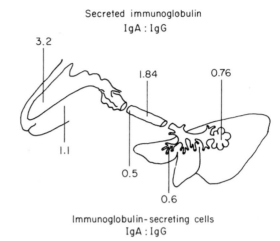

Secreted immunoglobulin
IgA : IgG

3.2

1.84   0.76

1.1

0.5

0.6

Immunoglobulin-secreting cells
IgA : IgG

Fig. 5.4. In ruminants, IgA predominates in nasal secretions and IgG predominates in bronchoalveolar secretions, although both immunoglobulins occur in these secretions. There is also evidence of active transport of IgG_1 across the lung alveolar epithelium. (Redrawn from Wilkie (1982), *J. Am. Vet. Med. Assoc.* **181**, 1074–1079, by permission.)

ruminants is IgG_1—reflecting the class of immunoglobulin which predominates in the colostrum of each species. In calves, the early preponderance of IgG_1 in secretions from the respiratory tract is, in time, slowly reduced in favour of IgA. Furthermore, experiments with adult pigs show that transfer of antibodies from serum to secretions does not readily occur, suggesting that any mechanism for concentrating serum immunoglobulins by respiratory tract epithelia in young animals, decreases with age.

The respiratory tract can, in general, be stimulated locally to produce antibodies of the IgA class with living but not killed microorganisms. Killed microbial vaccines do not readily stimulate local immune responses, but this can be influenced by the particle size introduced into the respiratory tract. Large aerosol droplets (>10 μm) mostly stimulate the nasal epithelium, but small droplets (0.5–3.0 μm) stimulate immune responses further down the bronchoalveolar tract. Both local and systemic immune responses may be stimulated, but local immunisation against respiratory diseases is not the usual route for vaccination because of the difficulty in controlling the dose rate.

However, an ingenious method has been developed for local immunisation of cattle against Infectious Bovine Rhinotracheitis (IBR) (Gerber *et al.*, 1978). A temperature-sensitive mutant of the IBR herpesvirus has been inoculated intranasally, and once there, it remains restricted to the lung because it cannot grow at the higher temperatures (38°C) found in the rest of the body. Therefore, the virus undergoes a limited replication in the lung, stimulating antibodies which provide both local and systemic immunity to natural infection with the virus.

Work has also been carried out in cattle with local immunisation against 'shipping fever' by direct infusion of vaccines into the lung. This has indicated that the protection is produced by antibodies against the bacterial toxins. A dichotomy exists in which antitoxins produce protective immunity but opsonising antibodies against cell wall components induce hypersensitivity, which enhances rather than minimises pneumonia. For this reason, it has been suggested by Wilkie (1982) that parenterally-administered vaccines against *Pasteurella haemolytica* are detrimental while local immunisation is beneficial because the locally-induced IgA is non-opsonising and does not stimulate Type III hypersensitivity in the lung tissue.

However, vaccines against respiratory diseases in other species, such as *Bordetella bronchiseptica* (causing 'kennel cough') in dogs can be carried out by intranasal instillation of avirulent live bacteria or parenterally with killed organisms in adjuvant. The adjuvant is especially important to stimulate immunity with the killed vaccine. A similar situation exists for Feline Rhinotracheitis and Calicivirus infections of cats. In sows, vaccination with killed *B. bronchiseptica* organisms protects newborn piglets via the colostrum against Atrophic Rhinitis or pneumonia. Experimental intranasal inoculation with an avirulent strain has also been effective in protecting pigs against this organism.

The cells in the secretions of the respiratory tract are a mixture of lymphocytes, alveolar macrophages and Type II epithelial cells. The alveolar macrophages differ from those of the peritoneal cavity in that the alveolar macrophages derive their energy from aerobic glycolysis while peritoneal macrophages derive their energy from anaerobic glycolysis. This point is of importance when the tissue culture of pig or sheep lung alveolar macrophages is attempted. In contrast to macrophages from other sites such as the peritoneal cavity or the mammary gland of the ewe, the alveolar macrophages must be kept in a well-oxygenated environment with a smaller column of liquid above them than with the other macrophages. If this is not done, the alveolar macrophages will not attach firmly to the floor of the tissue culture vessel and will eventually die.

The lymphocytes in bronchial mucus are mostly T-cells, but in the dog there also appears to be a high proportion of B-cells which have migrated into the alveoli from the blood. Some of these cells are in the process of producing specific antibody to microorganisms, although this has not yet been carefully quantitated. It is fairly clear that some specific antibody-producing B-cells migrate into the lungs of cattle. Evidence from immunisation against Contagious Bovine Pleuropneumonia shows that immunisation with virulent mycoplasmas in a subcutaneous site will provide protection against aerosol challenge of the lung. Both passive diffusion of serum antibodies and migration of B-cells with local production of the antibody are probably involved. Cattle have been experimentally immunised against Parainfluenza with aerosols containing the virus, and it seems likely that much of the specific antibody found in the mucus originated from B-cells which were stimulated locally in the lung interstitial tissues.

The alveolar macrophages of the sheep at least, appear to contain bacteriostatic substances which may be in addition to those normally found in macrophages from other sources. Certainly the lysosomal fraction from sheep alveolar macrophages is inhibitory to the growth of *Listeria monocytogenes* while the fractions from peritoneal or mammary macrophages are not. It is possible that lung macrophages acquire bacteriostatic substances from the mucus in which they are immersed. Surfactant from the lining of the alveoli is taken up and also the nuclei of dead cells, containing histones. Both surfactant and histones are potentially bacteriostatic, particularly in the low-pH environment of the alveolar macrophage phagocytic lysosome. However, it has yet to be proved if they are the reason for lung macrophages containing bacteriostatic lysosomes.

Also, it would appear that lung macrophages are generally in an activated state as a result of the antigenic stimulation from dust and microorganisms in the inhaled air. This does not prevent the establishment of facultative intracellular bacteria, such as *Mycobacterium tuberculosis,* since these organisms are resistant to activated macrophages. However, it does seem likely that diffusion of specific antibodies or migration of B-cells into the lung mucus can provide protection against the organisms such as those which cause Pleuropneumonia, 'shipping fever' and Parainfluenza in cattle and which are susceptible to opsonisation by specific antibodies, phagocytosis and intracellular killing by the alveolar macrophages. Many virus diseases, such as Infectious Laryngotracheitis (ILT) of chickens, are susceptible to neutralisation by specific antibodies, which have diffused from serum as a result of systemic, rather than local immunisation. Although local immunisation of the lung with antigens in aerosol is feasible, in practice it has been found that systemic immunisation by subcutaneous or even oral route, is easier, surer and less wasteful of antigen than by the aerosol method.

A particular case of oral vaccination against a lung infection is the vaccination of cattle against lungworms using irradiated *Dictyocaulus viviparus* larvae. These larvae are administered orally, go through their first exsheathment and burrow, to a limited extent, into the gut wall. However the irradiation inhibits their further development, and instead of migrating to the liver, into the blood stream and thence to the lung, they remain in the gut wall and eventually die. Nevertheless, they provide enough antigen to stimulate antibodies and possibly cells, and these protect calves against subsequent larval invasion by the wild strain of the parasite. In this case, as in the *Cysticercus ovis* vaccination of sheep, the cycle is broken at the point of entry in the gut, and the target organ, the lung, is not necessarily immunised by migration of B-cells or diffusion of antibody into the lung mucus.

5.6 LOCAL ANTIGENIC STIMULATION OF THE REPRODUCTIVE TRACT

Much of the work of veterinary interest on local immunity in the reproductive tract has involved disease causing infertility in cattle. It was shown by Kerr (1955) that the infusion of killed *Brucella abortus* into the reproductive tract, stimulated specific antibody in vaginal secretions of cattle. However, this did not become the normal route of vaccination against Brucellosis, because systemic vaccination with living Strain 19 was effective.

Local production of immunoglobulins has been detected in the reproductive tract on the basis of immunoglobulin ratios. Thus Duncan *et al.* (1972) demonstrated median IgG : IgA ratios from 10 heifers of 0.7 in vaginal, 21.9 in cervical and 13.0 in uterine secretions. In the vesicular and urethral fluids of bulls the IgG : IgA ratio was approximately 1.0 (Winter, 1982), suggesting that local synthesis of IgA occurs in the urogenital tract. With this method of assessing local synthesis of immunoglobulin, however, selective transport from serum cannot be excluded.

Experimental local vaccination and challenge with *Campylobacter fetus* of the bovine reproductive tract was carried out by Winter and colleagues. They found the predominant immunoglobulin after antigenic stimulation of the uterus to be IgG_1, but in the vagina there was a transient IgM response which slowly gave way to a long-lasting IgA response.

The persistence of the microorganisms in the reproductive tract, in the presence of specific antibody, is similar to that found with chronic staphylococcal mastitis. In contrast, *C. fetus* does not survive within phagocytes, and the presence of antibodies usually promotes resistance to challenge. The persistence of the *C. fetus* organism does suggest either a deficiency in the intracellular killing by phagocytes in the uterus or an adaptation by the organism so that it is not opsonised. A third possibility is that the IgA antibody is poor at opsonisation but interferes with normal opsonisation by IgG_1. The possibility of T-cell-directed macrophage cellular immunity has yet to be explored.

In general, the diseases of the reproductive tract of cattle have been controlled by systemic vaccination, and direct local vaccination of the reproductive tract has never been considered a practical alternative route for vaccination.

5.7 LOCAL ANTIGENIC STIMULATION OF THE EYE

Again, work on immunity in the eye has mostly been carried out in cattle in connection with vaccination against 'pink-eye' thought to be caused by a variety of microorganisms including *Moraxella bovis*.

Cannulation of the nasolachrymal duct of cattle was carried out by Banyard and Morris (1980), which allowed collection of tears which contained antibodies. An attempt to stimulate antibodies to keyhole limpet haemocyanin (KLH) by incorporation in eye ointment was unsuccessful. However, antibodies were induced in tears by subconjunctival injection of KLH antigen emulsified in Freund's incomplete adjuvant. Antibodies appeared in tears of vaccinated cattle 7 days after injection of antigen, the same time they appeared in serum. Since the titres of antibody in serum were higher than those in tears, there was no real evidence that the antibody in tears had not diffused from serum.

Therefore, systemic vaccination against pink-eye seems likely also to stimulate the appearance of antibodies in tears, and this supports attempts to vaccinate systemically against the disease. However, these attempts, using *Moraxella bovis* vaccine, have been relatively unsuccessful, even though animals which have recovered from infection are refractory to reinfection. Other factors are obviously involved, and sire effects in Hereford cattle have been reported by Pugh and colleagues (1982). Furthermore, Banyard and Morris (1980) found a difference between *Bos taurus* and *Bos indicus* cattle which favoured the *B. indicus* breed, which was more responsive to KLH than *B. taurus* after local immunisation of the eye.

At the moment, there is no effective vaccine against pink-eye, and prospects for local immunisation appear low. It seems more likely that systemic vaccination of cattle which have been bred to be responsive to antigenic stimulation will be the next approach to the problem.

5.8 GENERAL CONCLUSIONS

The stimulation of local immunity is only required when systemic vaccination is inadequate. This applies to the mammary gland, which responds to local infusion of antigen during the non-lactating period. This avoids depression of milk production and provides sustained stimulus to lymphoid cells within the gland. However, the vaccines against *S. aureus* are not yet good enough to provide adequate protection against chronic mastitis, and local vaccination is not used routinely in cattle.

The gastro-intestinal tract in calves and piglets can be stimulated to produce antibodies against pathogens such as *E. coli,* but colostral antibodies are also very effective and vaccination of the dam is more convenient than oral vaccination of newborn animals. The gut can also be used as a route of vaccination against respiratory viruses in chickens, Rabies in foxes and lungworms in cattle.

The respiratory tract and reproductive tract can be locally stimulated to resist bacterial and viral infections, but most vaccines work well with parenteral immunisation, using an adjuvant. There is no convincing evidence of local immunity in the eye.

Therefore, it appears that many apparent opportunities for local immunisation are not taken up because if there is an effective vaccine available, it can often be used parenterally to stimulate specific antibodies which are also protective for external body surfaces.

REFERENCES

Banyard, M. R. C. and Morris, B. (1980). *Aust. J. Exp. Biol. Med. Sci.* **58**, 357–371.
Beh, K. J., Husband, A. J. and Lascelles, A. K. (1979). *Immunology* **37**, 385–388.
Campbell, B., Porter, R. M. and Peterson, W. E. (1950). *Nature (London)* **166**, 913.
Curtain, C. C. and Anderson, N. (1971). *Clin. Exp. Immunol.* **8**, 151–162.
Dixon, F. J., Weigle, W. O. and Vazquez, J. J. (1961). *Lab. Invest.* **10**, 216–237.
Duncan, J. R., Wilkie, B. N., Hiestand, F. and Winter, A. J. (1972). *J. Immunol.* **108**, 965–976.
Gerber, J. D., Marron, A. E. and Kucera, C. J. (1978). *Am. J. Vet. Res.* **39**, 753–760.
Husband, A. J., Beh, K. J. and Lascelles, A. K. (1979). *Immunology* **37**, 597–601.
Kerr, W. R. (1955). *Br. Vet. J.* **111**, 169–178.
Larson, B. L. and Kendall, K. A. (1957). *J. Dairy Sci.* **40**, 659–666.
Lascelles, A. K. and McDowell, G. H. (1974). *Transplant. Rev.* **19**, 170–208.
Newby, T. J., Huntley, J., Evans, P. A. and Bourne, F. J. (1977). *Biochem. Soc. Trans.* **5**, 1574.
Paape, M. J., Wergin, W. P., Guidry, A. J. and Schultz, W. D. (1981). Phagocytic defense of the ruminant mammary gland. *In* 'The Ruminant Immune System' (J. E. Butler, ed.), pp. 555–578. Plenum Press, New York.
Pierce, A. E. (1955), *J. Hyg.* **53**, 247–260.
Porter, P., Kenworthy, R., Holme, D. W. and Horsefield, S. (1973). *Vet. Rec.* **92**, 630–635.
Pugh, G. W., Kopecky, K. E., Kvasnicka, W. G., McDonald, T. J. and Booth, G. D. (1982). *Am. J. Vet. Res.* **43**, 320–325.
Schnorr, K. L. and Pearson, L. D. (1984). *J. Reprod. Immunol.* (in press).
Schore, C. E., Osburn, B. I., Jasper, D. E. and Tyler, D. E. (1981). *Vet. Immunol. Immunpathol.* **2**, 561–569.
Scicchitano, R., Husband, A. J. and Cripps, A. W. (1984). *Immunology* **53**, 121–129.
Watson, D. L. (1980). *Aust. J. Biol. Sci.* **33**, 403–422.
Wilkie, B. N. (1982). *J. Am. Vet. Med. Assoc.* **181**, 1074–1079.
Winter, A. J. (1982). *J. Am. Vet. Med. Assoc.* **181**, 1069–1073.

6

Immunity
to Bacteria

In the veterinary field, the first vaccines developed against bacteria were among the most successful. In particular, the clostridial diseases of sheep and cattle could be effectively controlled by strategic vaccination of lambs and calves. The immunity depended on the production by the animal, of antibodies which neutralised the extracellular toxins produced by the bacteria while other antibodies opsonised the bacteria so that they could be phagocytosed and killed by leucocytes. For example, Pulpy Kidney of sheep caused by *Clostridium welchii* was controlled by antibodies directed towards the necrotising ε toxin as well as the somatic antigens. In horses and other domestic animals, an effective vaccine against Tetanus, another clostridial disease, was produced by including toxoided Tetanus toxin in the vaccine. In this disease, multiplication of *Clostridium tetani* produces tetanic spasms by means of a toxin which travels along nerve trunks to the spinal ganglia. Inactivated toxin, called toxoid, stimulated the appearance of circulating antibodies to the lethal toxin and also produced memory cells which provided virtual life-long immunity to the disease.

Not all bacterial diseases could be controlled by vaccines containing killed bacteria and inactivated toxins. For example, the gram-positive pyogenic staphylococci and streptococci were only partially effective used in killed bacterial vaccines or 'bacterins' against mastitis in cattle. The parenteral administration of these vaccines in cattle prevented the acute forms of the disease, such as gangrenous mastitis, but were ineffective in chronic mastitis. It was thought that the wide variety of staphylococcal strains made it impossible to produce a vaccine which contained all the possible antigens in a balanced formulation. However, possibly another factor was the low levels of antibody in the milk compared with blood, which resulted from the filtration by the mammary gland epithelium of serum proteins before they entered the milk.

The acid-fast organisms such as the *Mycobacteria* and *Nocardia* species presented a different problem. They appeared to be protected from the response of the host by a lipid coat or capsule, and attempts to vaccinate with killed organisms met with little success. This was thought to be due to the difficulty with which the microorganisms were killed even within phagocytic vacuoles inside cells and the ineffectiveness of antibodies in killing the bacteria in cells.

It also came to be appreciated that certain bacteria such as *Escherichia coli* had external structures called pili which enabled them to adhere to epithelial cells lining the mucous membrane of the gut, and once anchored, the bacteria could multiply and produce their pathogenic effects on these cells by release of their extracellular toxins. Another example of an organism with surface pili is *Bacteroides nodosus,* the cause of foot-rot in sheep; vaccines consisting of pilus protein antigen are highly protective against challenge with the same strain of bacteria used to prepare the vaccine (Stewart, 1978; Thorley and Egerton, 1981).

Vaccines against bacteria have therefore been carefully formulated to stimulate antibodies in the host which prevent attachment of the bacteria to mucous membranes, neutralise extracellular toxins and produce memory cells which provide long-term protection.

It is interesting that some diseases which were initially thought to be difficult to vaccinate against, could be controlled by vaccination at a key point in the disease transmission process. Vibriosis caused by *Campylobacter fetus,* is a disease causing infertility and abortion in cows. The problem of parenteral vaccination against the disease, which localised in the uterus, on the face of it appeared to be very difficult. However, vaccination of young bulls with a parenterally-administered vaccine, effectively immunised them against Vibriosis (Clark *et al.,* 1974). This was enough to break the transmission cycle from infected cow, to bull, to non-infected cow; and if combined with a two-herd system (infected and non-infected) was an effective means of controlling the disease. This approach has only been effective with Vibriosis, presumably because the number of pathogenic *C. fetus* strains is two at most, and production of antibodies against these strains protects the animals from a natural challenge infection (Clark *et al.,* 1977). Diseases such as Brucellosis which are mostly transmitted from cow to cow, rather than from cow to bull to cow again, have not been controlled by this method.

In the development of bacterial vaccines for use in cattle it has often been convenient to use a laboratory animal to test the effectiveness of the vaccine without the expense of using cattle. For example, a model system with the laboratory hamster has been used with the development of *Leptospira pomona* and *hardjo* vaccines in cattle. Guinea pigs have been used to test Strain 19 vaccines of *Brucella abortus* for use in cattle. Ultimately these vaccines must be used in cattle and their effectiveness in the field assessed indirectly by such criteria as calving rates, which measure protection against abortion.

Antibody titres may also be measured after administration of the vaccine, and this gives some idea of the immunogenicity of the batch of vaccine. Unfortunately it does not always give a measure of protection for individual animals, since some form of cellular immunity may be involved with diseases such as Leptospirosis or Brucellosis. Therefore the close examination of classes of immunoglobulin containing antibodies to the bacterial vaccine has been of diagnostic value in distinguishing antibodies produced by vaccination from those produced by active infection. However, it has been of little use in predicting the level of protection conferred by the vaccine against challenge with the organism.

6.1   CELLULAR IMMUNITY

One of the intriguing questions in immunity to bacteria has been the nature of the cellular resistance to microorganisms which survive within phagocytic cells. As mentioned in Chapter 2, facultative intracellular bacterial pathogens are often not accessible to circulating antibodies which may not even be present until the disease is established. Even prior vaccination with killed vaccines may not be effective in preventing establishment of the disease. In the case of Brucellosis of cattle, it was once thought that a living attenuated vaccine (Strain 19) was necessary to stimulate macrophage cellular immunity and provide effective protection against natural infection. However, with the demonstration that 45/20 strain organisms in oily adjuvant would protect cattle, the requirement for living vaccines became much less definite. This was also found with other vaccines against, for example, *Corynebacterium pseudotuberculosis* infection of sheep, in which a killed vaccine in oil adjuvant is now used (Burrell, 1978).

The concept of antigenic mass was also, at one stage, thought to be important with living attenuated vaccines, because it was thought that slow multiplication of bacteria within the host tissues eventually overcame the antigenic threshold of the cellular immune system and stimulated immunity. In addition, it was thought to provide a continuing stimulus for immunity which persisted for a longer time than with killed vaccines. To some extent, this may still be true with Strain 19 compared with killed 45/20 vaccine, since the latter requires at least two injections, with boosters at yearly intervals, while immunity from one injection of Strain 19 lasts several years.

Therefore, the experience with *Brucella* vaccines in cattle is that, attenuated vaccines are better than killed vaccines, which must be administered more often than living vaccines to obtain an effective level of protection. Balanced against this is the inherent danger to veterinarians of Strain 19, which produces a severe infection in vaccinators who are accidently infected.

Another facultative intracellular parasite is *Listeria monocytogenes,* which causes infertility and central nervous system (CNS) lesions in sheep. In the experimental work carried out in sheep, there is no evidence for protection with killed vaccines. Living attenuated bacteria or virulent bacteria administered by subcutaneous injection, appear to be necessary to protect sheep against infection (Njoku-Obi and Osebold, 1962). Certainly, intensive work with laboratory animals has failed to produce killed vaccines which protect against challenge infection with virulent organisms. In fact, Listeriosis has been used as one of the classical models for macrophage cellular immunity in immunological research. This work in mice has shown that immunity to *L. monocytogenes* infection can be adoptively transferred between inbred animals by lymphocytes. Furthermore, the active cells are the T-cells. The T-cells themselves are divisible into subpopulations as described in Chapter 2 on cellular immunology. A particular subpopulation produces delayed hypersensitivity (Tdh) when transferred from one inbred mouse to another, but it is not yet certain if this subpopulation is the one which transfers cellular immunity to *Listeria* infection. Certainly this subpopulation is a very good candidate for this function, since delayed hypersensitivity results in the production of lymphokines, among which are some which cause activation of macrophages and consequently more effective intracellular killing of bacteria. There is no comparable work in the sheep with which the work in the mouse may be compared because of the difficulty in carrying out lymphocyte transfer studies in outbred animals.

6.2 DELAYED HYPERSENSITIVITY

The phenomenon of delayed hypersensitivity is known to be the result of sensitisation of a population of lymphocytes which produce lymphokines rather than antibodies. This is because in diseases such as tuberculosis, the T-cells are stimulated in preference to the B-cells and the lymphokines produced in response to antigen cause increased permeability and inflammation at the site of deposition of the antigen.

The classical form of delayed hypersensitivity is the skin test for tuberculosis in cattle. In this test, a small amount of culture filtrate from heat-killed mycobacteria, termed 'tuberculin', is injected intradermally into the skin of the neck or into the caudal fold of the tail. Four days later, the skin injection sites are examined, and tuberculous cattle are found to have a swelling while the uninfected cattle do not.

The blood lymphocytes from infected cattle can also be induced to transform *in vitro* by addition of tuberculin to the medium, and the degree of lymphocyte reactivity can be measured by the incorporation of radioactive [^{3}H]thymidine into the lymphocyte deoxyribonucleic acid (DNA) (see Appendix).

This lymphocyte transformation test has been used extensively with cattle lymphocytes in research work on tuberculosis, Johne's disease and Brucellosis of cattle. The *in vitro* test corresponds well with the degree of delayed hypersensitivity in skin to intradermal injection with specific antigen (tuberculin, Johnin, Brucallergen) but not at all with resistance to experimental infection.

These results support the original findings in laboratory animals, that delayed hypersensitivity and macrophage cellular immunity could co-exist in the vaccinated animal but that they could also occur separately. Thus not all mice which exhibited delayed hypersensitivity to *Listeria* were resistant to challenge, and not all mice negative in the skin test, were susceptible to challenge (Osebold *et al.*, 1974).

Since no direct correlation between major histocompatibility complex (MHC) antigen type and resistance of mice to *Listeria* has been found (Cheers and Sandrin, 1983), it must be assumed that some other property of the immune cells is involved in resistance. Certainly it is possible that lack of delayed hypersensitivity in skin tests merely reflects an absence of antigen-reactive T-cells in the blood resulting from retention of the cells in the lymph nodes and spleen. Again, the idea of suppressor cells which control delayed hypersensitivity, can be put forward as a reason for negative skin tests. However, if Tdh lymphocytes are sequestered in central lymphoid tissue, or if they are actively suppressed by the suppressor cells, one would expect that animals would be very susceptible to challenge infection. This is not the case, and it is generally assumed that the macrophages of resistant animals are either normally more active than in susceptible animals or that they have become active as a result of a previous challenge which vaccinated the animal (e.g., *Brucella* Strain 19 in cattle).

It is not known if the bacteria themselves can slowly multiply in tissues and directly activate the surrounding macrophages. Certainly, examination of histological sections of tissue reaction around diffusion chambers, containing *Listeria,* which are implanted in the peritoneal cavity of mice, suggest that macrophages are actively involved in responding to soluble products released from bacteria contained within the chamber (Osebold and Dicapua, 1968). However, although these mice are well-protected against challenge infection, the best-possible immunity arises from direct injection of living bacteria subcutaneously, where there is direct interaction between macrophages and multiplying bacterial cells.

Experimental work in sheep (Njoku-Obi and Osebold, 1962) with vaccination against virulent *Listeria monocytogenes* strongly suggests that the route of vaccination has a strong influence on immunisation. A small dose of virulent bacteria, injected subcutaneously, provides long-term protection against intravenous challenge with a normally-lethal dose of virulent bacteria. In this case, it appears that a combination of circulating antibodies and activated macrophages in the spleen and liver is able to clear rapidly and to kill circulating bacteria.

6.3 THE ACTIVATED MACROPHAGE

Macrophages from sheep which are immune to challenge with *Listeria* have been examined with *in vitro* culture techniques. In this work, peritoneal macrophages were obtained from sheep and transferred to tissue culture containing immune serum or normal serum (Fig. 6.1). Virulent *Listeria* organisms were added at three concentrations, which were in a ratio of 5:1, 20:1 and 40:1 organisms per macrophage. Statistically-significant differences between immune macrophages and normal macrophages were found, particularly in the presence

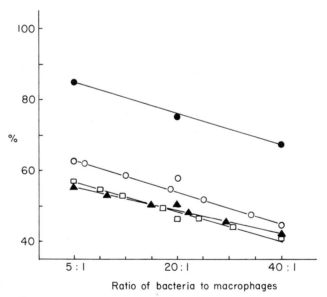

Ratio of bacteria to macrophages

Fig. 6.1. The figure shows the average percentage of sheep peritoneal exudate macrophages surviving *in vitro* at three levels of challenge with *Listeria monocytogenes* organisms at ratios of 5:1, 20:1 and 40:1 bacteria per macrophage. The greater the number of bacteria, the smaller the number of macrophages which have survived after 2 hours of incubation. The immune macrophages and immune serum combination (●——●) show the greatest resistance to the necrotic effects of the *Listeria* compared with the other three systems tested: ○——○, immune cells plus normal serum; ▲——▲, normal cells plus immune serum; □——□, normal cells plus normal serum. (Reproduced by permission from Njoku-Obi and Osebold (1962), *J. Immunol.* **89**, 187–194.)

of immune serum. These results provided strong evidence that in sheep, the peritoneal macrophages behaved the same as in small laboratory animals and became capable of greater intracellular killing of *Listeria* than macrophages from non-immunised control sheep.

The basis for this increased intracellular killing was closely examined, both in sheep and in the experimental mouse. It was assumed that the physical appearance of the activated macrophages reflected their ability to kill bacteria. Indeed, macrophages from immunised animals were larger than controls and contained more lysosomes than controls. The lysosomes were thought to be vital because they fused with phagocytic vacuoles containing *Listeria* and released enzymes which controlled growth of *Listeria* inside the cells.

The problem with this hypothesis was that most of the enzymes in macrophage lysosomes, such as lysozyme, were found to be totally ineffective in killing *Listeria* even at the lower pH found in the phagocytic vacuoles. *Listeria* organisms grew quite normally in enzyme combinations which were highly effective in controlling the growth of gram-negative organisms such as *Escherichia coli* (Outteridge *et al.*, 1972). Conversely, neutrophils contain cationic proteins which are effective in controlling growth of *Listeria,* particularly at pH 4, but macrophages contain no such cationic proteins, except those acquired by phagocytosis of degenerating neutrophils. Close examination of immune macrophages from sheep failed to demonstrate elevated levels of bactericidal substances in peritoneal macrophages and those obtained from the non-lactating mammary glands of sheep. Lung macrophages were inhibitory to the growth of *Listeria,* but this seemed not to be associated with active immunisation. Rather it appeared that nuclear histones from degenerating cells could have been taken up into lung macrophage lysosomes, and these highly charged molecules were responsible for inhibition of the growth of *Listeria in vitro.*

The present state of knowledge on the question of intracellular killing by macrophages is still inconclusive. Immunity to *Listeria* in mice can be transferred by T-cells. These T-cells have been shown to produce lymphokines, and these in turn have been shown to activate macrophages *in vitro.* The increased killing of facultative intracellular parasites has been attributed to halide ions in the presence of superoxide, an oxidising agent produced within the lysosomes for an extremely-brief period during phagocytosis of the organisms. It has also been attributed to fatty acids present in the plasma membranes of macrophages and in the lysosomal membranes too. However, the problem still remains, of how immune macrophages inhibit intracellular organisms over the long period of time required with these slow-growing, resistant microorganisms. Again it is possible that direct stimulation with intracellular phagocytosed bacteria provides an extra stimulus for production of inhibitors of bacterial growth.

The assay system of macrophages cultured *in vitro* with bacteria still appears to be the only real way to measure cellular immunity. Various combinations of immune cells and immune or normal serum can be used to test for immunity. This approach has also been used with *Toxoplasma gondii* to assess immunity in mice. In larger animals, the serial sampling of macrophages from the mammary gland of the ewe or cow offers one way of monitoring the response, at least in females.

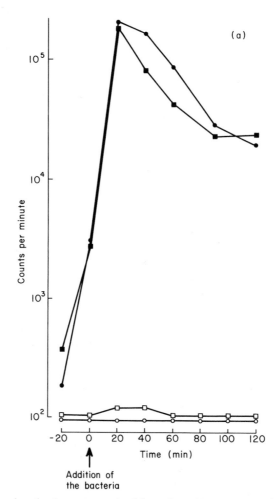

Fig. 6.2.   The chemiluminescence emitted from sheep (a) mammary polymorphs and (b) mammary macrophages during phagocytosis of killed, opsonised *Salmonella typhimurium* organisms. The assay was carried out using Luminol to enhance the chemiluminescence, which is shown in the graph as counts per minute against time in minutes after addition of the bacteria (↑). Two samples of polymorphs and macrophages are shown (■——■, ●——●) together with control cells with added bacteria but no Luminol (□——□, ○——○). (Reproduced by permission from 'The Ruminant Immune System', 1981, Plenum Press.)

6.4 CHEMILUMINESCENCE

The amount of superoxide released during phagocytosis of bacteria was discovered to be measurable by counting minute flashes of light from the cells in a scintillation counter. There are two ways of doing this: the first involves using the scintillation counter in the out-of-coincidence mode and keeping the vials in red light. The other method involves an amplification of the chemiluminescence using 'Luminol' as first described by Allen and Loose (1976).

The second method using Luminol is more convenient than the first, and the scintillation counter may be used in the normal coincidence mode with a wide window set for counting tritium. Both polymorphs and macrophages produce chemiluminescence during phagocytosis, but the polymorphs produce about 10 times as much chemiluminescence as the macrophages. An example of chemiluminescence responses during phagocytosis of bacteria by polymorph or macrophage suspensions from the sheep mammary gland is shown in Fig. 6.2.

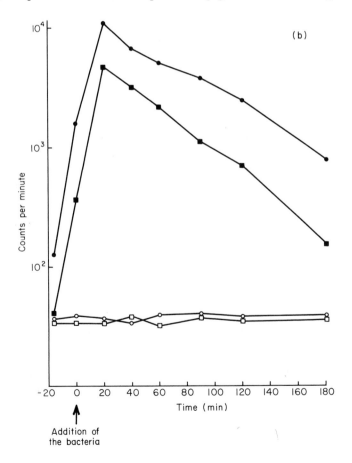

The method appears to measure the degree of phagocytic response by the cells, since different batches of opsonising serum used with the same bacteria produce varying levels of chemiluminescence in the same batch of phagocytes. If the opsonising serum is held constant, phagocytes from different individuals can be assessed for their phagocytic index. The method has been used in humans to assess individuals suspected of having lysosomal abnormalities in their poly-morphs. It has not proved useful for assessing the general level of macrophage cellular immunity in humans and has yet to be closely examined for this purpose in domestic animals. In mice, activated peritoneal macrophages have been shown to have increased chemiluminescence compared with normal control cells. The stumbling block with circulating monocytes is the difficulty in purify-ing them in sufficient numbers, uncontaminated with polymorphs, to allow them to be assessed for chemiluminescence. The consensus opinion appears to be that the method does not really measure cellular immunity to specific bacterial infec-tions but reflects the phagocytic index of cells obtained from individuals. As mentioned earlier, it appears that only the *in vitro* survival of bacteria within phagocytes is a possible correlate with cellular immunity to bacteria.

6.5 ANTIBODIES AND CELLS IN PARTICULAR DISEASES

6.5.1 Bovine Tuberculosis

The mechanism of immunity in tuberculosis has been the subject of research and considerable speculation. A vaccine for use in humans was developed from an attenuated bovine strain, Bacillus Calmette–Guérin (BCG). This was found to reduce the incidence of tuberculosis in human populations at risk, but it was not effective in populations with a very low incidence of tuberculosis resulting from an active public health campaign. In other words, the BCG was only a partially-effective vaccine.

It is interesting that BCG was developed from a bovine strain of mycobacteria, which points to the close similarity between *Mycobacterium tuberculosis* var. *hominis* and *Mycobacterium bovis*. The BCG vaccine has been used in cattle and found to be only partially effective in preventing infection with virulent strains. For this reason, BCG has not been used in eradication compaigns in cattle. The reason for the failure of this living attenuated vaccine to prevent tuberculosis, is unclear. It has been assumed that tubercle bacilli grow so slowly, that they are not susceptible to attack with short-term inhibitory substances such as lysozyme and superoxide. The organisms also possess a waxy coat which makes them resistant even to the effects of chemical disinfectants, although alcohol-based or phenol disinfectants eventually kill them. Therefore, the emphasis has always been on diagnosis and slaughter of infected cattle, rather than vaccination. It is fortunate that these organisms are particularly good at stimulating delayed-type hypersensitivity (DTH). As mentioned previously, this delayed hypersensitivity does not correlate with immunity, since mouse experiments have shown a divergence between DTH and immunity to experimental challenge with virulent organisms in BCG-immunised mice.

6.5.1.1 Delayed Hypersensitivity to Tuberculin

The property of tubercle bacilli to induce T-cell responses rather than B-cell responses results in delayed hypersensitivity to tuberculin. Antibodies to other components of tubercle bacilli do occur, but their occurrence in infected animals has proved to be too unreliable for them to be used in a diagnostic test. It is interesting that the intradermal injection of tuberculin is followed by the appearance of antibodies in infected herds of cattle, which were previously negative for serum antibodies. The longer-established the lesions, the higher the antibody titre, in this case, to mycobacterial polysaccharide which develops after tuberculin skin testing. However, it is the delayed tuberculin skin test which has been found to be the most effective test for tuberculosis in cattle, and this is the test used in the major eradication compaigns around the world. The ability of the tubercle bacillus to induce T-cell responses has been utilized in Freund's complete adjuvant, in which killed tubercle bacilli are incorporated in mineral oil. With this adjuvant, recipients of vaccinating antigens are stimulated to produce high titres of antibody and at the same time, delayed-hypersensitivity responses to the antigen are also often manifested. Freund's complete adjuvant is not used in cattle vaccines because of the danger of causing false-positive skin tests to tuberculin. Therefore, the 45/20 Brucellosis vaccine uses incomplete Freund's adjuvant added to killed *Brucella abortus* organisms.

6.5.1.2 Muramyl Dipeptide

The active principle of Freund's complete adjuvant has been examined by chemical analysis of the mycobacterial cell wall. It was shown that wax D could effectively replace whole mycobacteria in the adjuvant, and since then, the component causing enhanced stimulation of the immune response has been found. A water-soluble extract containing a portion of arabinogalactan linked to peptidoglycan was found, and it became clear that the key molecule was the peptidoglycan fragment *N*-acetylmuramyl-L-alanyl-D-isoglutamyl-*meso*-di-aminopimelic acid (Fig. 6.3). A synthetic molecule was produced, *N*-acetyl-muramyl-L-alanyl-D-isoglutamine, and this was known by the shorter name of muramyl dipeptide (MDP).

The synthetic adjuvant has been tested extensively in mice and found to enhance both antibody titres and delayed hypersensitivity to a wide range of antigens and bacterial vaccines. Because of its costliness, it has not been used in

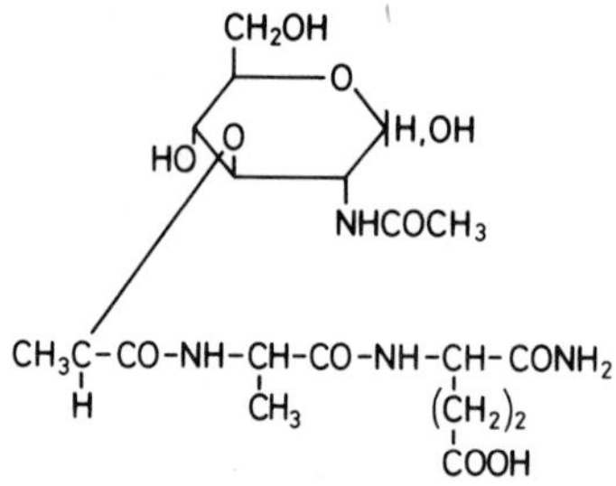

CH₂OH

    CH2OH
         |——O
   HO O   H,OH
              NHCOCH3

CH3C-CO-NH-CH-CO-NH-CH-CONH2
   | | |
   H   CH3   (CH2)2
                          |
                         COOH

Fig. 6.3. The formula for the adjuvant N-acetylmuramyl-L-alanyl-D-isoglutamine, or muramyl dipeptide (MDP), is shown. This molecule was synthesised after studies on mycobacterial cell walls isolated similar molecules with adjuvant activity.

domestic animals, except in isolated experiments. If it could be produced cheaply, the MDP molecule has the potential of enhancing immune responses in domestic animals without resort to the mineral oil so often used in adjuvants. However, it has yet to be seriously contemplated as an adjuvant in domestic animals because of its high cost.

6.5.1.3 Skin Reactions to Tuberculin

The measurement of delayed hypersensitivity can be accurately carried out using skin calipers. In this test, the tuberculin can be injected on the neck, a site shown to be the most sensitive of all sites in cattle. The double-skin thickness is measured at intervals after intradermal injection of tuberculin and compared with the pre-injection skin thickness. It is also possible to measure infra-red radiation emitted from the skin injection site during the course of the tuberculin skin reaction. This has been used as a research tool in investigations of tuberculin skin testing in cattle (Lepper et al., 1974) (Fig. 6.4). The time of appearance and the peak skin thickness are important measurements in the comparative tuberculin skin test used, for example, in the United Kingdom. In this, avian tuberculin is injected beside bovine or human strain tuberculin on the neck of the cow, and the reaction is measured at intervals afterwards. The cattle infected with atypical mycobacteria or the avian strain of *Mycobacterium tuberculosis,* usually swell much more rapidly at the avian tuberculin site than the mammalian tuberculin site. This is a sign for the veterinarian to look for superficial lesions caused by the atypical mycobacteria or *Mycobacterium avium,* which if found, classifies the infected animal in a separate category from the cattle with bovine tuberculosis, which are sent for slaughter.

In areas of the world where cattle are run under extensive grazing management, such as Australia or the Americas, the tuberculin skin test on the neck has proved to be impractical. Instead, cattle are injected in the fold of skin (caudal fold) where the tail joins the base of the spine. The injection of tuberculin into sensitised, infected cattle causes a swelling which can be palpated by the veteri-

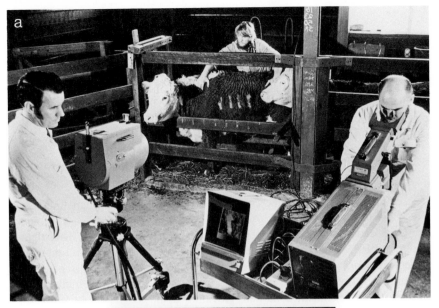

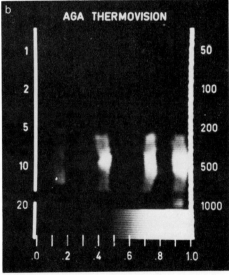

Fig. 6.4. (a) The emission of infra-red radiation from skin test sites is being measured in a cow reacting to tuberculin purified protein derivative (PPD) 24 hours after inoculation. The emission can be detected by a remote-sensing, image-forming device (Aga, Thermovision), which is able to detect minor differences between inflammatory sites and the surrounding skin which differ by as little as 2°C. (b) The Polaroid picture shows four sites: the extreme left site was not inoculated, but the next three sites from left to right received 0.5, 1.0 and 2.0 mg of tuberculin PPD, respectively. The progressive increase in reaction to the doses is reflected in the emission of infra-red radiation at the sites of inoculation. (Reproduced by kind permission of Dr. A. W. D. Lepper and the CSIRO, Division of Animal Health, Parkville, Victoria, Australia.)

narian from the side of the cattle race, by running his hand along the tail to its base.

Both methods of tuberculin injection have been used effectively in campaigns for eradication of tuberculosis. However, certain pitfalls in skin testing must be appreciated. The possibility of false-negative reactions in anergic cattle is one problem, and the possibility of false-positive reactions in non-specifically-sensitised cattle is another.

6.5.1.4 Sensitivity and Specificity of the Tuberculin Skin Test

A comparison between tuberculin skin testing and postmortem findings in cattle, has led to a simple division between sensitivity and specificity, a concept originally enunciated by Cochrane and Holland (1971) (Table 6.1). This method has been used, for example, to compare human- with bovine-strain tuberculin under trial conditions in the Northern Territory of Australia. It is also possible to determine the optimum dose for skin testing, as well as the type of tuberculin to be used under the climatic conditions prevailing at the geographical site of testing of the cattle. It should be emphasised that the results obtained in the cooler regions of Australia differed from those obtained in the hot northern regions (Lepper *et al.*, 1979). Factors affecting the test were the higher incidence of tuberculosis in the North and the much greater non-specific sensitivity due to saprophytic soil mycobacteria infecting northern cattle, compared with cattle from the cooler southern climate.

This apparent difference between tuberculin testing in different climates would most likely prevail in other parts of the world, and it would appear that local testing for fixing of the tuberculin test method, should be carried out.

In general, however, the tuberculin test with slaughter of reactors is very useful in reducing the incidence of tuberculosis to very low levels. At that stage of the eradication campaign, the cross-reactive *Mycobacterium avium, paratuberculosis smegmatis,* and so on, have to be distinguished as possible sources

TABLE 6.1

Formulae for Determining Sensitivity and Specificity of the Tuberculin Skin Test

Test result	Diseased	Not diseased	Total
Positive (*a*)	True positive (*b*)	False positive	*a* + *b*
Negative (*c*)	False positive (*d*)	True negative	*c* + *d*

$$\% \text{ Sensitivity} = \frac{a}{a + c} \times 100 \qquad \% \text{ Specificity} = \frac{d}{b + d} \times 100$$

of non-specific sensitisation. The use of specific tuberculins to distinguish these relatively non-pathogenic mycobacteria in cattle, is one direction that research may take in the future.

6.5.2 Bovine Brucellosis

The immunity against *Brucella abortus* is different from that of bovine tuberculosis, in that immunity to *Brucella* can be quite protective and last for several years. Brucellosis appears to occupy an intermediate position in the spectrum between cellular and humoral immunity. Antibodies are necessary for opsonisation of the bacteria, but macrophage intracellular killing is also required. Because of its fast growth, relative to the tubercle bacillus, antibodies are important in the clearance of *Brucella* organisms from the circulation. In humans, fluctuations in levels of bacteria in the blood, with antibodies rising and falling lead to undulant fever, especially in *Brucella melitensis* infection, and this can also be a particularly unpleasant symptom of accidental inoculation of veterinarians with Strain 19. Unfortunately, Strain 19 immunises only cattle and laboratory animals such as guinea pigs, but it causes the disease in humans. The advent of a killed vaccine (45/20) has substantially reduced the risk to veterinarians that Strain 19 vaccination presented. However, direct infection from wild strains of *Brucella abortus* is still possible. Again, vaccination of humans with 45/20 killed vaccine does not seem to be a solution, since it is not known if the immediate hypersensitivity produced, would be harmful or protective.

Comparisons between Strain 19 and 45/20 have been extensively studied in trials around the world. The conclusions are that Strain 19 is the yardstick against which killed vaccines are measured; Strain 19 requires only one inoculation to produce immunity for the lifetime of the cow. The killed 45/20 vaccine requires two doses for effective immunity, and booster doses are recommended each year.

The philosophy of current Brucellosis eradication campaigns is to reduce the incidence of Brucellosis to low levels by vaccination and then switch to test-and-slaughter for the final eradication phase. This approach has worked in countries with small, well-defined cattle areas (e.g., Denmark) or in islands such as New Zealand and Tasmania, but it has not worked very well in large countries such as the United States, Canada and Australia. Nor has it worked in areas of the world where effective animal management is difficult.

The problems appear to be twofold. Firstly, the vaccination does not produce 100% protection against natural infection. Protection is more like 80% in carefully-controlled trials on experimental farms. Secondly, vaccination produces antibodies which can be confused with those produced by infection with wild strains of *Brucella abortus*.

6.5.2.1 Antibody Tests for Brucellosis

Historically, the first test used in the diagnosis of Brucellosis was the simple agglutination test (SAT). This test detects a lipopolysaccharide antigen on the surface of phenol-killed *Brucella abortus* organisms. Efforts to improve this test have been directed towards purifying the lipopolysaccharide antigen and increasing the sensitivity of the test system. Sensitivity of the SAT does appear to be quite adequate for most diagnoses, but it has been the subject of considerable debate (Plackett and Alton, 1975) on where to draw the lower-titre limit for positive reactions (Table 6.2). The use of the complement fixation test (CFT) with *Brucella* lipopolysaccharide antigen increased sensitivity, but again, the lower limit for positive reactions had to be set. There was also the 'prozone' phenomenon, in which IgG_2 antibodies fixing complement only weakly themselves, interfered with the specific IgG_1 antibodies which fix complement strongly. The result was a false-negative test (Plackett and Alton, 1975).

The CFT was developed further by Plackett *et al.* (1976) into the indirect haemolysin test (IHLT). This test utilises guinea pig complement and the bovine antibodies to *Brucella* in the test serum, mixed with bovine red blood cells coated with lipopolysaccharide antigen. It suffers fewer 'prozone' reactions than the CFT, but its main contribution to the diagnostic problem is that it can help distinguish the antibodies produced by natural infection from those produced by vaccination with 45/20 vaccine. Extensive trials have shown that IHLT titres decline within 2 to 4 weeks after 45/20 vaccine inoculation, whereas the SAT can remain positive for at least 2 months after vaccine inoculation (Plackett *et al.*, 1980).

However, the most promising test developed so far is the enzyme-linked immunosorbent assay (ELISA). This test can be read with great accuracy using automatic photometry in microdilution trays (Fig. 6.5). Furthermore, acid treat-

TABLE 6.2

Relative Sensitivities of Tests Used in Diagnosing Brucellosis[a]

	Protein concentration (μg/ml)		
Serological test	IgG_1	IgG_2	IgM
Complement fixation test	10	—	5
Simple agglutination test	100	100	10
Rose–Bengal plate test	50	50	5

[a] From Allan *et al.* (1976), A quantitative comparison of the sensitivity of serological tests for bovine brucellosis to different antibody classes. *J. Hyg.* Cambridge Univ. Press.

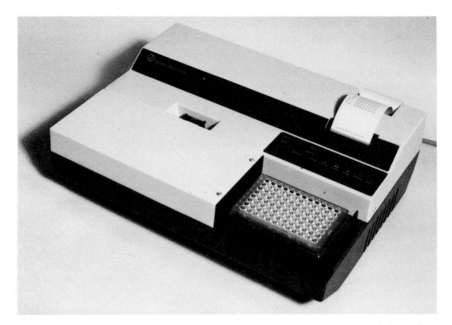

Fig. 6.5. The photograph shows a microdilution plate reader (Titertek Multiskan, Flow Laboratories, McLean, Virginia) which can automatically read the colour developed in the enzyme-linked immunosorbent assay (ELISA) carried out in these plates.

ment of the *Brucella* antigen improves its ability to detect positive reactions and at the same time reduces the number of false-negative results. The advantages of automatic reading, sensitivity and definition of the *Brucella* antigen, make this an attractive test for eradication campaigns for Brucellosis.

Finally there is a skin test for Brucellosis which utilises the delayed-hypersensitivity response to Brucallergen. This test is the same as the tuberculin skin test for tuberculosis, but care must be taken in obtaining a purified *Brucella* protein antigen for testing. This is because traces of lipopolysaccharide, which are unimportant in the tuberculin skin test, are very important to exclude from the Brucallergen skin test. The lipopolysaccharide from *Brucella abortus* induces a rapid Type III skin response, which appears at 6 hours and reaches a peak at 12 hours after injection into the skin. This is so in the Brucallergen skin test, because of the high titres of circulating antibodies to lipopolysaccharide, which are not found in comparable titres against the tuberculin polysaccharide. The Type III skin reaction masks the normal development of delayed hypersensitivity and can even lead to central necrosis at the skin injection site, due to the severity of the inflammatory response to the lipopolysaccharide antigen.

The skin test offers some advantages, in that the use of a laboratory is not necessary and the animal in the field can be classified as infected or uninfected without taking a blood sample. It is only used in parts of eastern Europe and Russia, and has not been adopted in western countries. The realisation that highly-purified protein antigen is necessary to obtain delayed hypersensitivity, without immediate hypersensitivity, makes this test attractive for further research as a field test in cattle, where laboratory facilities are not readily available.

6.5.2.2 Other Immune Phenomena in the Diagnosis of *Brucella abortus* Infection

Although Strain 19 vaccination is an effective method of immunising cattle against *Brucella abortus,* it causes difficulties with the diagnostic tests. This is because Strain 19 inoculation at a standard dose causes antibodies to persist long enough to interfere with the Rose–Bengal and complement fixation tests—the tests commonly used to diagnose the disease. The Rose–Bengal test is an adaptation of the simple agglutination test in which killed *Brucella* organisms are stained with Rose–Bengal stain, and used in a slide agglutination test, by mixing a drop of stained antigen with a drop of test serum. It has the advantage of being applicable in the field, without elaborate laboratory facilities (Alton and Jones, 1967).

Vaccination with Strain 19 causes antibodies to appear in the blood, which produce false indications of active infection. Even passively-acquired colostral antibody may transmit antibodies from heifers to calves, but this is not a general phenomenon, since serum titres are usually low by the time a heifer has her first calf.

The 45/20 killed vaccine, however, is often administered to adult cattle in extensive grazing areas where cattle are not easily mustered, and veterinarians prefer to vaccinate stock of all ages with the killed vaccine. In this case, passively-acquired colostral antibodies could well produce positive titres in calves which had not yet been vaccinated, and the time of last vaccination of the herd with 45/20 vaccine should be kept in mind during diagnostic procedures.

Two ways around the problem of persistent antibody titres have been explored. The first is to reduce the dose of Strain 19 vaccine and so, the time period which antibodies persist in serum. In this case the low dose is administered to adult cattle, since persisting passively-acquired antibodies in calves appear to interfere with the vaccine in the low dose. The low dose has been found to be as protective as higher doses but, of course, has the possible disadvantage of increasing abortion in pregnant cows. A compromise of low-dose vaccination of year-old non-pregnant heifers has been found to protect the cattle better than calfhood vaccination with the full dose of Strain 19 vaccine, but not as well as adult cattle vaccinated with the lower dose.

The other approach is to use the IHLT test as described earlier. This has proved to be the more practical of the two approaches, since it allows more accurate diagnosis than other tests, in the face of existing methods of vaccination of cattle with the full dose of Strain 19 and 45/20 killed vaccines.

It is interesting that killed 45/20 vaccine has been used experimentally to stimulate the appearance of antibodies in cattle, in herds known to have infection. This is done by vaccinating the herd with 45/20 vaccine and 2 weeks later, obtaining blood samples for testing in the laboratory. This procedure relies on the secondary immune response in *Brucella*-infected cattle producing titres, which are much higher than those in cattle developing antibodies in a primary immune response to the vaccine. This procedure has the advantage of stimulating antibodies in cattle which may otherwise show false-negative results, due to their being in the inactive phase of the disease. It has, as yet, to be fully evaluated as a reliable diagnostic procedure.

6.5.2.3   Limits to Accuracy of Diagnosis of Brucellosis

As with all diagnostic procedures, there are limits to the accuracy of antibody tests for Brucellosis which leave a residue of uncertainty about the status of negative cattle. Re-testing at close intervals or the stimulation of cattle showing falsely-negative results by 45/20 vaccination, then testing, are ways of reducing errors in diagnosis.

Past experience would indicate that, although the incidence of Brucellosis may be reduced to extremely low levels, constant vigilance and continuing high levels of testing are required in the latter stages of an eradication campaign. This is because of limits in accuracy of both diagnosis and the effectiveness of vaccination. A policy of no vaccination, with test and slaughter of reactors, has the disadvantage of producing herds which are highly susceptible to chance introduction of Brucellosis. The policy of strict quarantine between Brucellosis-free and suspect herds must be enforced, otherwise the eradication campaign will be jeopardised.

However, with the variety of tests now available (i.e., the SAT, CFT, IHLT, ELISA), sporadic positive-reactive sera in attested Brucellosis-free areas can be thoroughly examined to determine if the positive animals are, in reality, only cross-reacting to some other antigen related to *Brucella*. This does require the retention of specialists, whose skill in testing allows rapid checking of positive sera for several years after the disease has apparently been eradicated. Eventually however, the herds can be declared free of Brucellosis and further controlled by quarantine of cattle introduced from outside the country.

6.6   ANTIGENS IN IMMUNITY TO BACTERIAL INFECTIONS

Much of the present-day research into bacterial diseases of animals is directed towards purifying antigens for diagnostic tests or for immunisation of animals.

Many of the diseases are residual problems which have been recalcitrant to conventional approaches in diagnosis or vaccination. Considerable expertise has been developed in veterinary laboratories in diagnosis, not all of which has been published. Some examples of the problems which arise in vaccination against bacterial diseases are discussed next, as well as some of the methods devised for circumventing these problems.

6.6.1 *Staphylococcus aureus*

From a scientific point of view, *Staphylococcus aureus* presents a wide variety of challenges to vaccination of animals. It is a major cause of mastitis in cattle, goats and sheep, and there have been many attempts to vaccinate animals against the disease.

There are many strains of *S. aureus,* and these have been mostly classified using phage typing. However, phage types do not necessarily correspond to antigenic types measured by serological means, and there remains a need to classify the strains according to their surface antigens.

This is complicated by the occurrence, on some strains (e.g., Smith strain), of a loosely-bound antigen called protein A. This has the property of binding to the Fc fragment of IgG from many species (Table 6.3). However, this non-specific binding interferes with normal serological typing procedures, and bacteria must be carefully washed or partially digested with proteases to expose the other surface antigens which characterise the strain.

TABLE 6.3

Protein A Reactivity of Immunoglobulins from Various Species

Species	Immunoglobulin subclass bound	% Bound
Horse[a]	IgG	67
	IgM	16
	IgG (T)	20
Dog[a]	IgG	47
	IgM	36
	IgA	40
Pig[b]	IgG	94
	IgM	35
	IgA	23
Sheep[a]	IgG_1	2
	IgG_2	33
Cow[a]	IgG_1	26
	IgG_2	53

[a] Goudswaard et al. (1978).
[b] Bennell and Watson (1980).

The teichoic acids, incorporated in the wall of staphylococci, have been found to be important, both in typing and immunisation. These are linked to peptidoglycans, which form part of the structure of the bacterial cell wall and are also found in other families of bacteria such as streptococci and lactobacilli, and play an important role in serological classification of bacteria. Vaccines are known to require the presence of these antigens, which stimulate antibodies that opsonise the bacteria for phagocytosis. However, again the question of the large number of strains of staphylococci must be considered. It is difficult to include these antigens in sufficient variety in vaccines to cover every contingency. The antigens are usually included as killed organisms, and the formulation of a complete vaccine may require the inclusion of scores of strains of staphylococci. No doubt cross-reactions do exist, but there is no common antigen for all strains, against which the host can produce antibodies which opsonise all strains. Therefore, it is highly likely that antigenic competition will occur and antibodies to some important strains will not be produced in the high titre necessary for protection.

The extracellular toxins of staphylococci are a way by which the organisms increase their pathogenicity (Arbuthnott, 1970; Wiseman, 1970). These toxins are listed in Table 6.4 together with their main pathogenic effects and molecular weights. Some of these toxins have varying effects on different species. For example, leucocidin does not appear to have the same cytotoxic effects on ruminant leucocytes, that it has on human leucocytes. These toxins are often purified from culture filtrates, toxoided and added back to vaccines to bring their content up to an effective level. This is because some strains of staphylococci do not produce very much extracellular toxin *in vitro* during culture.

At one stage, it was thought that the division of staphylococci into those which

TABLE 6.4

Staphylococcal Exotoxins

Toxin	Molecular weight	Biological effects
α-Haemolysin	44,000	Dermonecrotic, leucocidal, lethal
β-Haemolysin	59,000	Not known except as haemolysin
δ-Haemolysin	68,000	Dermonecrotic, leucocidal
Leucocidin		
S	38,000	Leucocidal for human and rabbits but not ruminants
F	32,000	
Enterotoxin		
A	37,700	Enteritis, gastritis
B	35,300	Enteritis, gastritis
C	—	Enteritis, gastritis

produce coagulase and those which do not, provided a broad division of staphylococci into pathogenic and non-pathogenic strains. It is now realised that such a division is not reliable, because much of the work was based on culture of staphylococci *in vitro,* in which many toxins are not produced in the quantities that they are found *in vivo.* Experiments with diffusion chambers and semipermeable sacs have revealed with staphylococci and other species of bacteria, a wide variation between expression of antigens and toxins *in vitro* and those found *in vivo.* However, the practical advantages of killed staphylococcal vaccines of storage and safety, have caused a continuing effort to be mounted to formulate killed vaccines. Much work still needs to be done on staphylococcal vaccines, since the occurrence of antibiotic-resistant strains of bacteria is still a problem with treatment of bovine mastitis. The use of local immunisation with staphylococcal vaccines during the non-lactating period, as described in Chapter 5, is one avenue of research that would benefit from an effective staphylococcal vaccine.

6.6.2   *Streptococcus pyogenes*

At first sight, streptococcal vaccines should be much easier to produce than staphylococcal vaccines. The streptococci are less pathogenic, by virtue of having fewer toxins than staphylococci, and there are fewer strains which cause mastitis in cattle. However, there has only been one streptococcal vaccine produced commercially. This is the 'horse strangles' vaccine, produced from *Streptococcus equi.*

This is an effective vaccine in preventing severe swelling of the submaxillary lymph nodes in foals due to streptococcal infection—the so-called strangles syndrome. However, streptococcal vaccines have not been used against mastitis of cattle caused by *Streptococcus pyogenes.* Most strains of *S. pyogenes* are susceptible to antibiotics, and this has been the preferred mode of control.

Streptococcal vaccines have also been found to produce a great deal of Type III hypersensitivity. This is because of the large amounts of antibody produced during vaccination with the organism. It is not certain if this is an advantage or a disadvantage in the mammary gland. Local immunisation of sheep with streptococcal vaccine, followed by challenge with virulent streptococci, leads to the development of intense hyperaemia and swelling of the gland 6 hours after challenge. This leads to a rapid loss of milk production, and the question arises whether the low pathogenicity of many streptococcal strains, justifies the sensitisation of the gland by vaccine and loss of production during challenge. Streptococcal mastitis vaccines have therefore only been examined experimentally and not produced commercially.

6.6.3 Campylobacter fetus

Campylobacter fetus causes abortion and infertility in cattle and is a disease which is transmitted venereally from bull to cow. As was discussed earlier, vaccination of young bulls has proved to be an effective way of controlling the disease, when coupled with a two-herd management programme.

Campylobacter fetus occurs as only two main strains, and antibodies appear to be effective in controlling infection. Therefore, the approach in vaccination has been to boost titres using intramuscular injection of killed bacteria in oily adjuvant. The increased antibody titres in serum are accompanied by increased specific antibody in the external secretions. Local immunisation of the reproductive tract appears to be unnecessary and, being less convenient than intramuscular injection, has not been used in practical vaccination.

The antibodies produced in serum, appear to be mostly of the IgG_1 class, although IgG_2 is concentrated in external secretions relative to serum. The specific antibody in external secretions appears to be mostly IgG_1, and IgA immunoglobulin, specific for *C. fetus,* has not been found in high titre in external secretions.

The medium in which *C. fetus* is grown has been found to be important in vaccine production. Growth in liquid medium has been compared with growth on solid medium, and the vaccine produced from these two media gave different results. It was found that the vaccine grown in liquid medium gave less protection against experimental challenge than the vaccine grown on solid medium. This was particularly so in cattle vaccinated as calves at 5 to 8 months or at 12 months. In older cattle, the difference between vaccines was not evident (Clark *et al.,* 1972). Therefore, it appears that more of the protective antigens are produced by *C. fetus* organisms grown on solid medium than those grown in liquid medium. Considerations such as these are important for the commercial production of an efficient vaccine against Vibriosis of cattle and indeed for the production of vaccines against other bacterial diseases.

As an interesting aside to the *Campylobacter* story, the diagnosis of *Listeria monocytogenes* has been shown to be facilitated by treatment with trypsin of the heat-killed bacteria to be used in a simple agglutination test. The small amount of denatured protein deposited around the bacteria during heat treatment can be removed by digestion for a brief period with trypsin (Fig. 6.6). This has the effect of exposing fresh antigenic sites on the bacteria which improve the sensitivity of the test and remove some of the non-specific agglutination reactions (Osebold *et al.,* 1965). A further improvement in specificity can be obtained by depolymerising the IgM immunoglobulins in serum with 2-mercaptoethanol and testing the remaining IgG immunoglobulins, amongst which are specific antibodies to *Listeria* organisms (Osebold and Aalund, 1968).

138

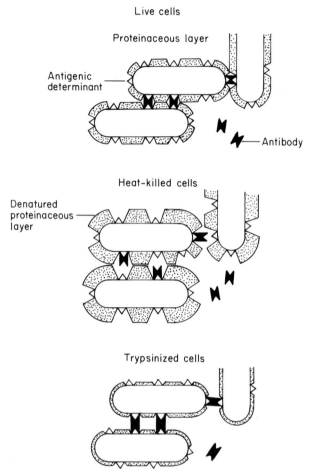

Fig. 6.6. The effect of trypsin treatment of heat-killed *Listeria monocytogenes* bacteria on the accessibility of antigenic sites for specific antibodies. The denatured protein is removed from the surface of the bacteria, allowing efficient cross-linking by antibodies. (Redrawn from Osebold, Aalund and Chrisp (1965), *J. Bacteriol.* **89**, 84–88, by kind permission of the authors.)

6.6.4 Clostridia

The clostridia are anaerobic spore-bearing organisms which are widely distributed in the environment and often infect wounds. Their mode of pathogenicity divides them into two groups. The first has little or no invasive ability but produces powerful toxins which cause tissue damage or general toxicity.

Examples are *Clostridium tetani,* which causes tetanus, and *Clostridium botulinum,* which causes botulism. The second and larger group, consists of species which have the ability to invade and multiply in tissue, and these are sometimes referred to as the 'gas gangrene' group. These organisms cause economic loss in cattle and sheep, and were the subject of successful early research into vaccination. The main organisms and the diseases they cause are listed in the accompanying tabulation.

Organism	Disease
Clostridium chauvoei	Blackleg in sheep and cattle
Clostridium welchii	Lamb dysentery and Pulpy Kidney disease
Clostridium septicum	Braxy and malignant oedema of sheep
Clostridium novyi	Black diseases of sheep and cattle
Clostridium haemolyticum	Red water in cattle

6.6.4.1 Immunity to Tetanus

Both passive and active immunity can be accomplished with tetanus. Since the organisms are present in the soil, animals are most often in need of passive immunity obtained by administration of 1500 units of tetanus antitoxin. This antitoxin is produced in horses, and repeated doses of antitoxin may result in anaphylactic shock due to injection of foreign protein. This also applies to horses which differ in their serum protein allotypes sufficiently for antigenic differences between horses to be recognised in passively-administered horse serum antitoxin.

Active immunity is started as soon as possible in animals with suspected infection of wounds with *C. tetani.* The immunising protein is Tetanus toxoid prepared by incubating highly-potent toxin with 0.4% formalin until toxicity has entirely disappeared. This is then adsorbed onto alum to make the product more antigenic. The vaccine is administered as two or three doses, separated by 3-week intervals, although a single dose will give appreciable immunity in animals at risk.

It is curious that horses rarely possess natural antibodies to tetanus, and this may be the reason for the high fatality rate of tetanus in the horse, whether treated or untreated. It may also reflect the much greater amount of poorly-immunogenic toxin required to stimulate natural antibodies than the amount required to produce toxic effects.

6.6.4.2 Immunity to Botulism

Since *Cl. botulinum* produces a variety of antigenic toxin types, it is usual to include the main types (A, B and C) in commercial polyvalent vaccines. Due to the sporadic nature of the disease in animals, passively-administered antitoxins are not used. The formalinised, alum-precipitated toxoids have been effectively used in sheep and cattle to protect them against botulism.

6.6.4.3 Immunity to Clostridia which Invade Tissues

Vaccines against these organisms have proved to be the most widely-used and effective vaccines in sheep and cattle. They are usually administered as a combined vaccine containing formalinised bacteria and toxins. It has been found that inclusion of strains, important to the area in which the vaccine is to be used, is a prerequisite for effective control measures.

Enterotoxaemia or 'Pulpy Kidney' of Lambs.   There is ample evidence that the symptoms of enterotoxaemia in lambs, caused by *Cl. welchii* Type D, is due to the ϵ toxin absorbed from the intestine. This is in contrast to *Cl. welchii* Type A infections in which it is not certain that the toxins produced play a dominant role in the pathogenesis of the disease.

The ϵ toxin occurs as a non-toxic prototoxin which is activated very rapidly by trypsin but not by pepsin. This means that all the ϵ toxin in intestinal contents of infected sheep is in the fully-activated form. High concentrations of ϵ toxin in the intestine for a period of 10 hours cause a rapid increase in permeability of the intestine. This is followed by absorption of large amounts of toxin and rapid death of the lamb.

Circulating antitoxin is very effective in protecting sheep against experimental enterotoxaemia. Even ileal contents containing between 10,000 and 20,000 mouse minimal lethal doses (MLD) per gram cannot produce the disease in the face of circulating antitoxin levels of 10 to 20 units/ml of serum (Bullen and Batty, 1957).

Passive protection of lambs can be produced by transmission of antitoxin via the colostrum to lambs from actively-immunised ewes and is effective for approximately 4 weeks. Passive immunisation of sheep with commercial hyperimmune horse serum, 2 ml for lambs and 5 ml for adult sheep, gives adequate protection for about 3 weeks. Active vaccination with *Cl. welchii* ϵ toxoid is used to follow up the passive immunisation and in some cases induces a secondary immune response because of previous sensitisation of the sheep by low doses of the ϵ toxin absorbed from the intestine.

Vaccines against *Cl. welchii* Type D, which causes the Pulpy Kidney syndrome in lambs and enterotoxaemia in both sheep and cattle, are usually carefully formulated to include toxoids of this strain. However, it has been found that the purified ε toxin deteriorates over a period of months, and therefore, vaccines against the clostridia also must deteriorate with storage. These vaccines should be administered before the expiry date on the label, to achieve effective protection.

Gas Gangrene.   Gas gangrene is caused by *Cl. welchii* Type A, and the lesion is a massive destruction of tissue, accompanied by severe toxaemia and shock. It is not certain whether the bacterial toxins α, θ, κ and μ are responsible for the invasive power of the bacteria. It has been found that of all the antitoxins present in *Cl. welchii* antisera, the anti-α toxin alone appeared to be responsible for protection. However, it was not equally protective against all strains of the bacteria, and some very invasive strains appeared to be weakly toxigenic. Thus in some circumstances the anti-α toxin gives very good protection and in others it does not.

A particular point of gas gangrene in human war wounds was that surgical extirpation of infected tissue was often found to be as important as the administration of antitoxin or penicillin. Thus severely-damaged muscle, lacking a proper blood supply, may be cut off from circulating antitoxin and penicillin. Experimental work in guinea pigs by Bullen and his colleagues has shown that antitoxin administered before experimental lesions are induced was only protective when adrenalin was administered simultaneously with the infective organisms. Therefore, the maintenance of the blood supply did promote the anti-invasive effects of the anti-α toxin. However, if tissue necrosis developed, no amount of antitoxin passively administered, prevented the spread of the infection, even though high levels of antitoxin could be measured in the lesion tissue.

6.6.5   *Bacteroides nodosus*

An anaerobic non-spore-bearing pathogenic bacterium, *Bacteroides nodosus*, is the major cause of 'foot-rot' in sheep. It is distinguished from another anaerobic organism called *Fusobacterium necrophorum*, the causative agent of foot-rot in cattle.

Attempts have been made with both organisms to vaccinate sheep and cattle against foot-rot. Considerable success has been achieved in trials on field stations, but the vaccines have not stood up well to testing in the field. There are break-downs in flocks of sheep vaccinated against foot-rot, and research is continuing into the best formulation for an effective vaccine. In Australia, eight strains of the organism have been incorporated into experimental vaccines. One of the problems is the reduced antigenic mass obtained for each component of the vaccine and the difficulty in obtaining suspensions concentrated enough to produce antigenic stimulation in the multivalent vaccine. There is also the increase in cost which accompanies the formulation of such a vaccine, and this is obviously a marketing problem.

Another problem which is found with the foot-rot vaccines is the rapid waning of immunity, 6–12 weeks after vaccination. Attempts have been made with various adjuvants, to boost serum titres of antibody, specific for the antigens of *B. nodosus*. Among these antigens is the bacterial pilus (Fig. 6.7), which can be purified from culture medium by differential centrifugation. Antibodies to the pilus antigens are highly protective and, in combination with oily adjuvants, can provide protection for 12 weeks—the seasonal period for which most sheep are at risk. However, the injection of oil subcutaneously into sheep often produces large reaction sites, with abscess formation. This is a problem with other vaccines such as the *Corynebacterium pseudotuberculosis* vaccine against Caseous Lymphadenitis. Therefore, other adjuants have been tried, such as aluminium hydroxide, but without success, since the period of immunity wanes even more rapidly than with oily adjuvant. These difficulties with oily adjuvants in sheep,

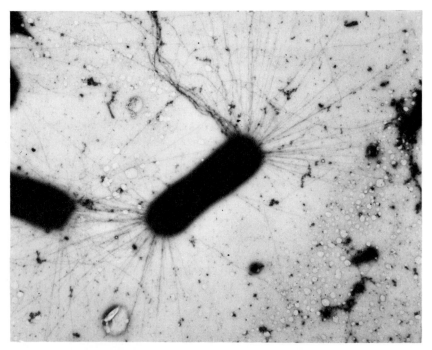

Fig. 6.7. An electron micrograph of *Bacteriodes nodosus*, the causative agent of foot-rot in sheep. The bacterial pili can be seen radiating from the surfaces of the bacteria. (Reproduced by kind permission of Dr. D. J. Stewart, CSIRO, Division of Animal Health, Parkville, Victoria, Australia, and the CSIRO Editorial and Publication Service.)

and indeed in cattle, remain one of the challenges in the vaccination of animals against bacterial disease.

6.6.6 *Corynebacterium pseudotuberculosis* (ovis)

This organism is a pyogenic diphtheroid bacillus which is the cause of 'Cheesy Lymph Node' in sheep. The accumulation of large numbers of neutrophil polymorphonuclear cells in the lymph nodes infected with *C. pseudotuberculosis,* leads to a characteristic greenish pus, a colour presumably due to the myeloperoxidase found in the leucocytes.

Inactivated vaccines have been found to give good protection against experimental infection. This type of vaccine is formulated to contain a high level of toxoid. Alum vaccine is highly effective, although the oily adjuvant causes the same problems of abscess formation as it does with the foot-rot vaccine. It is interesting that Freund's incomplete adjuvant, without added bacteria, produces very little reaction, demonstrating that the bacterial component in the vaccine causes the irritation to the injection site.

As mentioned in Chapter 2, a novel method of assaying the effectiveness of vaccination was developed by Burrell using the isolated popliteal lymph node challenge. This was followed by weighing the challenged and control lymph nodes at postmortem to assess objectively the degree of protection.

A diagnostic test for natural infection has been developed. This is a haemolysis inhibition test using *C. pseudotuberculosis* exotoxin and sheep red cells. The test carried out under optimum conditions, detects about 80% of natural cases. Positive tests from lambs suckling colostrum from ewes with high titres to this toxin can also be detected and may confuse diagnosis in young animals.

The two problems of diagnosis and vaccination in *C. pseudotuberculosis* infection of sheep, do appear to be soluble with developments in research. The vaccine is commercially available in Australia as a component of a 5 in 1 clostridial vaccine.

6.6.7 *Escherichia coli*

This is one member of the family Enterobacteriaceae which, among other things, has been used extensively in the new recombinant DNA techniques in biotechnology. There are, however, many strains of *E. coli* which are pathogenic for sheep, cattle and pigs. They have been isolated from cases of bovine mastitis, urogenital infections, abortions and diarrhoea of piglets and calves. This last appears to be the largest problem, and attempts to vaccinate animals have been directed towards protection of the gut mucosa.

There are natural barriers to the *E. coli* organism, amongst which is passively-acquired colostral antibody in newborn calves and lambs. Neonatal ruminants, deprived of colostrum, are particularly susceptible to *E. coli* scours. Vaccination of the cow against pathogenic strains does have the effect of passively protecting the calf through colostral antibodies.

Active immunity against *E. coli* scours has been achieved in piglets by means of feeding heat-killed organisms. In this case it appears that there is local production of specific antibody which interferes with the adhesion of the organisms to the gut mucosal epithelial cells. In addition, the gut secretions contain antitoxins against the enterotoxin of the *E. coli* organisms. In the first instance, it seems that the antibody is directed against the K antigens (K88 in pigs and K99 in calves) present on the pili which are involved in anchoring the organisms to the gut mucosa. In the second, the heat-stable enterotoxin can produce gut stasis and gas accumulation, but antitoxin present in the mucus, effectively neutralises this effect.

Modern research on *E. coli* vaccines is directed towards purification of the K88 and K99 antigens on pili and also towards isolation of the heat-stable enterotoxin. This is then injected parenterally as a vaccine or hopefully fed to the animal, so that protection at the gut mucosal surface can be effected.

It is interesting that the first commercially-available genetically-engineered vaccines anywhere, have been for scours in pigs caused by *E. coli*. The idea was developed to increase the yield of K88 pili by splicing the genetic material coding for the pili protein into a non-pathogenic strain of *E. coli*. This converted the protein-making machine of the bacteria into one for making pili of the K88 or the K99 strains. The pili were easily separated from the cell wall components such as endotoxin (lipopolysaccharide) and were used in sows as a vaccine.

Another recombinant DNA technique has been used with *E. coli* to produce an experimental vaccine. In pathogenic strains the enterotoxin consists of two proteins: protein A combines with receptors on the surface of the gut epithelial cells and protein B switches on the cyclic AMP in those cells. This leads to cell hyperactivity, diarrhoea, dehydration and even death of the host. A genetically-engineered vaccine has been prepared in which the genes responsible for expression of the protein B have been replaced by those from the plasmid of a non-pathogenic strain of *E. coli*. The new organism can still attach to the intestinal wall and provoke local antibodies without the toxic B protein producing pathogenic effects. This vaccine is still being examined in trials and has yet to become available commercially.

6.7 THE FUTURE OF BACTERIAL VACCINES IN DOMESTIC ANIMALS

Most of the bacterial infections of domestic animals have adequate vaccines, or if they do not, are the subject of continuing slow improvement resulting from research. In this, the veterinary field differs from the human immunological field in which research on bacterial diseases has been largely closed down. In the veterinary field the residual but still significant problems in diagnosis and vaccination against bacteria are still the preoccupation of present-day research.

Some likely directions for improvements are in the modification of the immune response so that cellular, rather than humoral immunity is stimulated by the vaccine. Secondly, the problem of detection of antibodies which confirm diagnosis without interference by antibodies from concurrent vaccination, may be solvable by close attention to immunoglobulin classes detected in the tests. Thirdly, alternatives to Freund's complete adjuvant need to be found, to alleviate the problem of abscesses produced at sites of injection of the vaccine, particularly in sheep.

REFERENCES

Allan, G. S., Chappel, R. J., Williamson, P. and McNaught, D. J. (1976). *J. Hyg.* **76**, 287–298.

Allen, R. C. and Loose, L. D. (1976). *Biochem. Biophys. Res. Commun.* **69**, 245–252.

Alton, G. G. and Jones, L. M. (1967). 'Laboratory Techniques in Brucellosis,' WHO Monograph Series, No. 55. WHO, Geneva.

Arbuthnott, J. P. (1970). Staphylococcal α-toxin. *In* 'Microbial Toxins: A Comprehensive Treatise' (T. C. Montie, S. Kadis and S. J. Ajl, eds.), Vol. 3, pp. 189–236. Academic Press, New York.

Bennell, M. A. and Watson, D. L. (1980). *Microbiol. Immunol.* **24**, 871–878.

Bullen, J. J. and Batty, I. (1957). *J. Pathol. Bacteriol.* **73**, 511–518.

Burrell, D. H. (1978). *Aust. Adv. Vet. Sci.* pp. 79–81.

Cheers, C. and Sandrin, M. S. (1983). *Cell. Immunol.* **78**, 199–205.

Clark, B. L., Dufty, J. H. and Monsbourgh, M. J. (1972). *Aust. Vet. J.* **48**, 376–381.

Clark, B. L., Dufty, J. H., Monsbourgh, M. J. and Parsonson, I. M. (1974). *Aust. Vet. J.* **50**, 407–409.

Clark, B. L., Dufty, J. H., Monsbourgh, M. J. and Parsonson, I. M. (1977). *Aust. Vet. J.* **53**, 465–466.

Cochrane, A. L. and Holland, W. W. (1971). *Br. Med. Bull.* **27**, 3–8.

Goudswaard, J., van der Donk, J. A., Noordzij, A., van Dam, R. H. and Vaerman, J.-P. (1978). *Scand, J. Immunol.* **8**, 21–28.

Lepper, A. W. D., Meharry, M. R. and Outteridge, P. M. (1974). *Aust. Vet. J.* **50**, 192–198.

Lepper, A. W. D., Carpenter, M. T., Williams, O. J., Scanlan, W. A., McEwan, D. R., Andrews, L. G., Thomas, J. R. and Corner, L. A. (1979). *Aust. Vet. J.* **55**, 251–256.

Njoku-Obi, A. N. and Osebold, J. W. (1962). *J. Immunol.* **89**, 187–194.

Osebold, J. W. and Aalund, O. (1968). *J. Infect. Dis.* **118**, 139–148.

Osebold, J. W. and Dicapua, R. A. (1968). *J. Bacteriol.* **95**, 2158–2164.

Osebold, J. W., Aalund, O. and Chrisp, C. E. (1965). *J. Bacteriol.* **89**, 84–88.

Osebold, J. W., Pearson, L. D. and Medin, N. I. (1974). *Infect. Immun.* **9**, 354–362.

Outteridge, P. M., Osebold, J. W. and Zee, Y. C. (1972). *Infect. Immun.* **5**, 814–825.

Plackett, P. and Alton, G. G. (1975). *Aust. Vet. J.* **51**, 374–377.

Plackett, P., Cottew, G. S. and Best, S. J. (1976). *Aust. Vet. J.* **52**, 136–140.

Plackett, P., Alton, G. G., Carter, P. D. and Corner, L. A. (1980). *Aust. Vet. J.* **56,** 405–408.
Stewart, D. J. (1978). *Res. Vet. Sci.* **24,** 14–19.
Thorley, C. M. and Egerton, J. R. (1981). *Res. Vet. Sci.* **30,** 32–37.
Wiseman, G. M. (1970). The beta- and delta-toxins of *Staphylococcus aureus. In* 'Microbial Toxins: A Comprehensive Treatise' (T. C. Montie, S. Kadis and S. J. Ajl, eds.), Vol. 3, pp. 237–263. Academic Press, New York.

7

Immunity to Viruses

The immunity to viruses has been traditionally held to be the result of a predominantly humoral immune response. The cellular responses to virus-infected cells do indeed exist, but the strategy of vaccination of animals has been to boost antibody titres so that initial attachment of virus to the target cell receptors is thwarted and the virus–antibody complex is removed by the reticuloendothelial system. This approach has been effective in most virus infections which undergo a viraemic phase, in which virus is found free in the blood before infecting the cells. In virus diseases involving external contact, such as Infectious Bovine Rhinotracheitis (IBR), a herpesvirus infection of cattle, there is a cell-to-cell transmission of the virus, in addition to the viraemia, and this makes the virus less accessible to neutralisation by specific antibody.

7.1 HUMORAL IMMUNITY

7.1.1 Virus Neutralisation Assay

The assay of antibodies to viruses is often carried out using tissue culture techniques. In these techniques, the virus is grown on a monolayer of cells such as a bovine kidney cell line, and dilutions of serum are added until the cytopathic plaques, due to virus, appear. The assay can also be carried out by inoculation of virus and antibody into the chorioallantoic membranes of embryonated eggs. In the *in vitro* assay, the dilutions are often conveniently carried out in multiple-well tissue culture trays which can be washed out, fixed and the cells stained for subsequent counting of plaques. Similar assays can be carried out *in vivo* with suckling mice using equal volumes of virus dilution and serum inoculated intraperitoneally into the mice. In the *in vivo* assay, newborn mice are used because their immature immune system makes them susceptible to viruses of all types, including those of non-murine origin which normally will not infect adult mice. Some care must be taken to ensure that maternally-transmitted antibody is not present against the virus to be assayed. The assay either involves measurement of the death rate of the suckling mice or culture of virus from the mouse tissues to assess the neutralisation.

7.1.2   Haemagglutination Inhibition Assay

Many viruses are capable of causing spontaneous agglutination of mammalian or avian erythrocytes. This serendipitous finding has been exploited in a haemagglutination inhibition assay, in which a fixed amount of virus is adsorbed to red cells in the presence of dilutions of serum antibody. The haemagglutination inhibition titre is calculated by multiplying the highest dilution which inhibits haemagglutination by the number of haemagglutinating units of virus used in the assay.

7.1.3   Enzyme-Linked Immunosorbent Assay

The enzyme-linked immunosorbent assay (ELISA) is being increasingly used to detect antibodies to viruses. The reasons are both the increased sensitivity compared with other assays and the convenience of not having to use a tissue culture system. Virus antigen is bound to the surface of the wells in polystyrene microdilution trays, often by just allowing the wells to dry after filling and emptying of the wells with the antigen solution. After fixation with methanol, the wells are washed with phosphate-buffered saline containing 3% bovine serum albumin, which prevents non-specific absorption of antibody to the plastic surface. Serial doubling dilutions of antiserum are added to the wells overnight at room temperature. Unbound antibody is washed off with water. The antigen–antibody complex is then reacted with a dilution of anti-immunoglobulin coupled with glucose oxidase, washed and a developer containing horse-radish peroxidase and a chromogen is added.

The colour developed, a yellow-brown, can be read by automatic scanners such as the Titertek, Multiskan, and this is an advantage in routine laboratory assays. Results are often expressed as the reciprocal of the serum dilution binding to 50% of the picomoles of antigen added to each well.

7.2 VIRUS ANTIGEN

Of course, virus antigen usually has to be isolated from tissue culture cells and their homogenates, and this antigen is often purified by further steps such as density-gradient centrifugation. Unpurified virus may be used in assays such as double diffusion in gel where some of the high molecular weight components are prevented from reacting because they do not diffuse out of the antigen well. However in general, it is preferable to purify the virus antigen to remove possible cross-reactions between antibody and tissue culture cells.

Virus is titrated so that its infectivity is known. This is usually done by limiting dilution techniques in tissue culture, but it may also be carried out with newborn mice or embryonated eggs. Virus is often inactivated using formalin or β-propiolactone (2-oxetanone) before being used as an antigen in assays such as the ELISA assay which do not require live virus. Often there is a problem in obtaining enough virus antigen for use in assays, and therefore microassays are often developed which do not use much antigen.

Subunits of virus, the protein components, can also be used for assays or vaccines if it appears to be necessary. Usually the labour involved in partial purification of virus from a large number of tissue culture samples is enough to discourage further purification of virus antigen, where the yield is small and losses during purification are high. Affinity column techniques are also possible using covalently-linked antibodies to virus coat proteins which selectively bind the virus. Again, the effort involved may discourage this purification step, if the antibody assay is not greatly improved.

The complement fixation test for assaying antibodies to viruses has been used as a convenient test for some virus diseases. The use of this test and others, such as the indirect fluorescence assay and gel diffusion, are described in detail in the *Manual of Standardized Methods for Veterinary Microbiology,* edited by Cottral (1978).

7.3 APPEARANCE OF ANTIBODIES TO EXOTIC VIRUSES

The sudden appearance of antibodies to previously-unrecorded viruses, or 'sero-conversion', can be taken to herald an outbreak of exotic virus disease. However, this is not always the case, and in a particular instance—the recent outbreak of Bluetongue in Australia—the antibodies to the virus were found in cattle, a species which is not susceptible to the pathogenic effects of the virus. Sheep were not found to have antibody titres to this relatively-mild strain of Bluetongue virus outside the cattle grazing areas, although antibodies certainly could be stimulated by experimental infection of sheep in isolation laboratories.

The distribution of animals with antibodies to virus is often dependent on the distribution of the insect vector; in the case of Bluetongue in Australia, the biting midge *Culicoides brevitarsis* was the insect vector. Virus was isolated from the insects before it was realised that it might be a strain of Bluetongue virus. Subsequent serological typing revealed that it was a subtype of Bluetongue virus. Retrospective examination of cattle serum then revealed antibodies which were found to change in their distribution through the cattle population from year to year in northern Australia. This waxing and waning of antibodies in cattle serum was assumed to parallel the distribution of the *Culicoides* spp., which varied according to the succession of wet and dry seasons normally occurring in northern Australia.

Retrospective searches of antibodies in stored sera from cattle helped to reveal the extent of another disease, Akabane virus infection. This was characterised by hydranencephaly and arthrogryposis of calves, but it was only by examination of serum from cattle in other areas that the extent of the outbreak could be mapped and correlated with the distribution of insect vectors. In both the Bluetongue and Akabane virus infections, the extent of the outbreak could be judged from the presence of antibodies in the serum of cattle. This has led to the establishment of 'sentinel herds and flocks', which are regularly bled and their serum assayed for antibodies to endemic viruses as well as being stored for later reference in future outbreaks.

7.4 LOCAL ANTIBODIES TO VIRUSES

The immunisation with attenuated live virus often has effects which are seen in the protection of mucous membranes from natural virus. The Sabin vaccine against poliomyelitis has been quoted earlier. This vaccine apparently provides a non-progressive infection of the gut mucosa with consequent production of specific antibodies by the plasma cells in the submucosa. On the other hand, the immunisation of chickens with the virus of Infectious Laryngotracheitis (ILT) via the cloaca or the gut appears to involve the migration of B-cells from the local infection site to the lungs where these cells produce protective antibodies against the natural virus infection.

In both cases, the local antibodies appear to be much more than just an adjunct to serum antibody and provide a barrier to the virus at its point of entry, the gut in poliomyelitis and the respiratory tract in Infectious Laryngotracheitis. Not all the virus diseases require the presence of locally-produced antibody to prevent infection. The Arabian foals with Severe Combined Immunodeficiency are protected from Equine Adenovirus infections of the lung for as long as maternal colostral antibodies remain at high levels. As soon as these antibodies wane, the virus causes increasing problems and many foals succumb to the virus infection by 3 months of age.

Antibody-forming cells can be demonstrated in lung tissue sections. These cells contain specific antibody of the IgA, IgM and IgG class with different immunoglobulin classes predominating in different species. The predominant class is often IgA, which is the most common antibody found in external secretions.

7.5 CELLULAR IMMUNITY TO VIRUSES

The ultimate removal of the virus–antibody complexes is by the phagocytic cells, which themselves can become infected with virus. These virus-infected phagocytes can become targets for immune attack by the cells of the reticuloendothelial system. Indeed, any somatic cells which are infected with virus and which express virus antigen on their surfaces are subject to attack by lymphoid cells of a different type.

7.5.1 Natural Killer Cells

Virus-infected cells can be attacked and destroyed by T-cells which have been sensitised to the virus antigen by previous exposure to the virus after vaccination or natural infection. There is also a non-specific attack by cells known as natural killer (NK) cells. These cells appear to be part of the T-cell population. They differ from the majority of the T-cells in being larger and less dense than the average and in their possession of cytoplasmic granules. Their entry into the peripheral circulation closely parallels the synthesis of interferon by somatic cells and also the activation of macrophages. These NK cells have been demonstrated in human, rat and mouse blood and more recently in cattle (Campos et al., 1982). For other domestic species, they have also been demonstrated in the chicken and the pig. In the pig, NK cells are not found in the circulation of the foetus before birth, but they appear after birth and steadily increase with time. Specific pathogen-free piglets have lower numbers of NK cells than conventional piglets, and the evidence points to the NK cell being one which is mobilised in response to virus infection and challenge. They have not been described in the blood of horses, dogs or sheep, but this is probably because they have not been looked for in these species. It seems likely that they will soon also be found in these species.

7.5.2 Killer Cells

Another system also operates with virus-infected cells which are coated with antibody, directed against the virus antigen. In this case, the antibody presents the Fc piece of the molecule for cells with Fc receptors, which attack and kill the

virus-infected cells. Cells with Fc receptors include neutrophil polymorphonuclear leucocytes, monocytes, macrophages and killer (K) cells. The K cells are
found as a small population in blood and appear to be distinct from either T- or
B-cells. They differ from NK cells in the possession of Fc receptors for IgG,
which are not present on the membranes of NK cells.

7.5.3 Antibody-Dependent Cell-Mediated Cytotoxicity

Collectively these cells with Fc receptors are known to participate in the
phenomenon of antibody-dependent cell-mediated cytotoxicity (ADCC). In cattle, these cells have been closely examined by Rouse *et al.* (1976), using the
Infectious Bovine Rhinotracheitis (IBR) herpesvirus for *in vitro* assay of cytotoxicity against bovine kidney cells infected with virus. An important finding was
that the neutrophil polymorphonuclear leucocytes were very effective in the
ADCC assay. These cells were obtained from the bovine mammary gland and
compared with the bovine mammary macrophages. The neutrophils were found
to be twice as effective as the macrophages in the release of ^{51}Cr from labelled
target cells. The neutrophils from the mammary gland were found also to be
twice as effective as those isolated from the blood. Peripheral blood lymphocytes
had virtually no effect on bovine kidney target cells.

In contrast, peripheral blood lymphocytes did cause release of ^{51}Cr, at about
one-sixth the rate of mammary neutrophils, from radiolabelled chicken red blood
cells. This assay is known to have a high background release of ^{51}Cr, and it is
conceivable that the activity of the peripheral blood lymphocytes is more accurately demonstrated by the release of ^{51}Cr from bovine kidney cells. In any case,
the peripheral blood lymphocytes released far less ^{51}Cr than either macrophages
or neutrophils, and this highlighted the importance of the neutrophil as a cell
mediating ADCC in the IBR virus infections of cattle and undoubtedly in other
species too.

On the other hand, in Canine Distemper, Ho and Babiuk (1979a) found that it
was the K-lymphocytes rather than the neutrophils and monocytes which destroyed virus-infected target cells. They made the point that this was only part of
the immune response to Canine Distemper, and in subsequent papers they demonstrated that serum antibodies prevented the intracellular and extracellular
spread of the virus (Ho and Babiuk, 1979b) and that serum complement was very
effective in the lysis of infected cells in the presence of specific antibody (Ho and
Babiuk, 1980).

7.6 GENETIC RESTRICTION

The attack by T-cells on virus-infected target cells, in particular Lymphochoriomeningitis (LCM) virus of mice, has been used in basic experiments to

demonstrate the importance of the major histocompatibility complex (MHC) in the immune response. Zinkernagel and Doherty in the 1970s used a mouse target cell system which involved cells from different strains of mice. In one set of experiments it was shown that lymphocytes from the strain of mouse with the H-2^k major locus type, would attack autologous virus-infected target cells of this H-2^k type but not the homologous H-2^b type (Fig. 7.1). This led to many other experiments in mice which have shown 'genetic restriction' of the immune response, and it is thought that a complex of virus and MHC antigens is recognised by the sensitised T-cells. With antigens which are not infective viruses, the macrophage is suggested to act as the passive presenter of antigen which is in a complex with the MHC antigen, and this acts as the sensitising group for T-cell responses.

In domestic animals genetic restriction has not been often reported because it is usually not accessible to experimentation with outbred strains of animals. An exception is perhaps the chicken, in which it has been shown that a particular MHC type ($B21$), is associated with resistance to Marek's disease virus. This kind of result has led to work which is attempting to correlate MHC types in

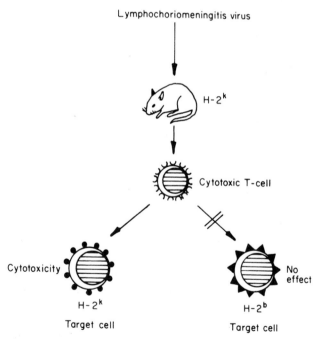

Lymphochoriomeningitis virus

H-2^k

Cytotoxic T-cell

Cytotoxicity

H-2^k

Target cell

No effect

H-2^b

Target cell

Fig. 7.1. Lymphocytes from a mouse strain with H-2^k major histocompatibility type will attack autologous virus-infected target cells of this type but not the closely-related homologous H-2^b type. This was described as 'genetic restriction' of the immune response by Zinkernagel and Doherty (1975).

ruminants and pigs with genetic susceptibility or resistance to infectious disease. This aspect is covered in greater detail in Chapter 10 on immunogenetics.

7.7 DELAYED HYPERSENSITIVITY

Delayed hypersensitivity to viral antigens has not been closely investigated. However, it was put to practical use in the dog, in which a close antigenic similarity between Human Measles virus and Canine Distemper virus was demonstrated using a skin test (Brown and McCarthy, 1974). Dogs sensitised with either Human Measles virus or Canine Distemper virus could be induced to produce a delayed skin reaction to the intradermal injection of either virus in the inactivated form.

However the involvement of delayed hypersensitivity in viral infection is not well-established, because some viruses have been shown to proliferate in activated lymphocytes. Thus although resting lymphocytes are unable to manufacture viruses upon infection, lymphocytes activated by specific antigens become capable of supporting virus replication.

This was the basis of a test for lymphocyte stimulation developed by Jiminez et al. (1971) in which plaque-forming cells to Vesicular Stomatitis virus of pigs were measured after in vitro infection of human lymphocytes proliferating in response to tuberculin purified protein derivative (PPD). The technique was complicated and not popular, but it did serve to demonstrate the peculiar problem with viruses, that in contrast to bacterial infections, the virus utilises the nucleoprotein-synthesising machinery of the cell and is not destroyed after phagocytosis by activated macrophages, stimulated by lymphokines. Indeed, the Infectious Bovine Rhinotracheitis (IBR) virus of cattle has been shown to replicate quite well in bovine macrophages.

7.8 LYMPHOKINES AND INTERFERON

It was found, however, that not all viruses grew within activated lymphocytes and that influenza and Coxsackie viruses were rapidly inactivated when they came into contact with stimulated lymphocytes. It also began to be appreciated that lymphocytes, in common with all other somatic cells such as macrophages, produced interferon. This molecule (MW 60,000) had long been known to inhibit replication of DNA and RNA viruses, but it was not appreciated that there might be several types of interferon. One type, called 'immune interferon', was produced by both T- and B-lymphocytes, after stimulation with antigen or mitogens such as phytohaemagglutinin (PHA). Indeed, this method was used to produce the first batches of human interferon for testing as a therapeutic agent in human cancer patients.

Immune interferon, or Type II interferon, differs from Type I interferon derived from other somatic cells. It is relatively unstable to low pH, while Type I interferons are stable to <pH 2 or >pH 10. This has been demonstrated in horses by Yilma *et al.* (1982). They identified an interferon from Newcastle disease virus (NDV) or polyinosinic:polycytidilic acid (poly-I:C)-induced equine fibroblasts, as an equine interferon β (based on the recommendation by the Committee for Interferon Nomenclature). A pH 2-stable and heat-labile interferon induced by NDV or poly-I:C from equine blood mononuclear cells was designated as equine interferon α. This was equivalent to the Type II interferon in the old nomenclature.

A third type of interferon was found, which was labile at pH 2 and after heating, and had slow activation kinetics (72 hours), in contrast to the other two interferon types, which had fast activation kinetics (24 hours). This interferon γ was obtained by PHA or concanavalin A (Con A) activation of equine blood mononuclear cells. It was also found to be deficient in Arabian foals with Severe Combined Immunodeficiency, but interferons α and β were not deficient.

The definition of these activities of the products from activated lymphocytes has led to some comparisons being made between the immune interferons and the lymphokine molecules. The lymphokines were also known to contain interferon activity, but it is still not known if the various biological effects of the lymphokines are due to interferon. This question is hard to answer because of the difficulty in obtaining enough of the lymphokines for detailed analytical experiments. At the moment, the lymphokines are regarded as a mixture of molecules with different biological effects. For example, 'skin-reactive factor' causes delayed-hypersensitivity skin reactions, 'mitogenic factor' induces the proliferation of lymphocytes and 'immunosuppressive factor' controls the proliferation of lymphocytes. Interferons have also been claimed to affect the proliferation of lymphocytes, and it may well be that the older 'lymphokine' nomenclature will have to be discarded in favour of terms such as interferon α, β and γ molecules. However, these questions and others will be answered when purified interferons from the recombinant DNA techniques are available for experimentation.

7.9 IMMUNISATION AGAINST VIRUSES

7.9.1 Foot-and-Mouth Disease

The most active area in virus immunisation in the veterinary field is the pursuit of effective vaccines against Foot-and-Mouth disease of cattle. As an example of a difficult problem, which is slowly being solved by effective research, Foot-and-Mouth disease must surely rank high.

Foot-and-Mouth disease virus has been the cause of one of the world's major animal diseases. It affects all artiodactyls and is a highly-infective virus which causes an estimated 25% loss of productivity in animals which become infected. The disease is controlled by vaccination in countries where it is endemic but by slaughter in countries in which it does not occur. It is estimated that over one billion doses of the vaccine are used each year, but the disease remains, even after 40 years of vaccination (Brown, 1981). Vaccines are prepared in tissue culture using bovine tongue epithelial cells or baby hamster kidney cells. The vaccines contain inactivated virus, and although they are quite effective they suffer from certain drawbacks. Firstly, difficulty is encountered in growing several strains of the virus in sufficient quantity to provide enough antigen for a vaccine. Secondly, the virus particle, even when inactivated, is unstable in acid pH, and the vaccine must be stored under refrigeration. This limits its use in

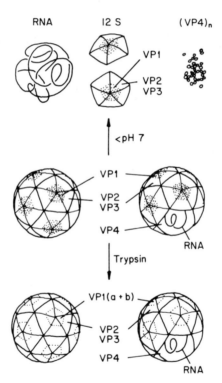

Fig. 7.2. The protein and RNA components of Foot-and-Mouth disease virus particles are shown after treatment with low pH or with trypsin. The lowering of the pH of the virus below 7 results in disruption of the particle into infectious RNA, the 12 S protein subunit and an aggregate $(VP4)_n$ of virus protein. Cleavage of VP1 with trypsin into VP1 (a + b) results in loss of infectivity. An important immunising protein appears to be VP1, and this protein can be synthesised by cloning techniques in *Escherichia coli*. (Reproduced by permission from Brown (1981), *Trends Biochem. Sci.* **6,** 325–327.)

tropical climates where refrigeration may not be available. Thirdly, there is the danger from improperly-inactivated virus, which has been the cause of outbreaks of the disease in Europe.

Seven serotypes of Foot-and-Mouth disease virus are known: O (Oise), A (Allemagne), C (Waldmann), SAT (South African Territories) 1, 2 and 3, and Asia 1. Animals which are infected and recover from one serotype are not protected from the others. In addition, subtypes of the major serotypes are known with some cross-immunity occurring beween subtypes. However, when immunity is waning several months after vaccination, infection with another subtype can occur.

Foot-and-Mouth disease virus belongs to the same family as the viruses that cause poliomyelitis and the common cold: the picornaviruses. It is in the shape of an icosahedron particle, about 25 nm in diameter, with one molecule of infectious single-stranded RNA and 60 copies each of four structural polypeptides. These are named virus proteins VP1, VP2, VP3 (MW 24,000) and VP4 (MW 14,000) (Fig. 7.2). The VP1 polypeptide appears to have an important antigenic role, because cleavage of this polypeptide with trypsin causes loss of infectivity and loss of immunising activity. Furthermore, VP1 possesses some immunising activity when isolated from the virus particle, whereas the others do not.

Although the immunogenic activity of the isolated VP1 polypeptide is much lower than that of the intact virus, this immunogenicity has encouraged research workers to investigate the possibility of producing the polypeptide by recombinant DNA techniques using the bacteria *Escherichia coli.*

7.9.2 Recombinant DNA Techniques

The use of recombinant DNA cloning involves the subversion of the bacterial DNA of a common bacterium, *E. coli,* to produce a particular polypeptide or protein, by substitution or 'splicing' a synthesised nucleotide chain into the circular DNA molecule of the bacterium. This recombination occurs naturally between different strains of a bacterial species and is the basis for the transfer of resistance of bacteria to antibiotics from resistant to susceptible strains. Recombinant DNA techniques also mimic natural transduction between bacteria in which DNA from a phage transmits genetic information from one bacterium to another, even when separated in laboratory experiments by a membrane which is impermeable to the bacteria.

The technique in the laboratory for this artificial transduction firstly involves the synthesis of the required DNA sequence which is complementary to the Foot-and-Mouth disease virus RNA. An enzyme called reverse transcriptase is used to effect this synthesis, and the DNA is then converted into the double-stranded form. This DNA can then be, for instance, annealed to a phage plasmid and the phage is used to insert the hybrid DNA into the *E. coli* bacterial cells.

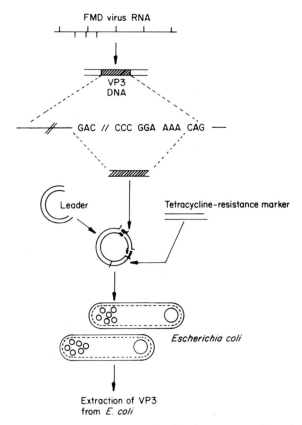

Fig. 7.3. A simplified diagram of the procedure for cloning Foot-and-Mouth disease (FMD) virus to produce a subunit vaccine. The virus protein specific complementary DNA (cDNA) is prepared using the known sequence of the virus RNA. The DNA is excised by endonucleases to produce a segment coding for the amino-acids of the virus protein. This segment is then incorporated into a plasmid having the correct leader, as well as a tetracycline-resistance marker. The insertion of this plasmid into the bacterium is carried out by increasing the permeability of the cell wall using $CaCl_2$. The bacterium grows and multiples expressing the gene product as virus protein, which usually has to be extracted from the bacteria and purified.

The addition of this hybrid DNA to the bacterial cell leads to it producing messenger RNA (mRNA), which is then translated by the bacterial ribosomes, which in turn synthesise the required polypeptide (Fig. 7.3). In the case of Foot-and-Mouth disease virus, at least 1000 molecules of the VP1 polypeptide are synthesised per bacterial cell. However, this expressed protein appears to be no more active weight-for-weight than VP1 produced from virus particles. There appears to be much more to be found out about the necessary structural features for effective immunisation with VP1, before it can be used as an alternative to inactivated virus particles.

However, in the course of the recombinant DNA technique, the DNA nucleotide sequence for the virus protein was analysed, and this has led to another approach in the preparation of the immunising VP1 polypeptide.

7.9.3 Chemical Synthesis of Peptides

The knowledge of the nucleotide sequence of the virus genome has allowed the primary amino-acid sequence of the VP1 polypeptide to be deduced. This is because the sequence of the nucleotide triplets necessary for each amino-acid has been worked out by molecular biologists. This has led to the synthesis of the VP1 polypeptide using chemical techniques on special resin, coupling the amino-acids in the required sequence, using a machine called a peptide synthesiser. These peptides were then coupled to keyhole limpet haemocyanin (KLH) as a carrier and injected into rabbits. These KLH-coupled peptides elicited antibodies to the peptide, and these antibodies were effective in the neutralisation of virus in the tissue culture test described earlier. Furthermore, guinea pigs were protected from experimental challenge with Foot-and-Mouth disease virus, when the animals were vaccinated first with the chemically-synthesised polypeptide in Freund's complete adjuvant (Bittle *et al.*, 1982). Some work in pigs and cattle has been reported, which shows that the synthetic peptide protects these species against experimental challenge.

At the moment, the prospects for a totally-synthetic polypeptide vaccine against Foot-and-Mouth disease virus are encouraging, but much more work remains in evaluating this vaccine for general use. Also much work has to be done in synthesising protective proteins from all the strains of the virus, and this should occupy research workers for several years to come.

7.9.4 Recombinant Virus Vaccines

Another approach to virus vaccines, which involves the use of genetic engineering, is the recombinant virus vaccine. It is possible to insert the coding sequence for Human Hepatitis B virus surface antigen into the vaccinia virus genome (Smith *et al.*, 1983). The host cells which are infected with these vaccinia virus recombinants, synthesise and excrete the hepatitis virus antigen, and vaccinated rabbits rapidly produce antibodies to this antigen.

This approach circumvents the high expense of manufacturing hepatitis B virus vaccine for humans and contributes a self-limiting vaccine with high immunogenic potential. This approach has yet to be used in veterinary virology, but it has obvious potential for vaccines which are difficult to prepare and where there is a requirement for immediate, high, specific antibody titres. Some cautious testing of such vaccines in high-security laboratories would be required before the vaccine is released into the field, in case a new strain of virulent virus is inadvertently manufactured.

7.10 MONOCLONAL ANTIBODIES FOR THE DETECTION OF VIRUS STRAINS

As described in Chapter 4 on immunoglobulins, monoclonal antibodies can be artificially produced by antibody-forming cells, fused with mouse myeloma cells. These 'hybridoma' antibody-forming cells can be screened for activity to virus coat proteins, and this has been of particular use in identifying strains of Rabies virus.

Rabies viruses isolated from different animal species were previously considered to be closely related. Some minor differences had been detected with conventional polyclonal antibodies, but it was only with the advent of monoclonal antibodies that conclusive evidence was provided for differences among the strains of several fixed and street Rabies viruses.

The concept of antigenic differences among Rabies virus strains was of special significance in vaccination against the disease. Vaccines for human use are derived from a rabbit-adapted strain originally isolated by Pasteur in 1882. It had been assumed that this had sufficient cross reactivity with field strains of the virus to protect individuals in different parts of the world. Unfortunately this was not the case, and occasional failures occurred even when prompt treatment was applied to exposed individuals. Antigenic differences were suspected to be responsible, but until the advent of monoclonal antibodies, there was no way to detect these differences.

In the work of Wiktor and Koprowski (1980), monoclonal antibodies were used to select antigenic variants of the CVS 11 strain of Rabies virus. In this technique, monoclonal antibodies, in excess of the amount required to neutralise the virus, are added one-by-one to the virus. Because of the fine specificity of the monoclonal antibodies, some variants do not react and can be grown up in tissue culture. In this technique the virus variant which does react with the antibody is unable to form virus plaques in tissue culture, while the unreactive variants do form plaques. A total of nine hybridoma antibodies were tested against the CVS 11 strain, and five variants were produced. Mice were immunised with the parent CVS 11 strain, and this immunisation provided protection against the parent strain and the variants. In contrast, mice immunised with the variant strains were protected only against the homologous variant strain but remained susceptible to the CVS 11 parent strain and the other variant strains. Examination of seven street Rabies virus strains using the monoclonal antibodies to the selected variants revealed cross-reactions. However, the challenge experiments with the street strains did not show a simple relationship between the monoclonal antibody specificity and induced protection according to virus strain. It remained unclear whether these apparently-minor antigenic differences in virus glycoproteins between strains accounted for the varying degrees of protection provided by the standard fixed Rabies virus vaccine.

This work, however, demonstrates the usefulness of the monoclonal antibody technique in detecting minor antigenic differences within an apparently homogeneous strain of Rabies virus. Further work will no doubt suggest improvements in the composition of Rabies virus vaccines which could be manufactured according to the geographical area in which they are to be used.

These techniques indicate an area for future research with viruses of domestic animals which might be explored as a means of improving the specificity of virus vaccines. The variety of canine and feline viruses which already are incorporated into vaccines may be a useful area for study to determine antigenic variation, if the vaccine in question has not reached its full potential.

7.11 VACCINATION AGAINST VIRUSES

The practical vaccination of animals against viruses usually depends on accurate isolation of the viruses followed by the adaptation to tissue culture. This adaptation is more successful for some strains than others, so that it is usually the easily-grown strain which is made into vaccine.

The original vaccines against Canine Distemper virus were grown in embryonated eggs, and this led to the unavoidable inclusion of some egg proteins in the vaccine. Revaccination of individual dogs could carry the risk of hypersensitivity reactions, and these days, in line with most human vaccines, the Distemper vaccine is grown in tissue culture.

7.11.1 Distemper in Dogs

The history of vaccination against Distemper in dogs illustrates the steady advance of knowledge and technique in vaccination against a virus disease. In early attempts, virulent virus was used with specific antiserum administered simultaneously to control the severity of the infection. This technique gave excellent immunity, but the margin for error was not wide and the possibility of producing a case of Distemper was always present using virulent virus vaccine.

Attenuated vaccines were therefore then produced in three main ways. The first was to adapt the virus in an atypical host, such as the ferret. Secondly, the virus was grown by passage in embryonated eggs until its virulence was reduced. Thirdly, the virus was also grown in tissue culture through numerous passages until an attenuated live-virus vaccine was produced. These vaccines have all been used with success in preventing Canine Distemper. The live-virus vaccines have been used in preference to formalin-killed vaccines because they have been shown to have far fewer breakdowns under normal field challenge than the killed vaccines.

However, it was appreciated for some time that the live vaccines might not work in puppies with circulating antibodies in their serum, which were derived from the mother's colostrum and by direct transfer via the placenta. In this case, the live vaccine does not multiply, and the puppies are fully susceptible to Distemper from 12 weeks of age onwards, when most of the maternal antibodies have been metabolised. Nomograms have been constructed to help the veterinarian decide the time at which the maternal antibodies are at a low ebb and the time at which the virus vaccine is most likely to grow in the tissues of puppies and provide a stimulus for active antibody synthesis. However, the practical approach has been to vaccinate puppies at 6 to 8 weeks of age with live vaccine and again at 12 weeks of age. This covers the period 6–12 weeks, during which the puppies may be at risk due to falling maternal antibody titres to Distemper virus.

Another interesting feature of the Distemper virus is its close antigenic relationship with Measles virus of humans and the Rinderpest virus of cattle. Both Measles and Rinderpest viruses are avirulent in dogs, but antibodies are produced by their inoculation which will protect dogs against Distemper. This has been put to practical use with an attenuated Human Measles vaccine being used in very young puppies at 3 weeks of age, where there is a risk even with attenuated Distemper virus. It also appears that the Measles vaccine is not appreciably inhibited by circulating maternal antibodies to Distemper virus because of the antigenic differences between them. However the period during which Measles virus protects the puppies is limited and subsequent vaccination with attenuated Distemper virus is required to provide a more specific stimulus in older puppies, and this is carried out at 14 to 16 weeks of age. A dual vaccine containing both Measles virus and Distemper virus is now used in puppies from 4 to 12 weeks of age.

7.12   LIVE VERSUS KILLED VACCINES

The use of live vaccine against Distemper virus carries the risk, admittedly very small, of reversion to the virulent form. However, live vaccine is often preferred to killed vaccine because of the better protection associated with the live vaccine than the killed one. Killed vaccines must be chemically inactivated with formalin or β-propiolactone and then checked to see that infectivity has been completely destroyed. Sometimes repeated testing is required, to be certain that no residual infectivity remains. Unfortunately, treatment with formalin denatures some protein, and some immunising activity of the vaccine may be destroyed also. As mentioned earlier, there may not be sufficient antigenic mass after loss due to inactivation, for effective vaccines to be produced economically or to produce sufficient immunity without an unacceptably-large dose, which causes tissue reaction. Therefore, this field is open to a great deal of improvement of genetically-engineered bacterial production of viral proteins or to actual chemical synthesis of the protective viral polypeptide.

Vaccines against viruses of domestic animals are probably best discussed on a species-by-species basis with attention drawn to features of particular vaccines.

7.12.1 Cattle

Two diseases of cattle, at either end of the scale of importance, in which killed vaccines are used, are Bovine Papillomatosis and Foot-and-Mouth disease. The Bovine Papillomatosis or wart vaccine is made up of ground-up warts from bovine skin, treated with formalin. A living vaccine using chicken embryo has also been prepared but is not used much. The Foot-and-Mouth disease vaccine has been described earlier in this chapter. Live vaccines are not used, because although they may be attenuated for cattle they may not be attenuated for pigs and may still cause the disease.

A living vaccine against the Bovine Herpesvirus which causes Infectious Bovine Rhinotracheitis (IBR) is available. This vaccine is not very effective against experimental challenge and is not considered to be satisfactory for use in cattle where latent infection is to be avoided. An interesting vaccine against IBR is a temperature-sensitive mutant. This virus multiplies at the lower temperature found in the nasal mucosa but not elsewhere, and provides a self-limiting stimulus for the production of antibodies locally in the respiratory tract.

Other live-virus vaccines used in cattle include those against Bovine Virus Diarrhoea (mucosal disease), Bluetongue, Rift Valley Fever, Rinderpest, Bovine Rotavirus and Bovine Coronavirus.

7.12.2 Horses

Killed vaccines used in horses include those against Equine Papilloma, Equine Encephalomyelitis virus, Japanese B-Encephalitis virus, African Horse sickness and equine influenza virus (subtypes 1 and 2). Living attenuated vaccines are available against Equine Herpesvirus (EHV) Types 1 to 3 and Equine Arteritis virus. An interesting disease phenomenon is found with Equine Infectious Anaemia virus, against which there is no effective vaccine. In the complement fixation test used to detect antibodies to Equine Infectious Anaemia, there is competitive inhibition of the IgG antibodies by IgG (T) antibodies. The IgG (T) antibodies do not fix complement and appear in the serum of horses 4–9 weeks after infection. A complement fixation inhibition test has been used to detect the presence of IgG (T).

The IgG antibody is able to neutralise the virus but the IgG (T) antibody is not. The persistence of virus in the circulation is thought to be due to the formation of virus–antibody complexes between the IgG (T) and virus particles which are still infective. The neutralising IgG antibody cannot bind to the complexes, and the virus persists. Glomerulonephritis occurs because of the deposition of the circulating virus–antibody complexes in the glomeruli of the kidney.

The IgG antibody participates in precipitation-in-gel against virus antigens, but IgG (T) appears to be non-precipitating. Antibody-dependent cell-mediated cytotoxicity (ADCC) has been demonstrated with IgG, but this is inhibited by IgG (T).

Vaccines against Equine Infectious Anaemia are not effective, presumably because of the immune complexes that may be formed between the virus and the IgG (T) antibody.

7.12.3 Pigs

Killed vaccines used in pigs include a crystal violet-treated Swine Fever virus vaccine which is only 60% effective. In some countries, simultaneous vaccination with antiserum of high titre and virulent virus, is still practised. The attenuated live-virus vaccines have not been found to be entirely safe.

Live and killed vaccines have also been developed for Porcine Herpesvirus Type 1 and Porcine Enterovirus subtypes 1–9. A living attenuated virus vaccine has been used against Transmissible Gastroenteritis virus of pigs. This vaccine is not effective if given parenterally, because, as with many mucous membranes, a local antibody component is required to protect the epithelial cells of the small intestine. In young pigs, IgA from colostrum provides protection, and it has been suggested that IgA antibody-forming cells migrate from the gut in the sow to the mammary gland where they produce IgA. However, selective concentration of circulating IgA antibody by the mammary gland is also likely.

Vaccination with attenuated live vaccine has been carried out in sows by the intranasal as well as the intramammary route, but results of oral vaccination of newborn piglets have not been encouraging.

The swine influenza virus has been shown to cross-react with human influenza virus, and people born before 1918 often have antibodies to the porcine virus. The great pandemic of human influenza in 1918 may have been caused by a swine influenza virus, but this has not been proven. More recently, swine influenza virus has been isolated from the lungs of a boy in 1974 and from several military recruits at Fort Dix, New Jersey in 1976. It is a Type A influenza virus, while Types B and C are exclusively found in humans. As in humans, there are no effective vaccines against the variety of strains of swine influenza virus.

7.12.4   Sheep

Inactivated-virus vaccines have been used against Sheep-Pox virus and against Louping Ill (Ovine Encephalomyelitis virus). Living attenuated vaccines have been developed against Bluetongue virus, but they should not be used in pregnant ewes because they can cause abortion, due to death of the lambs *in utero*.

A living virulent vaccine against Contagious Pustular Dermatitis (Scabby Mouth) is available. This virus is communicable to humans, and care must be taken by the operator during vaccination of sheep.

7.12.5   Dogs

Inactivated-virus vaccines are available for Canine Parvovirus and Canine Adenovirus. These vaccines have added adjuvant such as aluminium hydroxide. It has also been found experimentally that modified live Feline Panleucopoenia virus vaccine will immunise dogs against Canine Parvovirus (Pollock and Carmichael, 1983). A limited replication of the feline virus was found, but the virus did not spread on contact with other dogs or cats. This has yet to be evaluated as a potential commercial vaccine of dogs against Canine Parvovirus.

A formalin-killed vaccine is available for Canine Distemper virus, but living attenuated virus vaccines are usually preferred, often as a combined Measles virus and Distemper virus vaccine, as described earlier in this chapter.

Rabies virus vaccines are often derived from the 'fixed virus' originally obtained from the Pasteur strain by passage through rabbits about 100 times. Both killed and living attenuated live-virus vaccine are often derived from this fixed virus. Attenuated vaccines for dogs and cats have two levels of virulence. The virus is adapted to duck eggs, and the 'low egg passaged' (LEP) vaccines are more potent than the 'high egg passaged' (HEP) vaccines. Therefore, the HEP (Flury) or LEP vaccines are used in adult dogs, while only the HEP vaccines are used in puppies, cats and cattle.

7.12.6   Cats

Modified live-virus vaccines are available for the three main virus diseases of cats: Feline Panleucopoenia (Feline Enteritis), Feline Rhinotracheitis (Herpesvirus Type I) and Feline Calicivirus. These vaccines are also available as a combined inactivated vaccine. For Panleucopoenia, kittens are vaccinated at 9 to 10 weeks, followed by a second dose 2–6 weeks later. The intranasal or intramuscular route can be used, and immunity is supposed to develop within 3 days and be of life-long duration. Live attenuated vaccines are not recommended for pregnant females or kittens under 4 weeks of age.

7.12.7   Avian Viruses

Almost all vaccines for avian diseases are attenuated live viruses, although fully-virulent virus is used for Fowl Pox and Infectious Bursal disease virus. The attenuated live viruses of Infectious Bronchitis, Newcastle disease and Avian Encephalitis, can be administered by eye-drop or spray. They can also be administered in the drinking water from 4 days of age. The live vaccines against Marek's disease (Fowl Herpesvirus) is administered by subcutaneous injection into day-old chicks. The Infectious Bursal disease unattenuated virus is administered via the drinking water, while unattenuated Fowl Pox virus is administered subcutaneously into the wing-web or thigh.

There is a Pigeon Pox modified live-virus vaccine which is administered by feather follicle application on the breast or thigh.

7.13   CONCLUSIONS

The virus vaccine field is very active at this time, and a variety of vaccines can reasonably be expected to appear in the next few years. These will involve several new techniques such as recombinant DNA, virus recombinants and chemically-synthesised peptides, and all these new vaccines will have to be carefully evaluated first in the laboratory and then in the field.

The possibility of using virus strains from different species for immunisation, such as Feline Panleucopoenia virus against Canine Parvovirus, will continue to be explored. Finally monoclonal antibodies seem likely to be used with many viruses to distinguish strains and promote the production of more effective vaccines than are available now.

REFERENCES

Bittle, J. L., Houghton, R. A., Alexander, H., Shinnick, T. M., Sutcliffe, J. G., Lerner, R. A., Rowlands, D. J. and Brown, F. (1982). *Nature(London)* **298**, 30–33.

Brown, A. L. and McCarthy, R. E. (1974). *Nature (London)* **248**, 344–345.

Brown, F. (1981). *Trends Biochem. Sci.* **6**, 325–327.

Campos, M., Rossi, C. R. and Lawman, M. J. P. (1982). *Infect. Immun.* **36**, 1054–1059.

Cottral, G. E., ed. (1978). 'Manual of Standardized Methods for Veterinary Microbiology', Subcommittee on Standardized Methods for Veterinary Microbiology, National Academy of Sciences, National Research Council. Comstock Publishing Associates, Ithaca, New York.

Grewal, A. S., Rouse, B. T. and Babiuk, L. A. (1977). *Infect. Immun.* **15**, 698–703.

Ho, C. K. and Babiuk, L. A. (1979a). *Immunology* **37**, 231–239.

Ho, C. K. and Babiuk, L. A. (1979b). *Immunology* **38**, 765–772.

Ho, C. K. and Babiuk, L. A. (1980). *Immunology* **39**, 231–237.

Jiminez, L., Bloom, B. R., Blume, M. R. and Oettgen, H. F. (1971). *J. Exp. Med.* **133**, 740–751.

Pollock, R. V. H. and Carmichael, L. E. (1983). *Am. J. Vet. Res.* **44,** 169–175.
Rouse, B. T., Wardley, R. C. and Babiuk, L. A. (1976). *Infect. Immun.* **13,** 1433–1441.
Smith, G. L., Mackett, M. and Moss, B. (1983). *Nature (London)* **302,** 490–495.
Wiktor, T. J. and Koprowski, H. (1980). *J. Exp. Med.* **152,** 199–212.
Yilma, T., Perryman, L. E. and McGuire, T. C. (1982). *J. Immunol.* **129,** 931–933.
Zinkernagel, R. M. and Doherty, P. C. (1975). *J. Exp. Med.* **141,** 1427–1436.

8

Immunity to
Internal Parasites

Historically, the immunisation of livestock against bacterial and viral diseases
was carried out in parallel with attempts to vaccinate against internal parasites.
However, with some notable exceptions, these attempts were much less successful than those for the microorganisms. Various reasons for this relative lack
of success have been put forward. Foremost amongst these was the idea that after
a period of evolution, the parasites adapted to the host, causing the minimum
damage possible, but allowing survival and reproduction of the parasite.

What this meant in immunological terms was that parasites were often found
not to stimulate parasite-specific antibodies in high titre. If they did, the parasite
was not killed or even injured by the antibody response. There were however
certain points in the parasite life cycle known to be susceptible to attack by the
immune system. Usually these were found in parasites which had a larval stage
which migrated through the tissues where they were more susceptible to attack
than they were as adult worms in the gut lumen. The relative resistance of adult
parasites has been attributed, among other things, to their tough integument and
the dilution of specific antibody in the gut secretions.

Nevertheless, the knowledge gained over the years has led to some quite
successful vaccines against parasites. The use of irradiated-larvae vaccines has
been successful because such larvae can stimulate an immune response without
many of the larvae growing to adulthood. These vaccines are strategically directed towards stopping parasites establishing themselves at an early stage of

their life cycle. Model systems, using parasites from domestic animals, adapted to atypical hosts such as the mouse and the guinea pig, have given insights into possible mechanisms of immunity that might apply to the natural host. However, much remains to be learned about the ways in which resistant animals can reduce their parasite burdens below those of susceptible individuals. Ultimately the application of such knowledge will be of long-term benefit in producing strains of livestock which can be grazed successfully without the repeated use of anthelmintics which is now necessary.

8.1 VACCINATION AGAINST NEMATODES

8.1.1 Irradiated-Larvae Vaccines

The major success in vaccination against nematodes is that of the *Dictyocaulus viviparus* in calves. The larvae of this parasite migrate from the gut into the blood stream and are carried into the lungs, where they are impeded from further progress around the vascular system by the narrowness of the lung capillaries and venules. Once in the lung, the parasites migrate out of the lung capillaries into the alveolar spaces, to the bronchioles and trachea, where they reproduce and lay eggs. These are swallowed and traverse the gut to end up in the faeces and further contaminate the pasture. The arrival of large numbers of larvae in the lungs of calves can produce severe respiratory distress, due sometimes to the physical blockage of the airways by the developing worms. This can be a fatal infection in many calves, and anthelmintics are not effective because they kill the worms, which then remain in the lungs causing a hypersensitivity reaction which is triggered by the arrival of new worm larvae in the lungs from the blood stream. A successful vaccine against cattle lungworm was developed by Jarrett *et al.* (1959), and this has been the only commercially-successful vaccine against nematodes in domestic animals.

More recent work with lungworm of sheep (*Dictyocaulus filaria*) has shown that irradiated-larvae vaccines may work for this parasite too. For other strongyles, it appears that this approach of vaccination with irradiated larvae is only partially effective. Work with *Trichostrongylus colubriformis* by Dineen *et al.* (1978) has demonstrated partial effectiveness of irradiated-larvae vaccines in protecting lambs against experimental challenge. The basis of this partial effectiveness has been shown to be genetic variation of the host, and this is discussed later in this chapter. The importance of vaccinating lambs lies in the necessity of protecting young animals at a time before they have developed the immunity to *T. colubriformis* that they possess as adults.

It is essentially this problem, the lack of response by the lamb, which has prevented the use of irradiated-larvae vaccines against the barber's pole worm—

Haemonchus contortus. Irradiated *H. contortus* larvae vaccines, used in pen trials, are able to immunise lambs 8–12 months of age but not 3–5 months of age, and it is precisely during this period that a vaccine is required. Adult sheep are generally more resistant to *H. contortus* than lambs, due to natural immunisation from ingestion of larvae from the pasture. The reason for the lack of responsiveness could be genetic variation, as with *T. colubriformis,* or a general lack of maturity of the cellular immune response in the young lamb.

A similar situation is found with *Ostertagia* spp. in calves. Mature cattle do develop strong resistance, but this occurs from 14 to 18 months onwards. The use of irradiated-larvae vaccines at 3 to 4 months has been unsuccessful, presumably for the same reasons that apply with larvae vaccines in lambs. Irradiated-larvae vaccines against *Strongylus vulgaris* have been tried in foals, but they have provided no significant degree of protection. Hookworm in dogs, caused by *Ancylostoma caninum,* can be prevented using an irradiated-larvae vaccine. Indeed such a vaccine was placed on the market in the United States in 1973. However, it was withdrawn from the market 2 years later because of several adverse events, which were graphically summarised by Miller (1978). In aged, chronically-infected dogs, the larvae in the vaccine migrated to the lung, where they appeared to set off a hypersensitivity reaction causing excessive coughing several weeks after the vaccination. Although this usually resolved itself after a week, this syndrome led to the vaccine being contraindicated in adult dogs, even though many of them still gained benefit from the vaccine. Secondly, a number of dogs developed clinical disease during the vaccination period due to intercurrent natural infection. Thirdly, a proportion of vaccinated puppies were shown to have hookworm eggs in their faeces even though there was no clinical disease. Thus although the vaccine was effective in protecting dogs against hookworm (only 5 of 50,000 vaccinated dogs developed proven hookworm disease), the public did not accept the vaccine as being effective against hookworm. This led to falling sales of the vaccine and its eventual withdrawal from the market due to lack of profitability for the manufacturer. As was pointed out by Miller, who did much of the development work on the vaccine, there was the alternative of anthelmintic treatment, which meant that vaccination was not the only means of control.

The reasons for the success of the *Dictyocaulus* vaccine in cattle have been summarised by Urquhart (1977, 1980). These were firstly its high degree of efficiency in practical use, that is, a 95–99% reduction in lungworm infestation. Secondly, there was the inability of anthelmintics to ameliorate the clinical signs, since larvae which died in the lungs caused as much damage as living lung-worms, due to hypersensitivity reactions. Thirdly, there was an effective distribution of the vaccine directly to the farmers for administration by their veterinarian within 2 weeks of manufacture. This circumvented the short shelf-life of 2 weeks, which is encountered with irradiated-larvae vaccines. Finally, the vaccines solved a very real problem in northern England and Scotland where farmers were faced with 100% morbidity and 5–50% mortality due to lungworm, against which no anthelmintics were available and which could only be prevented by bringing calves indoors in mid-summer for hand feeding and convalescence—a very uneconomical procedure, as pointed out by Urquhart.

The procedure for making irradiated-larvae vaccines is a balance between damage to the larvae and allowing enough worms to remain which develop to maturity. An immunogenic effect is only found if a small number of parasites persist in the host to provide an antigenic stimulus as the parasites pass through their various stages of development. Too much irradiation prevents any of the worms developing, and the vaccine provides no antigenic stimulus. Too little irradiation fails to inhibit larval development, and a clinical case of lungworm ensues. By experimentation, it has been found that the larvae are best irradiated with 40 krad and administered as two doses, 1 month apart. Other variables which must be controlled during irradiation of the larvae are temperature, numbers of larvae and the oxygen tension in the suspension, and it is important that these are rigidly standardised. Above all, it should be remembered that being a living larval parasite vaccine, it has a shelf-life of only 2 weeks, and good distribution procedures are vital for its effectiveness.

8.1.2   Attempts to Immunise with Nematode Extracts or Metabolites

Most of the successful attempts to immunise with nematode extracts or metabolites have been carried out on laboratory animals such as mice, rats and guinea pigs. The worm antigens examined include crude worm homogenates, moulting fluid from different larval stages and purified proteins extracted from different larval stages (see review by Lloyd, 1981). These antigens have been mixed with various adjuvants such as Freund's complete and incomplete adjuvants, *Bordetella pertussis* and aluminium hydroxide. In the case of *Trichostrongylus colubriformis* infection of guinea pigs, for example, it was found that the best resistance was induced with aluminium hydroxide as an adjuvant.

None of these nematode extracts or metabolites when tested in sheep, have been found to protect them against challenge with *T. colubriformis* or *Haemonchus contortus,* and it must be concluded that killed-nematode vaccines prepared in this way are unlikely to be protective in the ruminant species.

8.2   VACCINATION AGAINST CESTODES

Irradiated metacestodes have been used to immunise dogs against challenge with *Echinococcus granulosus.* However, it was found that this technique is potentially dangerous because in some animals, the irradiated cestodes regenerated and grew to maturity, shedding large numbers of infective eggs. Another approach was to irradiate the eggs of *Taenia saginata* and vaccinate cattle, but difficulties were encountered in obtaining enough eggs and in endemic areas to vaccinate calves before they became naturally infected.

Cestodes do however stimulate strong immunity in ruminants (see review by Rickard and Williams, 1982), and if antibodies are transferred to infected animals before encystment of the parasites, many of them are destroyed. This suggested that if antibodies could be induced or transferred to neonatal ruminants before exposure to cestode eggs, the larval stages could be destroyed before they encysted. It was found that lambs could be successfully immunised against *Cysticercus ovis* by enclosing oncospheres from hatched eggs in Millipore diffusion chambers and implanting these chambers intraperitoneally into the animals (Fig. 8.1). The next step was to culture the oncospheres *in vitro,* where they grew for up to 2 weeks and released metabolic products which were antigenic in sheep. Intramuscular injection of concentrated culture supernates with Freund's complete adjuvant into 12-week-old lambs provided protection against challenge with *Taenia ovis* eggs 6 weeks later.

Another approach was to immunise the ewes 4 weeks before lambing, to boost titres of antibodies to *C. ovis* in colostrum by newborn lambs. The ingestion and absorption of these antibodies in colostrum by newborn lambs provided them with a high degree of protection from natural infection grazing on pastures which were heavily infected with *T. ovis* eggs. These lambs were then actively immu-

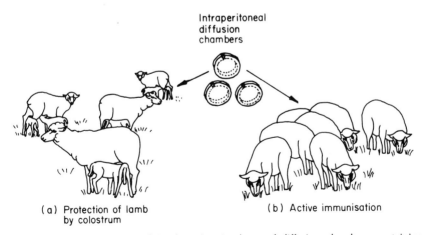

Intraperitoneal
diffusion
chambers

(a) Protection of lamb   (b) Active immunisation
    by colostrum

Fig. 8.1. The intraperitoneal implantation in sheep of diffusion chambers containing *Cysticercus ovis* oncospheres leads to the production of serum antibodies which either (a) protect newborn lambs via the colostrum or (b) directly protect sheep which are grazing pastures contaminated with parasite eggs.

nised at 2 months of age with culture supernates, when the colostral antibodies had largely been metabolised. However, the immunisation of dogs with the metabolic products from a closely-related cestode, *Cysticercus pisiformis*, had no protective ability against challenge with adult *Taenia pisiformis*. This is not the rule, however, and it was shown by Herd *et al.* (1975) that the metabolic products from adult *Echinococcus granulosus* maintained in culture and then administered to dogs, increased resistance to infection with *E. granulosus* and decreased egg production from the remaining parasites.

In cattle, there is a similarly high degree of protection against *Cysticercus bovis* provided by ingestion of colostrum containing specific antibodies. Oncospheres have been injected into the mammary gland to boost titres specific to *C. bovis* in colostrum. However, metabolic products of oncospheres can also be used to good effect for pre-partum immunisation of cows.

In summary, it seems that vaccination of sheep against *C. ovis* and cattle against *C. bovis* is quite practicable using the non-infective metabolic products of oncospheres grown in tissue culture. The immunisation of dogs against *E. granulosus* using metabolic products of adult cestodes also looks promising. However, so far, there are no commercially-produced vaccines against cestodes, although the potential for such vaccines would appear to be high.

8.3 VACCINATION AGAINST TREMATODES

Irradiated schistosomula of *Schistosoma matthei* and *Schistosoma bovis* have been used by Taylor *et al.* (1979) to immunise sheep and cattle against infection with schistosomes. The vaccine was given subcutaneously or intramuscularly in sheep and caused 60% reduction in the level of infection after challenge, compared with control animals, for a period as long as 55 weeks after immunisation. A most encouraging effect of vaccination was the significantly-higher growth rate in vaccinated animals compared with control animals, and this was also associated with lower faecal and tissue egg counts and lower adult worm counts. Therefore this vaccine clearly has economic advantages for animals in endemic areas despite a reduction of only 60% in adult worm counts in vaccinated animals.

Irradiated metacercariae of *Fasciola hepatica* have proved ineffective in immunising sheep and cattle against 'liver fluke' disease. Little natural resistance to reinfection of these hosts has been observed, so it is hardly surprising that irradiated vaccines do not work. Pigs appear to be naturally resistant to *Fasciola* infection, and vaccination would conceivably work in pigs. However, the hosts which would most benefit from a vaccine appear to respond only weakly to natural infection, and a vaccine for ruminants does not look promising.

8.4 MECHANISMS OF IMMUNITY TO INTERNAL PARASITES

The study of immunity to parasites contrasts with that of immunity to micro-organisms, in that the parasites are too large to be directly phagocytosed. Therefore, damage to the worms is mediated by antibodies or by soluble factors produced by the lymphoid and myeloid cells. The relative importance of these two kinds of responses varies with the parasite examined and the host to which it is adapted. For example, with guinea pigs infected with *Trichostrongylus colubriformis,* protective immunity can be passively transferred by mesenteric lymph node cells but not by serum containing antibodies (Wagland and Dineen, 1965). In contrast, lambs can be protected against the larval forms of *Cysticercus ovis* by transfer of colostral antibodies from the mother.

The mechanisms by which hosts rid themselves of parasites include most of the manifestations of the immune response, such as immediate hypersensitivity, delayed hypersensitivity and colostral antibody. These will be discussed in turn, with examples of particular parasites which involve these responses.

8.4.1 Immediate Hypersensitivity

In sheep, it was shown by Stewart (1953) that a 'self-cure' phenomenon could be demonstrated with *Haemonchus contortus.* This 'self-cure' phenomenon was found after ingestion of infective larvae, usually during the flush of pasture growth in the spring. Its effects were on adult worms in the abomasum, which were rapidly rejected and expelled. The reaction was blocked by treatment of sheep with anti-histamines, and this led to the idea of vaso-active amines, such as 5-hydroxytryptamine, being the effector molecules responsible for expulsion of the parasites from the sensitised sheep. The demonstration of homocytotropic antibody in sheep also provided impetus for examining immediate hypersensitivity in the gut, and attempts were made to correlate mast cell numbers in the gut submucosa with rejection of the parasites. In particular, it became evident that the so-called globule leucocytes were either degranulated mast cells or closely related to mast cells, and were associated with the rejection of worms by the intestinal mucosa.

However, in contrast to laboratory animals, 'self-cure' in sheep is not necessarily followed by protection against reinfection, and larvae which initiated the response can develop to maturity and cause severe infection. Thus the putative IgE antibody which initiates this reaction does not appear to provide long-term protection, even though prolonged production of IgE is characteristic of helminth infections in humans and animals. In particular, the *Ascaris lumbricoides* nematode which infects pigs, also infects humans and produces extreme immediate hypersensitivity to the components of the parasite, such as the coelomic fluid.

Indeed, Ascariasis of humans has been diagnosed using a serum test for specific IgE antibodies to *Ascaris* body fluid in the radioallergoabsorbent test (RAST). This is commercially available as the ^{125}I-labelled Phadebas anti-IgE test (Pharmacia, Uppsala, Sweden) and is carried out as a radioimmunoassay (O'Donnell and Mitchell, 1978). *Ascaris* antigen is adsorbed to aliquots of cyanogen bromide (CNBr)-activated Sepharose which has been pre-coated with serial dilutions of human serum containing IgE antibodies to the parasite. After washing the Sepharose, a standard curve is constructed by adding a standard amount of ^{125}I-labelled anti-IgE, washing and counting the Sepharose beads in the γ counter. A measure of non-specific binding is obtained by adding umbilical-cord serum, which should contain no IgE, and subtracting this background count from the standard curve counts.

This RAST assay works well for estimating specific IgE antibodies in human serum because the anti-IgE is specific for the human immunoglobulin. Although cross-reactivity between human and bovine IgE immunoglobulins has been demonstrated, there have been few quantitative studies with domestic animals on the IgE levels during parasitic infections. It would appear that boosting the levels of specific IgE antibodies is not necessarily beneficial for host resistance to parasites.

8.4.2   Delayed Hypersensitivity

Much of the evidence for delayed hypersensitivity in parasite infections comes from the detection of specific antigen-sensitive lymphocytes in the blood of parasitised animals. This has been demonstrated for *Haemonchus contortus, Ostertagia* spp. and *Trichostrongylus colubriformis* antigens in sheep. The test measures the uptake of [^{3}H]thymidine by blood lymphocytes *in vitro* in the presence of parasite antigen. Usually the worm antigen is a saline extract of homogenised worms or exsheathing fluid obtained from larval cultures. This material is passed through a Millipore filter to remove bacteria, but by its very nature, the worm larval antigen or saline extract cannot be freed of bacterial endotoxin. Therefore a strong possibility exists that some of the lymphocyte responsiveness to the parasite antigen is the result of B-cell stimulation by endotoxin. It is known that animals which are sensitised to bacterial endotoxin respond with transformation of B-cells and that in some species, unsensitised B-cells also respond.

Nevertheless, experiments have been conducted which show a rising level of responsiveness of lambs to repeated challenge with *T. colubriformis* larvae (Adams and Cripps, 1977), and this is most likely to be due to lymphocyte responsiveness to specific worm antigen. No reports are available on purified fractions of worm antigen, so it is not known which component of the parasite is responsible for lymphocyte stimulation. From results of IgE binding to separated

Ascaris components, it appears likely that the response is to multiple antigens, each producing a weaker stimulation alone than mixed together.

The involvement of the thymus in expulsion of worms has been demonstrated in *Nippostrongylus brasiliensis* infection of rats and mice. In these species, removal of the thymus or treatment with anti-lymphocyte serum, hinders the normal expulsion of parasites compared with controls. Although techniques for thymectomy in lambs and calves have been developed, this particular point of thymus dependency has not been examined in sheep or cattle.

Delayed hypersensitivity at the gut submucosa is difficult to measure, although it certainly does occur in cattle with *Mycobacterium paratuberculosis* (Johne's disease) infections of the gut. In sheep, cannulation of the intestinal lymphatics of parasitised sheep, allows collection of lymphocytes recirculating through the mesenteric lymph nodes. Among these lymphocytes are some which are reactive to the parasite antigen, measured *in vitro* by [^{3}H]thymidine uptake by the cells (Adams and Cripps, 1977). Therefore, reactive lymphocytes are present in close proximity to the gut, and it appears highly likely that delayed-hypersensitivity responses to parasite antigens take place in the gut submucosa.

The importance of delayed hypersensitivity in parasite immunity is really not known. The direct effects of lymphokines on parasites appear to be very little, and macrophage activation appears to be ineffective in the gut with parasites which are not phagocytosed. The larval stages of parasites do however seem to be susceptible to attack, and the oncospheres of taeniid worms stimulate a strong mononuclear cell reaction as they migrate into the tissues of immunised animals. Indeed it has been suggested by Rickard (1974) that the larval cestodes become coated with antibody and avoid attack by sensitised lymphocytes as the larvae migrate through the tissues.

In addition to lymphocytes, the tracks of larval parasites are often surrounded by eosinophils. These appear to be associated with hypersensitivity, but their exact function is not known. Considerable work has been carried out on larval schistosomes which have been coated with antibody and eosinophils experimentally in tissue culture. The eosinophils appear to inhibit the development of the larvae, but the mechanism is still not known. It has been suggested that hydrogen peroxide, eosinophil lysosomal basic proteins and arginase, all have a role in destruction of the schistosomula. Such mediators are produced by granulocytes and macrophages, but lymphocytes have also been shown to have a direct effect in destroying the schistosomula in tissue culture. Lymphocytes stimulated with phytohaemagglutinin (PHA) have an augmented ability to kill these parasites (Ellner *et al.*, 1982). There is increased binding of the lymphocytes to the schistosomula in the PHA-stimulated cultures compared with controls. This increased killing is not associated with activity in the culture supernates, and if lymphokines are involved, their effects must be very short-range at the interface between the lymphocytes and the surface of the schistosomula.

8.4.3 Antibody

As mentioned earlier, the only example of effective humoral immunity against parasites is that of the transfer of immunity to larval cestodes in the colostrum of sheep and cattle. This apparently prevents oncospheres from progressing past the gut submucosa and making their way to the liver. There are some larvae, however, which escape this humoral antibody barrier and eventually form cysts. The numbers of these cysts in passively-immunised animals is greatly reduced compared with unimmunised sheep. However, it has been postulated by Rickard (1974) that these larvae become coated with specific antibody and escape attack from the cellular response of the T-lymphocytes. This is because the antibody-coated larvae and cysts are not recognised as being foreign by the sensitised lymphocytes. Even this escape is only temporary, and ultimately cysts which have escaped initial immunological attack, seem to succumb and then degenerate, often to form calcified deposits at the site of the original cyst.

In nematode infections of sheep, high levels of total IgA, as well as specific antibody of the IgA class, have been induced in abomasal mucus with irradiated *Haemonchus contortus* larvae vaccines. Unfortunately immunity appears to work well only under experimental conditions. Lambs are well-protected against *H. contortus* experimental challenge, but in the natural field conditions there appears to be little immunity to *H. contortus* parasites throughout the life of the animal. Elevated IgA levels have been demonstrated in intestinal secretion of sheep infected with *Trichostrongylus colubriformis* and *H. contortus* in pigs infected with *Ascaris suum* and in rats infected with *Nippostrongylus brasiliensis*. However, evidence is lacking for a direct protective role of these IgA immunoglobulins, and the immunity found could equally be due to IgG immunoglobulins, lymphocytes and non-lymphoid effector cells, such as eosinophils, polymorphs and mast cells.

8.5 DIAGNOSTIC TECHNIQUES IN PARASITISM

For most parasite infections, faecal egg counts provide a direct diagnosis. However, in the case of hydatid cysts and the *Cysticercus* infections of sheep and cattle, no eggs are released in the faeces and the evidence of infection can usually only be found at postmortem. It would therefore be a useful procedure to be able to diagnose cysts in sheep and cattle to assess the extent of the problem before they are sent to the abattoirs.

The use of immunological techniques to diagnose *Echinococcus granulosus* in humans has been practised for many years. An intradermal test (Casoni test) has been used to detect immediate hypersensitivity to cyst fluid antigen in humans. This is a sensitive test but not a very specific one. Evidence from a number of sources suggests that the cyst fluid is anti-complementary and activates serum complement spontaneously, causing a high incidence of non-specific reactions in the skin. The skin test has been contemplated, but not used, in the diagnosis of hydatid disease in sheep.

A complement fixation test has also been used in human patients, but again this gives a high proportion of false-positive results in patients with hepatic, pulmonary and other systemic disorders. An indirect fluorescent antibody test has also been used, and this is extremely sensitive. However, it also suffers the problems of false-positive reactions. An indirect haemagglutination test has been developed for the diagnosis of hydatid disease in humans. In this test, sheep hydatid cyst fluid is attached to sheep or human red cells using tannic acid, and the test is easily carried out in Microtiter plates.

The indirect haemagglutination test has been used in New Zealand with cyst fluid of *Taenia hydatigena* or *E. granulosus* to diagnose experimental cestode infection of sheep (Blundell-Hasell, 1969). Sheep reared in a tapeworm-free environment were mostly lacking in antibodies to either antigen. Following ingestion of eggs of *T. hydatigena,* these sheep developed antibody to the homologous antigen. A problem was found with naturally-infected sheep in that, although no cysts were found at postmortem, there had been a previous contact from ingestion of eggs or resolution of a few cysts and this was enough to stimulate serum antibody. Furthermore, the presence of cysts was not associated with the higher range of haemagglutination titres. The conclusion was that neither the parasite species of the cysts nor their viability could be predicted by the higher titres to the homologous cyst fluid antigen compared with the heterologous cyst fluid antigen.

This approach was developed further by Craig *et al.* (1981), using the monoclonal antibody technique. Crude extracts from cystic larva or adult tapeworm stages of *T. hydatigena, T. ovis, T. saginata* or *E. granulosus* were administered to mice, and after the acquisition of serum antibodies, spleen and lymph node cells were harvested for fusion with myeloma cells in the standard hybridoma technique. A solid-phase radioimmunoassay or enzyme-linked immunosorbent assay (ELISA) was used to detect antibodies in sheep serum by competitive inhibition of binding. Sera from sheep exposed to *T. hydatigena* eggs were positive, but sera from sheep infected with *T. ovis* were also positive. However serum from *E. granulosus*-infected sheep were negative. This suggests that a similar monoclonal antibody test could for example be used, in cattle to distinguish those infected with *Fasciola hepatica* or *E. granulosus* from those infected with *T. saginata.* This is a highly-welcome increase in specificity, because previous work has shown that these three parasites strongly cross-react in other tests.

For sheep, it appears that even with the high degree of specificity of hybridoma antibodies, *T. ovis, E. granulosus* and *T. hydatigena* may sometimes still strongly cross-react in this test. Therefore, work is continuing, using an affinity-binding technique to purify specific parasite antigens for use in the test to increase its specificity. These attempts may well be successful, but the question of non-progressive infection in sheep which causes the appearance of specific antibodies in serum, appears likely to remain.

8.6   GENETIC RESISTANCE TO PARASITE INFECTION

The existence of differences within species of animals in resistance or suscep- tibility to parasites has been known for some time. The knowledge of the herita- ble nature of the resistance raises the possibility of selectively breeding lines of animals which have a clearly- defined range of responses to a particular infection, so that the mechanisms of resistance can be studied. However, a potential obsta- cle which may arise in domestic animals is the necessity for parasite resistance to be linked to normal rates of wool growth, milk production and meat production. This point has yet to be explored and evaluated adequately. Nevertheless, these inherited traits, conferring resistance to nematode parasites for example, are only now being explored as a possible alternative to the continued use of anthelmin- tics. This has been stimulated particularly by the emergence of anthelmintic- resistant strains of helminth parasites which threaten to cause considerable eco- nomic loss, particularly in sheep production.

Sheep have been bred for resistance or susceptibility to *Haemonchus contor- tus, Ostertagia circumcincta* and *Trichostrongylus colubriformis*. In the case of *H. contortus* the resistance is inherited as a simple dominant characteristic. At one stage this was thought to be due to the inheritance of the particular haemo- globin type (Hb/A) which conferred resistance, while inheritance of another haemoglobin type (Hb/B) was associated with susceptibility. It was thought that the possession of Hb/A increased the ability of sheep to withstand the effects of blood loss due to *H. contortus* and in particular, to maintain normal haematological values for packed-cell volume and haemoglobin content of the erythrocytes. More recent work suggests however, that the ability of these sheep to resist infection is due to the development of brisk hypersensitivity reactions which lead to 'self-cure'. This is thought to reflect a general ability of the Hb/A- type sheep to mount an immune response to parasites which regulates the devel- opment of worm populations. There are breed differences however, and it is possible that the ability to mount a 'self-cure' reaction is due to breed rather than haemoglobin type. Nevertheless within breeds, the Hb/A type is still associated with resistance to *H. contortus*.

This association between haemoglobin type and resistance has not been found with other parasites of sheep such as *T. colubriformis*. Sheep can be bred for resistance to this parasite and at the same time exhibit resistance to another parasite, *O. circumcincta,* but not *H. contortus.* Dineen and his colleagues have bred sheep on the basis of the observed bimodal distribution of *T. colubriformis* faecal egg counts in randomly-bred young lambs. If animals are selected on the basis of faecal egg counts, they can be segregated into 'high responders' with low egg counts and 'low responders' with high egg counts (Fig. 8.2). Assortative mating of high-responder ewes with high-responder rams produces progeny which are also high responders (Windon *et al.,* 1980). Heritability of resistance is high and has been calculated to be 0.35. Similarly, susceptibility in a low-responder line of sheep has been calculated to have a heritability of 0.51.

The immunological basis for the resistance of the high responders is not known, but it appears that the activity of the reticuloendothelial system may be higher in these sheep than in the low responders. The antibodies to *T. colubriformis* antigen, which develop after vaccination with irradiated larvae and challenge with normal larvae, appear earlier and reach higher titres in the high responders

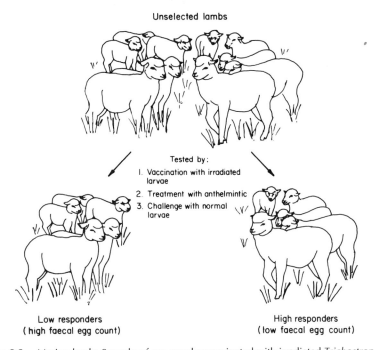

Fig. 8.2. Merino lambs 8 weeks of age may be vaccinated with irradiated *Trichostrongylus colubriformis* larvae, which protects about half of them from experimental challenge with 20,000 normal larvae at 12 weeks. This natural division into high and low responders is heritable, and the progeny from matings of high-responder rams with high-responder ewes are also high responders. The same holds for the low-responder rams and ewes. In this way sheep can be bred to be responsive to vaccination against a helminth parasite.

than in the low responders. However, a most interesting finding is that the ovine lymphocyte antigens (OLA) of the high responders contain a particular type (SY1) in a frequency of 70%, compared with 22% in the low responders. Thus, the response to this parasite may involve a particular *Ir* gene allele which is selected in the resistant sheep. The possibility is discussed in more detail in Chapter 10 on immunogenetics.

For cattle, a similar segregation of Friesian calves into high and low responders has been achieved with *Cooperia oncophera* infections by Kloosterman *et al.* (1978). Using an indirect fluorescent antibody test, a low but significant correlation between increased antibody titre and resistance was found. Breed differences have also been found, and it is known that resistance is often associated with the *Bos indicus* contribution in cross-breeding with *Bos taurus*. However, within both purebred *B. indicus* and *B. taurus* breeds, there appears to be a distribution from highly-susceptible to highly-resistant individuals. The possibility of the bovine lymphocyte antigens (BoLA) being involved in resistance or susceptibility of cattle to parasites has yet to be closely examined.

For other species, such as laboratory rodents, there are many examples of strain differences in resistance to parasites. For example, certain strains of mice and rats have been bred which are highly resistant to *Trichinella spiralis,* and strains of guinea pigs which are resistant to *Trichostrongylus colubriformis*. Again, in the guinea pig, resistance to *T. colubriformis* has been linked with an *Ir* gene locus. However, in other domestic species such as dogs and horses, little or nothing is known about innate resistance or susceptibility to parasites.

8.7 GENERAL CONCLUSIONS

From the work described herein it can be concluded that the best immunity is stimulated in domestic animals to parasites using irradiated-larvae vaccines. These living vaccines have their drawbacks, such as short shelf-life and production difficulties. The ideal vaccine would be a killed vaccine or an extract of the parasite which stimulated protective immunity.

In the past, such an approach seemed unlikely to succeed because of the difficulty in obtaining enough antigen from the parasites for vaccination of large numbers of sheep or cattle. With the advent of recombinant DNA techniques for production of proteins in *E. coli* organisms, it now seems very likely that the protective antigens against parasites will be produced in sufficient quantity for field trials to be carried out on a large number of animals.

The hope for the future is that these genetically-engineered antigens could be put to use in vaccinating animals which have been selected for responsiveness to vaccination against the parasite. There is the prospect that with this two-handed approach to the problem, results will be produced which will lead to vaccines for livestock against parasitic infections.

REFERENCES

Adams, D. B. and Cripps, A. W. (1977). *Aust. J. Exp. Biol. Med. Sci.* **55,** 509–522.

Blundell-Hasell, S. K. (1969). *Aust. Vet. J.* **45,** 334–336.

Craig, P. S., Hocking, R. E., Mitchell, G. F. and Rickard, M. D. (1981). *Parasitology* **83,** 303–317.

Dineen, J. K., Gregg, P. and Lascelles, A. K. (1978). *Int. J. Parasitol.* **8,** 59–63.

Ellner, J. J., Olds, G. R., Lee, C. W., Kleinherz, M. E. and Edmonds, K. L. (1982). *J. Clin. Invest.* **70,** 369–378.

Herd, R. P., Chappel, R. J. and Biddell, D. (1975). *Int. J. Parasitol.* **5,** 395–399.

Jarrett, W. F. H., Jennings, F. W., McIntyre, W. I. M., Mulligan, W., Sharp, N. C. C. and Urquhart, G. M. (1959). *Am. J. Vet. Res.* **20,** 522–526.

Kloosterman, A., Albers, G. A. A. and Van den Brink, R. (1978). *Vet. Parasitol.* **4,** 353–368.

Lloyd, S. (1981). *Parasitology* **83,** 225–242.

Miller, T. A. (1978). *Adv. Parasitol.* **16,** 333–359.

O'Donnell, I. J. and Mitchell, G. F. (1978). *Aust. J. Biol. Sci.* **31,** 459–487.

Rickard, M. D. (1974). *Z. Parasitenkd.* **44,** 203–209.

Rickard, M. D. and Williams, J. F. (1982). *Adv. Parasitol* **21,** 229–296.

Stewart, D. F. (1953). *Aust. J. Agric. Res.* **4,** 100–117.

Taylor, M. G., James, E. R., Bickle, Q., Hussein, M. F., Andrews, B. J., Robinson, A. R. and Nelson, G. S. (1979). *J. Helminthol.* **53,** 1–5.

Urquhart, G. M. (1977). *Colloq.—Inst. Natl. Sante Rech. Med.* **72,** 263–274.

Urquhart, G. M. (1980). *Vet. Parasitol.* **6,** 217–239.

Wagland, B. M. and Dineen, J. K. (1965). *Aust. J. Exp. Biol. Med. Sci.* **43,** 429–438.

Windon, R. G., Dineen, J. K. and Kelly, J. D. (1980). *Int. J. Parasitol.* **10,** 65–73.

9

Immunity to
External Parasites

The immunity to external parasites primarily involves reactions to the attachment of the parasites to the skin. The protozoal diseases that these parasites transmit, on the other hand, are usually blood-borne and involve humoral and cell-mediated immunity similar to that found with bacterial infections.

In domestic animals, the major external parasites are ticks, fleas, lice, mites and blow-fly larvae. In many of these infestations no appreciable immunity has been demonstrated, and animals are fully susceptible to reinfestation after removal of the parasites with insecticide treatment. The insect bites do, however, produce hypersensitivities, and these can be of direct concern to the veterinarian in treating pets such as dogs and cats with the condition of 'summer eczema'.

The question does remain, are these hypersensitivity reactions a form of immunity, which could be directed by strategic vaccination towards reducing the external parasite burdens in domestic animals? At the moment, this question has yet to be answered, but the bulk of the evidence suggests that skin hypersensitivity can be more disadvantageous to the host than to the parasite.

9.1 SKIN HYPERSENSITIVITIES

The early classification of skin hypersensitivities into immediate and delayed hypersensitivity—which reached peaks at 6 hours and 48 hours, respectively—

proved to be inadequate for the classification of very early immediate-hypersensitivity reactions at 30 minutes and those intermediate reactions which reached a peak between 12 and 24 hours—the so-called Jones–Mote reactions.

Therefore Coombs and Gell in 1963 proposed a classification of skin reactions into four types, and this has gained wide acceptance and helped to clarify a previously-confused perception of skin reactions.

9.1.1 Type I Hypersensitivity

The classical wheal (oedema) and flare (erythema) reaction observed in human skin, which appears after only 30 minutes from the time of injection of the eliciting antigen or 'reagin' is known as Type I hypersensitivity. It was early work by Prausnitz and Kustner in 1921 which demonstrated that the human forearm could be passively sensitised by the intradermal injection of serum from an antigen-sensitive donor. The subsequent injection of the same sites 24 hours later (the P–K test), provoked an immediate wheal-and-flare reaction. The basis of the hypersensitivity has subsequently been shown to be the IgE antibodies in the serum from the sensitised donor. These IgE antibodies attach to tissue mast cells in the skin. Contact with antigen causes the release of histamine, which in turn, causes the increased capillary permeability, oedema and inflammation found in the skin reaction.

The mechanism by which this is accomplished is not precisely known, but intracellular proteases and phospholipases have been suggested to cause the release of the histamine from the mast cell granules. The initial membrane event, which is the signal for the release of histamine and leukotriene C (formerly slow-reacting substance of anaphylaxis), has been attributed to adenyl cyclase, which converts adenosine triphosphate (ATP) to cyclic adenosine monophosphate (cAMP). This cAMP may initiate glucose oxidation, lipolysis and an increase in lysosomal membrane permeability, releasing the histamine and leukotrienes. This mechanism has yet to be proven to be the correct one.

9.1.2 Type II Hypersensitivity

Type II hypersensitivity is primarily a cytotoxic reaction of antibodies which combine with cell receptors or with antigen adsorbed to cells, in the presence of complement. Transfusion reactions and haemolytic disease of the newborn are both Type II reactions.

With protozoan diseases it has been suggested that the severe haemolytic episodes which occur in malaria in humans or in Babesiosis of cattle may involve Type II reactions. There is some evidence that the parasite antigens are adsorbed to red cells, which then become the target of attack by leucocytes or subject to direct lysis by serum complement. Certainly in the case of Theileriosis there seems to be antibody-dependent cell-mediated cytotoxicity (ADCC) directed towards transformed lymphocytes, which are assumed to have parasite antigens expressed on their surfaces.

9.1.3   Type III Hypersensitivity

Type III hypersensitivity is the one which is represented classically by the Arthus reaction. This reaction is found in humans or animals which have been transfused with foreign serum proteins. In the case of the human, it was usually the horse serum component of tetanus antitoxin. The reinjection intravenously of the foreign protein some time later, leads to the formation of antigen–antibody complexes and even aggregates which are trapped in the peripheral capillaries and venules as they circulate through them. Complement is activated and the C3 component bound, and this attracts neutrophils from which lysosomal enzymes and cationic proteins are released near the basement membranes of the capillaries. The resulting oedema is due to the increased capillary permeability of these blood vessels. There is no appreciable fixation of antibody to mast cells, since IgG, not IgE, is involved in the reactions. Nevertheless, it is thought that the FcG receptors on the neutrophils are involved in the attachment of the complexes to the neutrophils, with their subsequent phagocytosis and degranulation of the neutrophils.

Immediate-hypersensitivity reactions can also occur after subcutaneous injection of bacterial, viral or parasite antigens, and these normally reach a peak 6 hours after injection. They can also occur in the mammary glands of sheep and cattle which are sensitised to streptococcal and staphylococcal antigens and which subsequently become infected with these bacteria. Although not the only cause of neutrophils in milk, the migration of these cells into milk in the early stages of mastitis can be in response to the formation of antigen–antibody complexes between the bacteria and the specific antibodies in the milk.

9.1.4   Type IV Hypersensitivity

Classically a mononuclear cell reaction, Type IV hypersensitivity occurs as a delayed reaction in cattle skin, for example, which reaches a peak at 48 to 72 hours after injection of tuberculin into hypersensitive cattle. The histology of the injection site shows an initial accumulation of neutrophils during the first 12 hours, but the cells infiltrating the site gradually change in type towards the mononuclear cell. Both selective migration into the site and lymphocyte proliferation appear to be involved in this accumulation of cells. Lymphocytes release a migration inhibition factor which is thought to inhibit the migration of macrophages and perhaps polymorphonuclear leucocytes from the site. This migration inhibition factor can be assayed *in vitro* by measuring migration of macrophages out of a capillary tube, and during the early 1970s a considerable amount of work was carried out to see if this could be used as an *in vitro* test for delayed hypersensitivity. However, it was found that the initial response of lymphocytes to tuberculin could be far more conveniently measured using [³H]thymidine uptake, and the macrophage migration inhibition test is now used only for research purposes.

At the same time as they release migration inhibition factor, lymphocytes also release a so-called skin-reactive factor which in an isolated form, can elicit skin reactions on its own. This has been shown in guinea pigs, but at the moment there are no reports on experiments with skin-reactive factor in domestic animals. Similarly a 'lymph node permeability factor' has been demonstrated with guinea pigs but has yet to be studied in domestic animals. It is possible that the thickness of the bovine skin would preclude detection of the relatively-weak response to the skin-reactive factor, although histological studies would confirm or deny this possibility.

Delayed hypersensitivity has been demonstrated in dogs to the oral secretions of fleas such as *Ctenocephalides canis* and in guinea pigs to the bite of ticks such as *Dermacentor andersoni*.

9.2 ALLERGIC RESPONSES TO FLEA BITES

The allergic response to the oral secretions of fleas was studied by Feingold, Benjamini and Michaeli (1968). They obtained the oral secretions by a novel technique, which was to allow thousands of fleas to feed through membranes on warm distilled water. The intradermal injection of this distilled water, containing the flea oral secretion, elicited skin reactions in previously-exposed guinea pigs. The allergen could only sensitise guinea pigs if it was injected with Freund's complete adjuvant; if injected alone, the allergen could not induce sensitivity.

So it was suggested that there was a hapten effect in which the oral-secretion antigen (MW 2000–6000) bound to the host protein, becoming more antigenic in the process. Something like this was needed to explain the natural hypersensitivity which fleas themselves could induce. It was found that collagen bound some of the oral secretion and that this acid-soluble hapten derived from skin biopsies could itself induce hypersensitivity without Freund's complete adjuvant. A low molecular weight component, which was obtained from the fluid surrounding a dialysis sac containing the hapten of collagen and oral secretion, could only induce hypersensitivity with Freund's complete adjuvant. The haptenic complex was only formed at acidic or basic pH, not at neutral pH.

Experiments with guinea pigs exposed to flea bites showed that no reactions occurred until the fifth day, when previously-bitten sites flared up. Thus it seemed likely that the hapten remained at the bite site and was available as an

antigen for stimulation of sensitised lymphocytes or for combination with reaginic antibodies.

This phenomenon could also explain the summer eczema and flea-bite dermatitis in dogs in which only one new flea bite is required to trigger old flea-bite
sites—years after the initial sensitisation.

9.3 DESENSITISATION TO FLEA BITES

It has been noted by veterinarians that hypersensitivity is mostly encountered
in dogs infested with only a relatively small number of fleas or in dogs that are
regularly treated with an insecticide to remove fleas. In stray dogs, with large
numbers of fleas, the hypersensitive condition is relatively rare.

Therefore, it appears that dogs can become desensitised naturally but at the
cost of having large numbers of fleas in their coat. Attempts have been made to
desensitise dogs artificially by the repeated injection of oral secretions from
fleas. This is not always effective, perhaps because of the difficulty in standard-
ising the powdered flea extract used for desensitisation. In some dogs, the
hypersensitivity becomes worse than before desensitisation was attempted. However, in other hypersensitive dogs, intradermal injection of this flea antigen
induces hyposensitivity for 5 to 6 weeks and in some cases, up to 6 months.
There is unfortunately no way of permanently desensitising dogs to flea bites.

9.4 INTRADERMAL ALLERGY TESTS IN DOGS

The flea-bite allergy is, of course, very important in dogs, but allergies to
other antigens are also of considerable importance. It was work by Halliwell *et
al.* (1972) which showed that there is a close antigenic relationship between
human IgE and canine IgE. Furthermore, dogs closely parallel humans in their
predisposition to allergy, which appears to be inherited as an autosomal gene
mutation controlling histamine release (Fig. 9.1).

It was also observed in the course of this work that a spontaneously ragweed-
sensitive dog produced anti-DNP (dinitrophenol) IgE reaginic antibody following the injection of DNP–ragweed pollen. In contrast, the repeated exposure to
DNP–canine serum albumin, failed to do so. Thus it appeared that the pollen
carrier was a crucial factor in the induction of hypersensitivity to this hapten.

Dogs become hypersensitive to a wide variety of allergens such as housedust,
housedust mites, animal dandruffs, fleas, grasses, pollens, trees and fungi. In
fact, commercially-available allergy-testing kits for the human can be used for
testing allergy in dogs (Willemse and Van den Brom, 1982). The test carried out
is an intradermal injection of antigen followed by measurement of the wheal

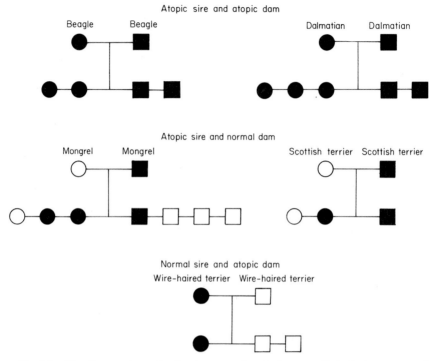

Fig. 9.1. The diagram shows the development of atopic hypersensitivity in the progeny of atopic dogs after a natural exposure to environmental allergenic materials. ● Atopic female; ■ atopic male; ○ normal female; □ normal male. (Reproduced by permission from Schwartzman, Rockey and Halliwell (1971), *Clin. Exp. Immunol.* **9**, 549–569.)

diameter (Type I hypersensitivity) 20–30 minutes afterwards. Standard reactions to dilutions of histamine diphosphate in dog skin have been used to grade responses to the allergens. The term 'histamine-reactive value' (Rh) has been used to express skin reaction intensity. Another standard used to measure the amount of allergen injected is the protein nitrogen unit (PNU), which is defined as 1 unit = 10.5 mg nitrogen precipitated with phosphotungstic acid in 1 ml. Another unit which is used is the Noon unit, which is 1 ml of extract made from 1 mg of pollen in 1 litre of extracting fluid.

These differing units reflect the problem of standardisation in allergy tests which is the result of not knowing the exact nature of the eliciting reagin. The determinant group of each allergenic compound may only be a very small component of the whole, and this makes difficult the standardisation of amounts for injection as a skin test allergen.

As with flea-bite allergy, atopic reactions to other allergens, such as housedust in dogs, are usually only of diagnostic value, and attempts to desensitise dogs permanently have generally been unsuccessful.

9.5 CONTACT ALLERGY

Contact allergy to ragweed pollen is found in dogs in the United States and Canada. However, it is in the pig that an experimental system has been set up by Balfour and her associates, to investigate the basis for contact sensitivity.

Pigs may be made hypersensitive to the dinitrophenyl (DNP) chemical group by painting the skin with dinitrofluorobenzene (DNFB). The progression of the allergen from the skin to the regional lymph node has been examined by the cannulation of the afferent lymphatics in pigs at a site draining a skin patch painted with DNFB (McFarlin and Balfour, 1973). The DNFB was found to bind strongly to serum proteins and also to mononuclear cells, which are found floating free in the afferent lymph. In particular the DNFB binds to large mononuclear cells in the skin known as Langerhans cells. These cells resemble macrophages in most respects except that they are relatively non-adherent cells which do not have some of the surface antigens associated with monocytes. They are adapted for movement along afferent lymphatic vessels to the regional lymph nodes where they are filtered out and presumably become part of the population of dendritic cells in the node. It is thought that these Langerhans cells provide an antigenic focus in the lymph node for DNFB-sensitised lymphocytes. It is known that human Langerhans cells have large amounts of the *HLA-D* locus antigen on their surfaces, and this would make them ideal for presenting antigen associated with a major histocompatibility complex (MHC) gene product in the way that is thought to be required for many immune responses.

Endothelial cells in the walls of capillaries also have large amounts of *HLA-D* on their surfaces, and it has been suggested that these cells too may provide a focus for antigenic stimulation of lymphocytes in the skin. Confirmation of these findings in humans for domestic animals has not been made, but it seems that this might be a useful avenue for research into the skin diseases of animals.

9.6 IMMUNE RESPONSES TO TICKS

The resistance of cattle to ticks such as *Boophilus microplus* has been closely examined by Australian workers such as (Roberts and Kerr, 1976; Wagland, 1975, 1978a,b, 1980; Willadsen *et al.,* 1978). They investigated the known difference between the Zebu or Brahman (*Bos indicus*) and European (*Bos taurus*) breeds of cattle. It was found by Wagland that similar numbers of ticks matured on previously-unexposed cattle for both breeds, although the development of larvae into mature engorged females was slower on the *B. indicus* than on the *B. taurus* cattle. Resistance could be transferred by serum from one cow to another, which led Roberts to conclude that immunological mechanisms were involved. There was also a correlation between the level of resistance in the host and the amount of larval tick antigen required to elicit a Type I hypersensitivity reaction. As was pointed out by Willadsen, the more resistant the animal, the more sensitive it is to small amounts of antigen in the skin test.

The basis for this apparent resistance must be examined closely in the case of the cattle tick, because the grooming and physical removal of the tick larvae can be taken as a manifestation of resistance. It has been suggested that the increased hypersensitivity of resistant animals also increases the frequency with which they groom, because of the skin irritation around the attachment site. Some cattle of both Zebu and European type had decreased larval counts after being restrained from grooming, and this may represent a true difference in resistance between individual cattle, which may be immunologically mediated.

A delayed-type hypersensitivity to ticks has been reported with guinea pigs infested with *Dermacentor andersoni*. Injection of antigenic material produced a Type IV reaction, and the same antigen could stimulate sensitised lymphocytes to transform *in vitro*. However, similar results have yet to be reported for the cattle tick. The histological examination of the skin reaction site to tick bites in guinea pigs reveals a striking accumulation of basophils (Allen, 1973). Thus, the reaction in guinea pigs to the tick bites may be a mixture of Types I and III hypersensitivity together with Type IV delayed hypersensitivity. A complicating factor for interpretation is the presence of larger numbers of eosinophils at the tick attachment site. Eosinophils are rare in Type IV reactions but are common in hypersensitivity to tick bites, so that the skin reaction elicited by injection of the tick antigen is obviously different from that around a tick attachment site.

Immunity to ticks has been transferred in guinea pigs using lymphocytes from cervical, axillary and prescapular lymph nodes. No conclusions have been drawn as to the type of lymphocyte subpopulation responsible for the transfer. It is still possible that transfer of IgE-forming cells is responsible for resistance in the recipients. In this connection, the transfer of resistance in cattle by serum seems almost certain to be due to the transfer of IgE or IgG antibodies, which initiate Type I and Type III hypersensitivity reactions in response to the tick bite.

9.7 IMMUNISATION AGAINST TICKS

Again, the guinea pig has been used as a model system for immunity to *Dermacentor andersoni*. Whole-tick homogenates, as well as dissected midguts of ticks, have been successfully used to vaccinate guinea pigs (see review by Willadsen, 1980). If all internal organs of ticks are used in the vaccine, there is a dramatic effect on egg production and fertility in attached female ticks, presumably because of antibodies directed towards the tick reproductive organs.

Although immunised guinea pigs affected the ticks by inducing them to lay non-viable eggs, this appeared not to be the case with immunised cattle. Further experiments seem to be necessary in cattle to see if tick salivary glands, midgut or reproductive organs can immunise them against ticks. Obviously, the problem exists in obtaining sufficient antigen, and this limits these experiments to small groups of cattle.

Chemical characterisation of tick antigens still requires identification of the important antigens. Immunofluorescence staining with serum from infested animals has shown up antigens in the digestive system, as well as the salivary gland of the tick. Three antigens secreted from *Boophilus microplus* have been described. One is a hydrolytic enzyme, serine esterase, and another is an inhibitor of proteolytic enzymes. The inhibitor of proteolytic enzymes affects both blood coagulation and complement-mediated cell lysis. The function of the third antigen is unknown. None of these antigens appear to be protective when used in a vaccine against cattle tick.

Perhaps the final point could be made that there is substantial susceptibility of cattle to reinfection with ticks. This may be an evolutionary adaptation by the parasite to the host, so that an immune response is not usually stimulated.

9.8 BREED DIFFERENCES IN RESISTANCE TO TICKS

The assessment of cattle breed differences in resistance to ticks is complicated by the problem of demonstrating convincing immunity to ticks. As mentioned before, Brahman cattle in Australia acquire a higher degree of resistance than European cattle to *Boophilus microplus*. However, similar numbers of ticks mature on previously-unexposed cattle of both breeds. The Brahmans usually acquire resistance more rapidly and to a higher degree than European cattle. Grooming by both breeds can affect the persistence of larvae, but if cattle are restrained from grooming, some Brahman cattle have a high loss of nymphs during the experimental period.

The conclusions to be drawn from such studies are that both European and Brahman cattle develop resistance but in Brahman cattle it develops more rapidly than in European cattle. Within both breeds there are individuals which are highly resistant and some which are highly susceptible. The basis for this resistance could quite simply be the intensity of physical grooming by individual cattle and removal of larval ticks.

The cellular reaction around the tick-bite site is often more intense in Brahman cattle than in European cattle, but there is no convincing evidence that this reaction is relevant to immunity. In this connection, the response of the sheep to keds (*Melophagus ovinus*) feeding on skin, appears to be one of rapid reduction in blood supply, which results from a local release of histamine by mast cells at the hypersensitive skin site. No direct immunological mechanism has been found with resistance to keds, although experiments with louse-infested skin grafts on nude, T-cell-deficient mice, suggest that T-cells are required to maintain resistance to lice (Bell *et al.*, 1982)—presumably by continuing T-cell collaboration with B-cells which produce IgE antibodies to the parasite.

Similar problems apply to the cattle tick, in that, if an immune response is involved, the evidence suggests that this is a Type I or III hypersensitivity reaction mediated by antibodies rather than T-cells. In an attempt to assess potential resistance to cattle ticks, the animals have been typed for MHC antigens of the bovine lymphocyte antigen (BoLA) system. Some encouraging results have been obtained which suggest that particular lymphocyte antigens are associated with either resistance or susceptibility to ticks. This aspect is discussed in more detail in Chapter 10.

9.9 THE DOG PARALYSIS TICK—*IXODES HOLOCYCLUS*

The occurrence of an ixodid tick of bandicoots in Australia provides an excellent example of a problem of adaptation by the tick to new hosts. The tick, *Ixodes holocyclus,* is known as the 'paralysis tick' on the eastern seaboard of Australia, because it secretes a toxin back into the host, such as a cat or dog, which causes an ascending, flaccid muscular paralysis. This usually culminates in acute respiratory distress, and the condition may be complicated by aspiration pneumonia and cardiovascular involvement.

The toxin is very potent, since only one adult tick attached and feeding is enough to produce the paralysis. Humans are not immune, and babies have been known to be severely affected by attachment of the tick.

The toxin has been isolated from the tick salivary gland, and it is proteinaceous in nature (Stone and Wright, 1979). An *in vivo* assay in suckling mice has been used by Stone and his associates to evaluate antitoxic antibodies. One antitoxic unit is defined as that amount of antitoxin which will cause 50% neutralisation of one standard paralysing dose of tick toxin when 100 µl of antiserum are incubated with 40 µl of toxin solution at 37°C for 45 minutes and then injected into 4- or 5-gm suckling mice.

In practise, antitoxin is prepared in dogs which become hyperimmune after prolonged attachment of the ticks. There is an initial 'priming' stage of 14 weeks with one tick, followed by progressively-increasing numbers of ticks up to 40 weeks, when maximum antitoxin titres are attained. After removal of the ticks, the serum antitoxin titres drop to about one-third of the peak levels, but these can be restimulated by reattachment of progressively-increasing numbers of ticks for another 10 weeks (Fig. 9.2).

The prolonged course of the immunisation schedule makes the production of the antiserum quite expensive. However the use of the antitoxin in paralysed dogs has highly-dramatic effects, with apparently moribund dogs returning to life again a few hours after the administration of the antitoxin. Unfortunately, dogs can be left too long before treatment, and if the respiratory paralysis has set in, the antitoxin treatment is often not effective in saving the animal.

Because of the expensive nature of the antitoxin and the defined nature of the toxin, there is good reason for developing a vaccine. However, high doses of toxin antigen are required to immunise dogs naturally and for the preparation of a toxoided vaccine. The problem at the moment is to obtain enough tick salivary gland toxin to produce sufficient doses to test a toxoided vaccine in dogs or cats. Thus, the production of a vaccine may have to be postponed until the chemical

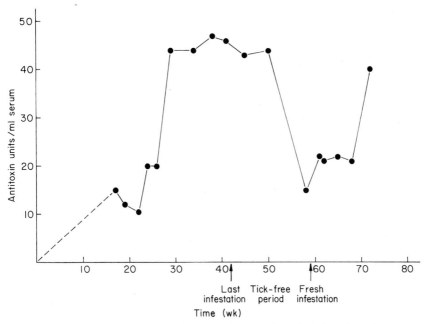

Fig. 9.2. The antitoxin response in the serum of dogs with *Ixodes holocyclus* ticks attached is shown. The initial priming stage is 14 weeks with the attachment of one tick, followed by increasing numbers of ticks up to 40 weeks. After removal of the ticks, the serum antitoxin titres drop, but they may be restimulated by attaching more ticks. In Australia the hyperimmune serum is used for intravenous administration to dogs with tick paralysis. (Redrawn from Stone and Wright (1979), *in* 'Ticks and Tick-borne Diseases' (L. A. Y. Johnston and M. G. Cooper, eds.), by kind permission of the Australian Veterinary Association.)

sequence of the protein toxin is known and it can be synthesised artificially for vaccine production.

Tick paralysis is also known in dogs and cats in North America to be caused by *Dermacentor andersoni*. It differs from *I. holocyclus* in that removal of the tick is usually enough to allow the animals to recover, while the toxin from *I. holocyclus* can still kill the animal even after the tick has been removed. It also seems that several *Dermacentor* ticks are required to cause paralysis in the dog, while only one *Ixodes* tick will produce the same effect.

The toxin is an unfortunate side-effect of the tick salivary gland secretion, which is primarily directed towards promoting the right conditions for growth and maturation of the tick, than in killing the host.

9.10 IMMUNITY TO TICK-BORNE DISEASES

The tick-borne diseases of domestic animals mostly involve diseases of cattle in the tropics. Obviously there are rickettsial diseases such as Rocky Mountain Spotted Fever, which affects dogs as well as humans, and this is transmitted by the dog tick *Dermacentor variabilis* or the sheep tick *Dermacentor andersoni*. Also, there is Q-Fever, which is caused by *Rickettsia burnetii* and which is transmitted to humans and livestock by the faeces of cattle ticks feeding on infected cattle. However, the diseases of economic importance which are transmitted by ticks are mostly protozoal diseases of cattle.

9.10.1 East Coast Fever

Occurring in Africa, East Coast Fever is caused by the protozoan *Theileria parva* and is transmitted by the tick *Rhipicephalus appendiculatus,* which ingests the erythrocytic piroplasm stage of the parasite while feeding on infected cattle. During the moulting phase of the tick life cycle, after it has dropped off the cow, the parasites migrate to the salivary glands of the tick. When a new host is bitten, the parasites are inoculated, and 4 days later, macroschizonts are present in the lymphoblasts of the regional lymph nodes.

It is of particular interest that, like some viruses, the parasite multiplies in lymphoid cells throughout the body. This leads to blast transformation of the lymphocytes, which in turn become the targets for attack by the cytotoxic T-cells that appear in the blood of convalescent cattle. The cytotoxic response appears to be genetically restricted, and work by Emery and Kar (1983) with continuously-grown *Theileria*-infected lymphoblasts, has suggested that *Theileria* antigen is associated with MHC antigens in the cell membranes.

Fourteen days after infection, the macroschizonts change into microschizonts and invade the erythrocytes again. From the tenth day onwards the host develops fever and almost invariably dies from 16 to 26 days onwards.

Since survivors are immune to reinfection, at least with the same strain, it has appeared possible that a vaccine might be developed. Suspensions of infected lymphocytes have been used, but the collection and preservation of macroschizonts from infected cattle on a large scale has proved a formidable task. However it was found possible to obtain infective particles by harvesting them from tick salivary glands directly, and these were readily standardised and preserved by freezing in liquid nitrogen.

It was initially thought that a low dose of infective particles would provide an immunising dose without a high rate of clinical infection. However, this proved difficult to achieve, and attempts were then made to attenuate the infective particles by X irradiation. Again, problems were encountered, with a narrow margin being demonstrated between protection on the one hand and over-attenuation on the other hand.

The simultaneous injection of a tetracycline antibiotic and the infective particles was then tried and found to produce solid immunity to *Th. parva* in experimental cattle. In the field, however, another protozoan, *Theileria mutans,* was found still to cause sporadic outbreaks, and there was also a fear that ticks feeding on vaccinated cattle might introduce new strains of *Th. parva* into particular areas.

At the moment, tissue culture vaccines from bovine spleen cells are being explored as a means of producing infective particles. Obviously the characterisation of the protective antigens would seem an area for exploration to develop a genetically-engineered 'safe' vaccine.

Natural immunity does exist in cattle which have been reared for generations in endemic areas. Resistance appears to be by selection and not to be the result of transmission of specific colostral antibody to calves.

9.10.2   Babesiosis

Babesiosis is primarily known for its importance as a disease of cattle, although horses, dogs, cats, sheep and pigs all have specific *Babesia* parasites. The disease in cattle is caused by *Babesia bovis* and to a lesser extent by *Babesia bigemina* transmitted by the tick *Boophilus microplus*.

Immunity can be induced in calves by the inoculation of a living vaccine, containing several strains of *Babesia* parasites, which is prepared by passage through splenectomised calves (Callow and Dalgliesh, 1979; Wright and Mahoney, 1979). The removal of the spleen is necessary in the donor calves to allow multiplication of the parasite in the blood stream without filtering by the spleen. In Australia, the parasites are suspended in a diluent from which the erythrocytes have been removed. This is done because repeated injection of the calf blood vaccine into pregnant cattle, may lead to haemolytic disease in newborn calves due to transmission of antibodies against erythrocytes in the colostrum. This finding is at variance with experiments described earlier in Chapter 3 on the immunology of reproduction. In those experiments, deliberate immunisation of cows with blood from bulls to which they were mated, did not lead to haemolytic disease in newborn calves. This discrepancy may merely reflect a range of antibody responses, the most active of which only shows up with the inoculation of thousands of cattle with incompatible erythrocytes.

The vaccine has a shelf-life of about 14 days, which is long enough for distribution by modern transportation methods. This method of vaccine production and distribution has been used in Australia since the 1890s and has been very effective in preventing the outbreaks of Babesiosis in cattle at risk. Paradoxically, the effective control of cattle ticks results in the development of susceptible cattle which must be protected by vaccination against an upsurge in the tick population. Again, the experience in Australia would suggest that the use of a virulent *Babesia* vaccine does *not* perpetuate the disease, and this is because of two factors. Firstly, the successive passages through the splenectomised calf donor has reduced the virulence of the vaccine strains, and secondly, the infectivity to ticks appears to have been greatly reduced at the same time. The protection observed has been found to be 1% of vaccinated cattle becoming clinically sick with Babesiosis, compared with 18% of unvaccinated cattle under natural challenge exposure.

Living vaccines have been used chiefly because of the ease with which large numbers of parasites can be grown for vaccine production. The separation of *Babesia* antigen completely from the erythrocytes to produce a killed vaccine has proved too arduous to be of value in a practical vaccination scheme. The use of irradiation to attenuate the parasites has been tried, but there is a narrow margin between killing the parasites and allowing them limited survival to stimulate immunity in the host. Nevertheless, work is continuing on the preparation of dead vaccines suspended in Freund's complete adjuvant which provide good protection against experimental challenge. These findings challenge the earlier concepts of 'premunition' in which the survival of a few parasites was necessary for prolonged immunity. Attempts have also been made to isolate the messenger RNA which codes for *Babesia* antigens and then to produce the antigens in bacteria by recombinant DNA techniques. At the time of writing, this technique was still at the experimental stage with laboratory rodents and was still to be tested in cattle. It would have to compete with the tried and tested method of preparing living vaccine in calves.

The mechanism of immunity to Babesiosis appears primarily to involve antibody, since there are reports indicating that passive transfer of antibodies is protective in calves. The phagocytes in the spleen and liver are obviously important in the removal of the opsonised parasites, although serum complement may well be capable of causing lysis of opsonised parasites. The presence of activated macrophages has not been reported in Babesiosis of cattle, but it seems likely that lymphokines could activate macrophages, since rats have been protected against *Babesia rhodaini* by passive transfer of lymphoid cells. The situation may be similar to another intracellular protozoan parasite, *Toxoplasma gondii*, which has certainly been shown to stimulate macrophage cellular immunity as a result of lymphokines released from sensitised lymphocytes *in vitro*.

Serological tests for Babesiosis include the fluorescent antibody test, the complement fixation test, passive agglutination test, bentonite flocculation test, capillary agglutination test, card agglutination test, parasitised erythrocyte agglutination test, the gel precipitation test and the enzyme-linked immunosorbent assay (ELISA) (Zwart and Brocklesby, 1979). The multiplicity of tests indicates the unsatisfactory nature of serological tests for Babesiosis, but the complement fixation test and fluorescent antibody test appear to be the most useful.

9.10.3   Anaplasmosis

The rickettsial parasites *Anaplasma marginale* or *Anaplasma centrale* are often included in *Babesia* vaccines. A vaccine prepared in Australia has been used successfully in Southeast Asia and South America. Forty-five years of experience with vaccines containing *A. marginale* or *A. centrale* in Australia indicate that the vaccine does not increase in virulence and does not spread the disease. Nevertheless, the use of *A. centrale* vaccine in some countries is not allowed because of the fear of spread by vaccination.

Vaccination against Babesiosis and Anaplasmosis has proved useful in Australia, but the manufacturers of the vaccine are alert to the possibility of contamination with virus diseases such as leukaemia, ephemeral fever, Infectious Bovine Rhinotracheitis and mucosal disease. Donor calves are constantly screened for these diseases and other, less common protozoan infections, so that the final vaccine contains only those infectious agents that it is intended it should contain.

9.11   TRYPANOSOMIASIS

A protozoan disease, Trypanosomiasis, is of course not transmitted by ticks but by the tsetse fly in central Africa. Many attempts have been made to vaccinate against trypanosomes, but the fundamental problem is the apparently-unlimited antigenic variation of the parasite as it multiplies in the host.

This has been of fundamental interest to molecular biologists who have postulated a 'hot-spot' area in the chromatin of trypanosomes which allows rapid recombination and coding of the variable surface antigens. Considerable work is being carried out at the International Laboratory for Research in Animal Diseases (ILRAD) in Nairobi, Kenya. Work has centred predominantly on *Trypanosoma brucei*, although other species such as *T. congolense* and *T. vivax* also cause disease in cattle.

It has been found that each antigenically-distinct strain of *T. brucei* possesses a unique glycoprotein which covers the entire surface of the organism. These surface antigens are strongly immunogenic and result in the production of high titres of antibody by the host. This would, at first glance, appear to be detrimental for the trypanosome, and indeed most parasites are opsonised and suffer complement-mediated lysis or are phagocytosed by the reticuloendothelial system. Townsend and Duffus (1982) have shown that bovine neutrophils, eosinophils, monocytes and macrophages are cytotoxic to trypanosomes in the presence of antibody but lymphocytes are not.

Paradoxically this strong immunogenicity of the trypanosome antigens may benefit the parasite by allowing survival of the host. It is also a selective pressure on the remaining parasites which encourages antigenic variants in low frequency, to multiply and displace the original variant. Thus, there are successive waves of parasitaemia resulting from successive changes in the parasite antigens.

The surface glycoproteins have been the subject of close chemical analysis in an attempt to find an antigenic determinant common to all variants. However, since there is little natural immunity, the production of a vaccine does not appear imminent. The puzzle of what causes the antigenic variation may be solved by basic research on the parasite, which can be grown in the laboratory. Vaccination against the parasite will have to compete with chemotherapy, which is very effective in controlling natural infections.

A method of controlled infection using chemotherapy, to produce so-called non-sterile immunity has been demonstrated in eastern Africa by Wilson and colleagues (1976). Calves and cattle were treated on an individual basis and only when clinically ill or when their packed-cell volume fell below 20%. A chemotherapeutic agent was used, which was almost completely curative. It was found that the period between drug treatments could be increased and that eventually the drugs could be withdrawn. The animals survived and continued to gain weight at the same rate as those given routine therapy. This type of immunity may be the result of non-specific macrophage activation, which is enough to keep all antigenic variants at levels which are controllable by the host.

There is a breed of cattle, the Ndama breed, which appears to have a natural tolerance to trypanosomes. This breed may be the result of intensive natural selection which has produced a particular bovine MHC type, resistant to trypanosomes. Ultimately the breeding of resistant cattle may depend on the selection of cattle from among the introduced breeds, with a particular MHC type associated with resistance. The acquisition of non-sterile immunity with the persistence of parasitaemia may be the answer with cattle at risk. The other long-term solution is to alter the environment so that it is unfavourable for tsetse flies. Without the insect vector Trypanosomiasis would be rapidly controlled by quarantine and slaughter methods.

9.12 GENERAL CONCLUSIONS

Immunity to external parasites is very often manifested by hypersensitivity reactions in the skin of the host. These reactions appear to have only a minor effect on the survival of the external parasite, although efforts to direct the immune response against the vital organs of the parasite may ultimately be rewarded with success.

The hypersensitivity to flea bites is often very difficult to control, and attempts to desensitise dogs with flea antigens are not always successful. A particular problem with the tick *Ixodes holocyclus* in Australia has been met by producing specific antiserum in dogs to the tick salivary gland toxin.

Immunity to diseases transmitted by external parasites is usually incomplete, although successful vaccines against *Anaplasma* and *Babesia* parasites have been in use for many years. The remaining major problems are the protozoal diseases of cattle in Africa, such as East Coast Fever and Trypanosomiasis. An intense effort is being mounted to isolate protective antigens from these parasites using techniques such as the raising of monoclonal antibodies to the coat proteins of stages in the life cycle of the parasites. From the knowledge obtained on the protective antigens, it is hoped that these can be cloned and produced in bulk by recombinant DNA techniques to be incorporated into vaccines for testing in the field.

REFERENCES

Allen, J. R. (1973). *Int. J. Parasitol* **3**, 195–200.
Bell, J. F., Stewart, S. J. and Nelson, W. A. (1982). *J. Med. Entomol.* **19**, 164–168.
Callow, L. L. and Dalgliesh, R. J. (1979). The development of effective, safe vaccination against Babesiosis and Anaplasmosis in Australia. *In* 'Ticks and Tick-borne Diseases' (L. A. Y. Johnston and M. G. Cooper, eds.), pp. 4–8. Australian Veterinary Association, Sydney.
Coombs, R. R. A. and Gell, P. G. H. (1968). Classification of allergic reactions for clinical hypersensitivity and disease. *In* 'Clinical Aspects of Immunology' (P. G. H. Gell and R. R. A. Coombs, eds.), pp. 575–596. (1st edition published in 1963.)
Emery, D. L. and Kar, S. K. (1983). *Immunology* **48**, 723–731.
Feingold, B. F., Benjamini, E. and Michaeli, D. (1968). *Annu. Rev. Entomol.* **13**, 137–158.
Halliwell, R. E. W., Schwartzman, R. M. and Rockey, J. H. (1972). *Clin. Exp. Immunol.* **10**, 399–407.
McFarlin, D. E. and Balfour, B. (1973). *Immunology* **25**, 995–1009.
Prausnitz, L. and Kustner, H. (1921). *Zentralbl. Bakteriol., Parasitenkd. Infektionskr., Abt. 1: Orig.* **86**, 160–169.

Roberts, J. A. and Kerr, J. D. (1976). *J. Parasitol.* **62**, 485–488.

Schwartzman, R. M., Rockey, J. H. and Halliwell, R. E. W. (1971). *Clin. Exp. Immunol.* **9**, 549–569.

Stone, B. F. and Wright, I. G. (1979). Toxins of *Ixodes holocyclus* and immunity to paralysis. *In* 'Ticks and Tick-borne Diseases' (L. A. Y. Johnston and M. G. Cooper, eds.), pp. 75–78. Australian Veterinary Association, Sydney.

Townsend, J. and Duffus, W. P. H. (1982). *Clin. Exp. Immunol.* **48**, 289–299.

Wagland, B. M. (1975). *Aust. J. Agric. Res.* **26**, 1073–1080.

Wagland, B. M. (1978a). *Aust. J. Agric. Res.* **29**, 395–400.

Wagland, B. M. (1978b). *Aust. J. Agric. Res.* **29**, 401–409.

Wagland, B. M. (1979). *Aust. J. Agric. Res.* **30**, 211–218.

Willadsen, P. (1980). *Adv. Parasitol.* **18**, 293–313.

Willadsen, P., Williams, R. G., Roberts, J. A. and Kerr, J. D. (1978). *Int. J. Parasitol.* **8**, 89–95.

Willemse, A. and Van Den Brom, W. E. (1982). *Res. Vet. Sci.* **32**, 57–61.

Wilson, A. J., Paris, J., Luckins, A. G., Dar, F. K. and Gray, A. R. (1976). *Trop. Anim. Health Prod.* **8**, 1–12.

Wright, I. G. and Mahoney, D. F. (1979). Babesia bovis infections: New concepts in vaccination. *In* 'Ticks and Tick-borne Diseases' (L. A. Y. Johnston and M. G. Cooper, eds.), pp. 11–13. Australian Veterinary Association, Sydney.

Zwart, D. and Brocklesby, D. W. (1979). *Adv. Parasitol.* **17**, 50–113.

10

Immunogenetics

It has long been appreciated that the mortality to infectious diseases of animals is usually not 100% and that a proportion of animals quickly develop immunity and survive the epidemic. This is obviously a mechanism of natural selection for resistance, and in wild animals it forms the basis for natural immunity, for example of African artiodactyls to Trypanosomiasis in the face of constant challenge by the tsetse fly vector.

A possible inkling of the mechanism of this genetically-transmitted resistance has been provided by basic studies in immunogenetics, using first the mouse and then the chicken, in the study of transplantation antigens.

10.1 TRANSPLANTATION ANTIGENS

As their name implies, the transplantation antigens are found on the cells of animals and constitute a barrier to the transfer of organ grafts from one animal to another. They are glycoproteins (MW 36,000) embedded in the plasma membranes of all cells and are unique to each individual, apart from identical twins. They are under genetic control of a segment of DNA on the short arm of chromosome 6 in the human and on chromosome 17 in the mouse. The antigens in the cell membrane are associated with another protein, β_2-microglobulin, which in the human is encoded separately on chromosome 15 (Fig. 10.1).

The localisation of these segments of DNA as those which control the expression of the cell membrane transplantation antigens presents a fascinating

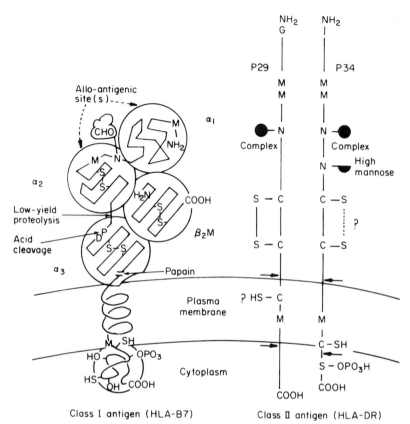

Class I antigen (HLA-B7)   Class II antigen (HLA-DR)

Fig. 10.1. The two major histocompatibility glycoprotein classes found in the plasma membranes of human lymphocytes are shown. The Class I lymphocyte antigens (e.g., HLA-A, -B) are composed of two chains. The larger α chain has a molecular weight of 41,000 and traverses the cell membrane. The smaller chain, β_2-microglobulin (β_2M), has a molecular weight of 11,500 and is non-covalently associated with the larger α chain. The Class II antigens (e.g., HLA-DR) are found predominantly in B-cells. They consist of two polypeptide chains, both traversing the cell membrane, with an α chain of 34,000 MW (P34) and a β chain of 29,000 MW (P29) tightly linked in a non-covalent complex. (Reproduced by kind permission from Strominger (1980), *in* 'Immunology 80: Progress in Immunology IV' (M. Fougereau and J. Dausset, eds.), pp. 541–554. Academic Press, New York.)

story in molecular biology. Both recombinant DNA and cell fusion techniques have been separately used to provide this information. The messenger RNA which codes for the isolated transplantation antigens has been prepared and, using radiolabelling techniques and DNA–RNA hybridisation, the segment of DNA which codes for it has been localised on particular chromosomes. The more direct technique of cell fusion has shown that the loss of certain chromosomes during the fusion process is accompanied by the loss of the transplantation antigens from the surface membrane of the cell. The identification of the missing chromosomes is carried out by chromosome spreads from dividing cells, which are stained and identified under the microscope.

Transplantation of organs such as kidneys, liver, heart and skin in humans is of obvious importance in the human field, but is rarely attempted in the clinical field of veterinary surgery. Nevertheless, much is known of the transplantation antigens in the dog and the pig because they have been used as experimental models for transplantation in the human. Similarly, Rhesus monkeys and chimpanzees have been used as models, and their transplantation systems are well-characterised. The other domestic species are less well-characterised, except perhaps for the chicken, because there has been no reason to study their transplantation antigens (Fig. 10.2). The best-characterised species is the mouse, and it was in this species that a connection between transplantation antigens and disease resistance was first examined on a molecular basis.

10.2 TRANSPLANTATION ANTIGENS AND DISEASE RESISTANCE OR SUSCEPTIBILITY

Transplantation antigens have been studied in the mouse to such an extent that Klein (1975) estimated that several hundred different H (histocompatibility) loci exist. However, these consist of one strong or major locus and many weak or minor loci. The significance of this division is that incompatibility for the major locus between donor and recipient leads to early rejection of surgically-transplanted organs, which is difficult to alter by induction of tolerance or immunosuppressive treatment with drugs. On the other hand, in the presence of minor locus differences, transplanted tissues survive for a prolonged period, tolerance is more readily induced and further prolongation of the graft survival can be achieved by immunosuppression.

The connection between this diverse system of tissue antigens and resistance to infectious disease was suggested by the work of Zinkernagel and Doherty in the mid-1970s using inbred strains of mice. These strains had been developed in the preceding two decades to the stage of being congenic by multiple brother–sister matings over many generations. These congenic strains often differed from each other by only one transplantation antigen, and, apart from their use in defining the H-2 locus antigens, were being used extensively in basic immunological research because of their uniformity of immune response and their usefulness in cell transfer studies in the work on T- and B-cell populations.

Zinkernagel and Doherty (1975) looked at the transfer of cellular and humoral immunity to Lymphochoriomeningitis (LCM) virus between mouse strains differing by only one histocompatibility antigen and found that this was an effective barrier to cell cooperation in resistance to the virus. As mentioned in Chapter 7 on immunity to viruses, they found that lymphocytes from the mouse strain with H-2^k major locus type, would attack autologous virus-infected target cells of the H-2^k type but not the homologous H-2^b type. This was termed 'genetic restriction' and led to work which concluded that for optimum cooperation between helper T-cells and B-cells, the helper T-cells had to recognise both the virus antigen and the histocompatibility antigen, either as a complex or each separately, in order to mount an immune response.

Not all immune responses were subsequently found to be equally affected by genetic restriction, but because this phenomenon had been demonstrated with an infectious disease of mice, it suggested to many research workers that transplantation antigens might have a particular function in disease resistance and that their very heterogeneity ensured that not all individuals would be susceptible to an epidemic of an infectious disease to the same degree and that some would survive.

10.3   THE IMMUNE RESPONSE (*Ir*) Locus

The transplantation antigens of the major histocompatibility complex (MHC) have been assigned or 'mapped' to regions of the chromosome, which in the human consist of four loci (A, B, C and D) (Fig. 10.2) and in the mouse also of four loci (K, I, D and L). One of these loci has been linked with immune responsiveness, and in the mouse this is called the I locus. In the human it is the D locus which is the apparent equivalent of the mouse I locus. Evidence has been obtained that the human D locus is coded by a section of DNA which is outside that for the other three loci. Conversely, in the mouse it is coded by the I locus, which is within the K, D, L regions. In this, the mouse appears to be the exception, since most mammals including the rat, dog, pig, goat and cow, appear to have the equivalent of the D locus, as in the human, located some distance from the other loci.

The significance of this is not really known, but although the mouse is the best-characterised of the species studied, research workers are cautious about extending findings in the mouse to other species. Nevertheless the mouse has provided information on the possible organization of the I-region equivalents in the other species.

The Ir genes of the mouse control the Ia antigens on the lymphocyte surface and have been further subdivided into IA, IB, IJ, IE and IC regions of DNA chromatin. The tissue distribution of the Ia antigens is the surface of macrophages, B-cells and activated T-cells; normal resting T-cells express little or no Ia antigens. The significance of this latter finding is that careful experiments have suggested that the IA region is associated with helper cell activity and that

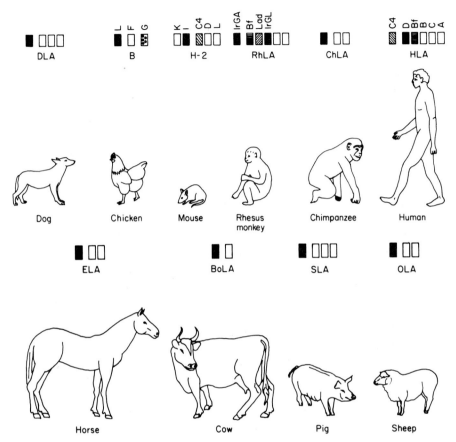

Fig. 10.2.   The current knowledge on the lymphocyte MHC antigens for several domestic species is compared with that for laboratory animals and primates. The mouse has the best-characterised MHC region. □ Class I antigens; ■ Class II antigens. Various other loci, such as the chicken *G* locus and the serum complement loci, are represented by cross-hatching or dots. Generally, the knowledge of the MHC complex in domestic animals is poorer than that for laboratory animals and primates.

of the *IJ* region with soluble suppressor cell factors, both functions of subpopulations of T-cells. The functions of the other three regions, *IB*, *IE* and *IC*, have not been clearly determined.

In the human, the *HLA-DR* locus appears to be the equivalent of the *IE* locus in the mouse. Sequence studies have shown considerable homology in amino-acids in the antigens under the control of these two regions, and it is assumed that they function in a similar fashion by providing a control of the immune response.

Whether this is true or not, considerable effort is being made to define further the *HLA-D* locus of the human as a means of exploring immune responsiveness. Two techniques have been used; first, the mixed-lymphocyte reaction (MLR) between lymphocytes from unrelated individuals is used. The lymphocytes are grown in tissue culture and react to the HLA-D antigens rather than the other antigens (HLA-A, B, C) by undergoing blast transformation and synthesising DNA, which can be measured by [^{3}H]thymidine uptake. Secondly, the same or very similar lymphocyte antigens can be measured by microcytotoxicity testing. The terms lymphocyte determined (LD) and serologically determined (SD) have been coined, and the distinction confirmed by naming the LD *Ir* gene products HLA-D and the SD products HLA-A, B, C. Another set of terms used for the same entities is Class I (SD antigens) and Class II antigens (LD antigens), which describes the same integral cell surface glycoproteins as the other terms used. A Class III has also been created for components of the complement system, which although coded by loci on the same chromosome in the mouse and close to the other MHC loci, are not found as membrane components.

Since humans cannot be challenged with pathogens experimentally, the association between lymphocyte type and disease resistance or susceptibility has centred on surveys of patients admitted to hospital and for whom disease histories are available. This has meant that patients with chronic disorders have tended to be much more closely examined than those with acute infections. Thus, a close association has been found between *HLA-B27* and Ankylosing Spondylitis and *HLA-DR3* and Coeliac disease. As can be seen from the code numbers, each *HLA* locus consists of many alleles which have been determined by comparisons between laboratories at International Workshops. The suffix *W* is used to denote a provisional identification of a new allele which is to be confirmed at a subsequent workshop. Similar workshops have been started for the BoLA (bovine lymphocyte antigen) system to compare lymphocyte specificities, mostly as serologically-determined (SD) types by microcytotoxicity testing.

10.4 TRANSPLANTATION ANTIGENS IN DOMESTIC ANIMALS

The state of knowledge for each of the domestic species is shown in Fig. 10.2. Compared with the human, mouse and ape, it is obvious that the domestic species are poorly characterised except perhaps for the dog and the chicken.

Cross-reactions do exist between HLA antigens and those on lymphocytes of other primates and those of more phylogenetically-distant species. A distinction can be drawn between highly-specific antibodies to 'private antigens', which are found on individuals, and the broadly-specific antibodies to 'public antigens', which are found on a high proportion of the population. It has been shown that broadly-polymorphic antibodies show considerable cross-reactivity with other species while highly-specific antibodies do not. Therefore, it has been suggested that the private or highly-specific antigens are the result of recent evolution, while the public or broadly-polymorphic determinants are older parts of the molecule (Brodsky and Parham, 1982).

In practise, this means that antibodies to HLA antigens do cross-react with those species which are phylogenetically distant, such as cattle, goats and dogs, but they react in low frequency and in a haphazard fashion. With phylogenetically-close species such as the chimpanzee and gorilla, there are frequent cross-reactions between species across the spectrum of antibodies to the human lymphocyte antigens.

As a consequence, there are no broadly cross-reactive human antisera which can be used for domestic animals, and each species must be typed by panels of antisera which are painstakingly collected or prepared and sorted into recognisable gene loci and their alleles for the respective MHC antigens. This is logical when one considers that the lymphocyte antigens of the human associated with resistance to disease are most likely to be quite unrelated to those which have emerged in domestic animals as a result of quite different selection pressures.

10.4.1 Chicken Lymphocyte Antigens (*B*-locus)

The chicken is discussed first because its MHC antigens have been carefully studied and found to be in close linkage with resistance to Marek's disease. The chicken is also unique, in that antisera prepared against the nucleated erythrocytes of the birds, also agglutinate lymphocytes. In the 1960s, Schierman and Nordskog (1963) found that lymphocytes lacked the antigens of three blood group systems: A, E and D-L. Antibodies specific for these three systems did not agglutinate homologous lymphocytes, while antibodies specific for the B and C systems agglutinated both lymphocytes and erythrocytes.

It was further demonstrated that the *B* blood group locus was the major histocompatibility locus in the chicken. Skin grafts from closely-related birds having a B antigen not present in the recipient cells, survived for a significantly shorter time than those from a *B* locus-compatible donor. The *C* locus appeared not to have as strong an influence as the *B* locus, since in one inbred line, grafts from donors incompatible at the *C* locus survived as long as grafts that were compatible.

There appear to be at least three regions of the *B* locus or MHC, and these are called *F*, *L* and *G* regions, which code for the corresponding F, L and G antigens or antigenic complexes. The Class I or SD antigens are represented by the F antigen, which is composed of two polypeptide chains with molecular weights of 40,000–43,000 and 11,000–12,000. The large chain is a glycoprotein, non-covalently linked to a small chain, apparently the avian equivalent of β_2-micro-globulin. The F antigen is present on most somatic cells and on all peripheral blood lymphocytes and erythrocytes.

The Class II or LD antigens are coded by the L region, which includes the equivalent of the I and HLA-D regions in mouse and human lymphocytes, re-spectively. The molecular weight of these antigens is approximately 30,000, and the molecules are composed of two non-covalently-associated polypeptide chains. The L antigen is found on a proportion of blood lymphocytes, of which 10% are T-cells and 90% are B-cells. It is also found on cells of the monocyte–macrophage series.

The Class III antigens, which in other species are controlled for example by the HLA-$C2$ locus, have yet to be demonstrated in chickens.

A unique set of Class IV antigens, the G locus, has been found in chickens but not in other species. It has two chains, with apparent molecular weights of 31,000 and 42,000 under reducing conditions, but under non-reducing condi-tions, the molecular weights are 135,000 and 160,000. This G antigen is not associated with molecules resembling β_2-microglobulin.

10.4.2   Dog Lymphocyte Antigens

The study of dog lymphocyte antigens (DLA) has closely paralleled that of the human. Those of the dog were studied because this species was used as a model for techniques in the surgical transplantation of organs, later to be used in humans. Vriesendorp initially identified two and later three SD loci for which multiple alleles were found. The loci were named DLA-A, DLA-B and DLA-C.

Using the mixed-lymphocyte reaction (MLR), an LD locus was found and named DLA-D. This was further divided to give DLA-E, another LD antigen. As in the human, it is thought that the DLA-C locus is located between the A and B loci on the chromosome, while the D locus is outside this group.

Using chemically-synthesised co-polymers of amino-acids (e.g., L-glutamine, L-alanine), it was shown that the immune response against these antigens segre-gated in families of dogs in parallel with the DLA complex. Therefore the canine equivalent of Ir genes are also found within the MHC region as in other species.

The equivalent of the mouse Ia antigens have also been demonstrated for the dog (Deeg et al., 1982), and the concentration of the antigen was found to be greater on B-cells and macrophages than on peripheral T-cells, as for other species.

The use of cross-matching of DLA-A and B for renal transplants between outbred dogs has led to a doubling of survival time for the grafts. However, as was pointed out by Bull (1982), cross-matching is not the complete answer in itself, since immunosuppressive therapy is also required to maintain the graft for longer periods of time (Fig. 10.3).

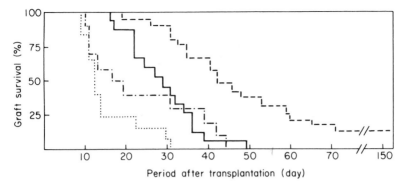

Fig. 10.3. The percentage survival of kidney allografts in different groups of donor–recipient pairs of beagles. It can be seen that even siblings with identical DLA types are not matched for all transplantation antigens, since many grafts are rejected. ——— DLA-Identical nonsiblings; - - - - - - - DLA-identical siblings; -·-·- DLA—one haplotype different siblings; ······ DLA—two haplotypes different siblings. [Reproduced by kind permission from Bijnen et al. (1980)].

10.4.2.1 Tumour Immunity in Dogs

A Canine Venereal Sarcoma is transmitted by sexual contact, and after a period of rapid growth, most tumours regress spontaneously in adult dogs. However, in immunologically-incompetent dogs or in puppies, the tumour progresses and metastasises, eventually killing the host.

It appears that the normal immune response of the dog to this tumour is in the nature of a graft rejection. This is because the tumour is transmitted by intact tumour cells which grow into the epithelial surfaces of the external genitalia of both sexes. This tumour has been very useful in experimental studies on tumour immunity directed towards identification of tumour-associated cell antigens (Palker and Yang, 1981).

Immunotherapy of Canine Lymphoma, usually in unison with chemotherapy, has been carried out (Theilen and Hills, 1982). The survival rates of the treated dogs are markedly longer than those for dogs given chemotherapy alone, but a complete cure has not been achieved with this treatment.

10.4.2.2 Grey Collie Syndrome

A lethal hereditary disorder associated with grey-silver hair colouration in collies, Grey Collie syndrome, is associated with abnormalities in the cell cycle of bone marrow cells, particularly mature neutrophils, and severe neutropoenia occurs at intervals of about 12 days. The episodes of neutropoenia are followed by fever, diarrhoea, gingivitis, respiratory infections and lymphadenitis.

It has been possible to cure collies completely of the disease by bone marrow transplants from litter-mates, matched for Class I and Class II DLA antigens (Yang, 1978). The recipient is lethally irradiated and then reconstituted with bone marrow from the donor litter-mate. Recovery of the normal coat colour in collies which have been cured by the bone marrow transplantation occurs about 2 years later.

10.4.3 Feline Lymphocyte Antigens

Very little has been published on the feline MHC, but a report by Pollack *et al.* (1982) described some unusual features for this species. In contrast to most other species, lymphocytotoxic antibodies were not usually detected in the serum of multiparous cats or in cats which had received blood transfusions. It also appeared that the mixed-lymphocyte reactions to Class II antigens were very weak between unrelated cat lymphocytes compared with other species such as the human. If this report is confirmed, the results point to a rather limited polymorphism in the feline histocompatibility system.

10.4.4 Pig Lymphocyte Antigens

Pig lymphocyte antigens (SLA) have been studied in some detail, because the pig has also been used as a model for transplantation surgery with organs such as kidneys and liver (Calne, 1973; Sachs *et al.*, 1976). The work of Vaiman and colleagues has established that there are three Class I loci and one Class II locus. According to the convention used in humans, these have been named *SLA-A*, *SLA-B* and *SLA-C* for the Class I antigens, and *SLA-D* for the Class II antigen. A further splitting of the *SLA-D* locus has been suggested from experiments in which fluorescent antibodies to two SLA-D determinants formed caps which moved independently in the membrane.

It is interesting that interspecies cross-reactivity of antibodies against Ia determinants in the mouse was first shown for the rat and then for the pig. It has now been shown that antibodies to mouse IE antigens are the ones responsible for the cross-reactivity in rat, guinea pig, human, pig, horse, dog and cat (Shinohara and Sachs, 1982). The conservation of the IE antigen by so many species suggests that the molecule is vital for the survival of all these species.

Biochemical analysis of the SLA proteins has shown that there are molecules of 42,000 MW which are the SD antigens, molecules of 31,000 and 25,000 MW corresponding to a molecule resembling mouse Ia and a small molecule of 11,000 MW corresponding to β_2-microglobulin. Treatment of the Class I antigens with papain produces a heavy chain of 28,000 MW and a light chain of 11,000 MW, which is β_2-microglobulin (Lunney and Sachs, 1978).

In work with hens' egg-white lysozyme, Vaiman *et al.* (1978) showed that the primary immune response to this antigen in pigs was under the control of the MHC genes. Individual pigs, heterozygous for two lymphocyte antigens, had a higher response than homozygous animals. This suggested that a complementation phenomenon can occur between several genes, amongst which there is at least one linked to the SLA loci. Therefore it seems likely that pigs also have the *Ir* genes equivalent to those in other species. Without the highly-inbred strains available for mice and chickens, the presence of *Ir* genes in pigs may be difficult to prove unequivocally. Nevertheless, these data on pigs were the first to be described for large domestic animals.

10.4.5 Bovine Lymphocyte Antigens

The study of bovine lymphocyte antigens (BoLA) has been surrounded by some controversy, since it has been difficult to prove conclusively that they are under the control of more than one locus. In extensive studies, Stone and his colleagues could find no conclusive evidence for more than one SD locus (Amorena and Stone, 1980), but their studies with the MLR technique in bovine lymphocytes suggested two linked LD loci. Spooner and colleagues initially suggested that there were two SD loci (Spooner *et al.*, 1978), but withdrew from this position when it proved difficult to exclude cross-reactions between lymphocyte types. Stear and colleagues (1982) found as many as five independently-inherited alleles in some cattle, and the evidence at the moment suggests that there are indeed two SD loci and possibly more. Quite large breed differences in frequencies of BoLA specificities have been observed (Oliver *et al.*, 1981).

The designation of the bovine MHC loci and their alleles has yet to be agreed upon, but international BoLA typing conferences are being held to reach some agreement on the possible organisation of the BoLA antigens. Recombinants appear to be very rare, and it is possible that the Class I and Class II loci are very close together on the bovine lymphocyte chromosome which controls them.

There are no reports on biochemical analysis of the bovine lymphocyte antigens. However, bovine β_2-microglobulin has been shown to have 75% sequence homology with human β_2-microglobulin. Evidence has also been obtained that bovine β_2-microglobulin has binding sites for HLA-A, B and C heavy chains (Church *et al.*, 1982). However in the absence of well-characterised BoLA heavy chains, no work has been carried out on the homologous system.

10.4.5.1 Tumour Immunity in Cattle

Bovine ocular squamous-cell carcinoma ('cancer eye') has been treated by vaccination of cattle with a phenol–saline extract of allogeneic cancer cells (Hoffmann *et al.*, 1981). The results were encouraging, since 77% of the carcinomas responded favourably, in varying degrees, to the treatment. The immunising activity of the vaccine appears to be associated with proteins of MW

19,000–34,000, which may prove to be altered transplantation antigens from the tumour cells.

10.4.6 Sheep and Goat Lymphocyte Antigens

In the sheep and the goat, there have been two allelic loci recognised: *OLA-A, B* and *GLA-A, B*. The work of Millot (1979) has established that there is another factor (*OLA-X*) which segregates on the same chromosome as *OLA-A, B*, and another (*OLA-Z*) which is independent and may be on another chromosome. As was found in cattle, there are large differences in OLA antigen frequencies between different breeds of sheep (Cullen *et al.*, 1982).

In the goat there is some evidence obtained by van Dam for the existence of Class III (*C′*) regions within the MHC genes. Goat Class II antigens appear to be on the same chromosomal region as the Class I antigens (van Dam *et al.*, 1981). There are no reports of cross-reactions between the lymphocyte antigens of goats and sheep. Also there has been no biochemical characterisation of the sheep or goat MHC antigens.

10.4.7 Equine Lymphocyte Antigens

Limited published work is available for the equine lymphocyte antigens (EL-A). The evidence of Mottironi *et al.* (1981) suggests that there is only one genetic locus controlling the equine MHC, but obviously much more work needs to be done. Up to 10 antigens have been identified to be under the control of one autosomal chromosome region. An attempt to correlate the MHC antigens in horses with the incidence of Severe Combined Immunodeficiency (SCID) in Arabian horses has not been successful.

It was found by Swift and Mottironi (1982) that the Class II locus appeared to be separate from the Class I locus, as in other species. It was also observed in Arabian horses that the number of unidentified or 'null' alleles was very low, suggesting that the modern Arabian horse is descended from a limited foundation stock.

Again, since they are relatively poorly characterised, there has been no bio-chemical analysis of equine MHC antigens.

10.5 THE PRODUCTION OF ANTISERA AND MICROCYTOTOXICITY TESTS

10.5.1 Antisera

Antisera to lymphocyte antigens can be produced in four ways: lymphocyte immunisation, skin grafts, the collection of sera from pregnant mothers and the production of monoclonal antibodies.

Immunisation with lymphocytes is usually carried out with or without Freund's complete adjuvant and produces antisera which are complex due to antibodies against minor histocompatibility antigens as well as major antigens. These antibodies therefore usually have to be absorbed with lymphocytes which do not have common major antigens.

Skin grafts, or indeed any organ graft, can also be used and the titres obtained in the recipient are usually very high, but again, some absorption may be necessary to remove unwanted antibody specificities. The degree of response in the recipient depends on the quality of the skin graft, and it seems important that a blood supply is re-established and the skin graft survive until first-set rejection, in order to obtain the highest titres possible. In humans, antibodies are often produced in the recipients of blood transfusions, and this has been used in cattle also to produce antibodies to erythrocytes and lymphocytes simultaneously. However, the impression can be gained that this is a far less reliable method than skin grafts. The high titres in serum of recipients of skin grafts have the added advantage that extensive absorptions can be carried out with several lymphocyte suspensions, without the danger of complete loss of antibody activity. One final point can be made that experience with liver and kidney organ grafts in pigs indicates that these grafts do not produce high titres of antibodies to Ia antigens. Rather it appears in the pig and other species that skin is the organ which is rich in Ia antigens and the organ of choice for their production by grafting.

Reciprocal skin grafts between mother and offspring can reduce the complexity of the antiserum, since each is only reacting to antigens controlled by one chromosome half or haplotype. In the case of the mother, she reacts to the contribution of the sire to the lymphocyte antigens of the offspring, but not to her own contribution. This is the method of choice for producing anti-lymphocyte serum of high titre and high specificity.

Pregnancy sera have the advantage of reduced complexity, because the antibody response is to the paternal haplotype. It is curious that the peak titres in cattle are usually 3 months after calving. Re-mating to the same bull produces higher titres in subsequent pregnancies, but there is no certainty that the same haplotype will be inherited by the offspring. In general, subsequent pregnancies produce antisera of higher titre than the first pregnancy, but of increased complexity. Therefore, antisera from primiparous animals is the most useful, especially when one bull can be mated to about 40 heifers, which then produce antibodies to either one or the other of his haplotypes.

The main disadvantage of pregnancy sera is the low titre of 1 : 2 to 1 : 8 in the sera of primiparous animals, which makes absorptions difficult, due to complete loss of antibody activity. An advantage is that absorptions are frequently not necessary, and panels of antisera can be rapidly produced by mating a large number of dams to one sire.

Not all dams produce antibodies, and the incidence in sera of primiparous animals such as heifers is about 35%. The incidence increases to about 66% after several pregnancies. The type of placentation does not appear to affect the incidence of antibodies, although a very high incidence (84%) has been reported for horses by Mottironi *et al.* (1981).

Monoclonal antibodies would appear at first sight to be the answer to the production of highly-specific antibodies to the MHC antigens. However, despite intense activity in the human field, not more than about nine specificities have been produced from a potential of about 66 alleles. The problem appears to be that the mouse mostly recognises the more accessible public specificities on the human lymphocytes rather than the private specificities so easily demonstrated in human pregnancy sera. It may well be only a matter of time with the slow accumulation of useful clones to replace ultimately the use of pregnancy sera with monoclonal antibodies. However, there is another problem with monoclonal antibodies, in that a considerable proportion of them do not fix complement and cannot be used in the conventional microcytotoxicity assay. Monoclonal antibodies to bovine MHC antigens have been reported in the literature, but these are not available commercially. It is interesting that monoclonal antibodies to membrane IgM of bovine B-cells and β_2-microglobulin are often produced in these experiments.

The production of antibodies to the chicken MHC obviously cannot be carried out by collection of pregnancy sera, but the chicken has the advantage that erythrocytes share MHC antigens with lymphocytes, and cross-immunisation with erythrocytes between lines of chickens can produce high titres of highly-specific antisera. Strategic absorptions of antisera with either lymphocytes or erythrocytes can produce antisera highly specific for single loci for exclusively-erythrocyte or exclusively-lymphocyte antigens.

Finally it should be mentioned that in mammals the Ia antigens are not found on platelets, and suspensions of these can be used to absorb all antibodies to the other loci, leaving antisera to the Ia antigens exclusively.

10.5.2   Microcytotoxicity Testing

This is usually carried out in multi-well microcytotoxicity plates (Terasaki plates) under oil to prevent desiccation of the droplet. A 1-μl volume of test serum and 1 μl of lymphocyte suspension (2000 cells/well) is mixed and left for 30 minutes at room temperature. Then 5 μl of fresh rabbit serum complement is added and the plates left for a further 1-hour period. Then 5 μl of filtered aqueous eosin Y solution is added and 2 minutes later 5 μl of neutral buffered formalin. The eosin allows the differentiation of killed from live cells, and the formalin preserves them until they can be examined under the microscope.

The test plates are left overnight in the cold to allow the cells to settle completely into the bottom of each well, and the tests are read on an inverted microscope. The details of scoring the results are to be found in the Appendix of Methods.

Testing of human antisera for anti-Ia antibodies has been reported to involve a longer period of 2 hours after addition of the rabbit complement and before addition of the eosin Y and formalin for best results.

10.5.3 Analysis of Results

Computer programs are available which have been developed primarily for analysis of microcytotoxicity test results. These perform cluster analysis and χ^2 statistical analysis to allow sera of similar specificity to be grouped for further testing and verification. However, for small amounts of data it is preferable to examine the clusters by eye, using a chequerboard of antisera against lymphocyte samples.

10.6 ANTIBODIES TO ERYTHROCYTES

There is an extensive literature on erythrocyte typing of domestic animals which goes back to the early 1900s. In fact, contrasting with knowledge on bovine lymphocyte antigens, the knowledge on bovine erythrocyte antigens is the most extensive of all domestic species (Stone, 1967: Saison and Bull, 1976). There are bovine erythrocyte-typing laboratories set up in the United States, the United Kingdom, Canada, Australia and other countries, and they have accumulated extensive panels of antisera for typing the major erythrocyte groups. Unfortunately this extensive effort has not led to the expected insights into linkages between erythrocyte types and production characteristics, such as milk and meat production. More unfortunately, unlike the chicken, the erythrocyte-typing facilities cannot be used to type lymphocytes in mammals, since the erythrocytes do not possess the MHC antigens.

The knowledge of erythrocyte types has proved very useful in the resolution of doubtful paternity of stud cattle because of the large number of polymorphic blood group systems available. In fact, it has become mandatory for all registered bulls to be blood-typed, so that cases of doubtful paternity can be easily resolved. The vast number of alleles (>1000 for the bovine B system) make it highly improbable that two animals will have identical blood types. In horses too, blood-typing is also necessary for paternity exclusion rather than verification, because mares may be bred to more than one stallion during their heat period. Not as many alleles are recognised for horses as in cattle, and consequently the accuracy of the paternity testing is reduced. The blood groups of horses have also been used to test for potential cases of haemolytic disease of the newborn, which can be detected by testing mares before parturition.

In dogs, the blood groups have been studied because of the use of dogs in experimental transplantation studies. Dogs generally do not have iso-antibodies to other blood groups unless there is a history of previous transfusion. The exception is DEA 7, which is similar to the A antigen of the human ABO system. Dogs lacking DEA 7 will respond to the A substance in the environment and develop antibodies to the human blood group A, which cross-reacts with DEA 7. In this case, it is not possible to transfuse DEA 7-positive blood into DEA 7-negative recipients without a transfusion reaction (Bull, 1982).

In cats, Auer *et al.* (1981) have demonstrated an AB blood group system which is important for successful blood transfusion. The group A cats occasionally have anti-B, which is a weak agglutinin but strong haemolysin. However, all group B cats have high titres of anti-A, which is a stong agglutinin and haemolysin. Group AB cats contain neither anti-A nor anti-B and can be used as recipients for either group A or group B blood (Fig. 10.4).

Cross-matching of blood samples for both dog and cat is carried out in an agglutination test by mixing serum and red cells in tubes or on slides. A method for cross-matching of blood is described in the Appendix of Methods.

The other test for antibodies to erythrocytes is the haemolysis test, which appears to be more reliable than the agglutination test. It is interesting to note that an early test for lymphocyte antigens was carried out using an agglutination test as for erythrocytes. This test was very subject to spontaneous agglutination and

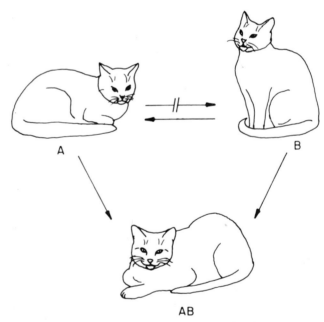

10.4. The AB blood group system in cats allows transfusion of group A cats with group B blood but not vice versa, because group B cats usually have high natural titres of anti-A, which is a strong agglutinin and haemolysin. Group AB cats have neither anti-A nor anti-B, and can be used as recipients for both types of blood.

was soon replaced by the Terasaki two-step microcytotoxicity test in the early 1960s.

10.6.1   Neonatal Isoerythrolysis

Known also as haemolytic disease of the newborn, this condition has been well-reviewed by Stormont (1975), and is essentially the result of destruction of red cells brought about by the action of iso-antibodies or allo-antibodies. In the horse the antibodies are acquired from the mother by the ingestion of colostrum by the newborn foal. Destruction of red cells can take place in the blood stream, but most of it occurs in organs such as the liver and spleen. A feature of neonatal erythrolysis is the grossly-enlarged spleen which appears black at postmortem.

The disease can be induced artificially in cattle as a result of the use of *Anaplasma* or *Babesia* vaccines, which contain bovine erythrocytes pooled from several donors. This produces a multiplicity of antibody specificities, and appropriate absorption analysis may show iso-antibodies which do not react with the erythrocyte antigens of the sire of the calf suffering the condition. Furthermore, steers as well as heifers have erythrocyte antigens as a result of vaccination.

A similar condition was found in the late 1940s following the use of the so-called crystal violet vaccine against 'hog cholera' or Swine Fever. The numbers of cases dramatically declined with the decreasing use of this vaccine.

Naturally-occurring neonatal isoerythrolysis is almost exclusively a disease of horses. Very rarely do ruminants have the disease, and attempts to produce it artificially in these species have surprisingly, been unsuccessful. This is despite the evidence that erythrocytes of lambs can become highly sensitised with antibodies which reach the circulation after ingestion of colostrum, without apparent effect on the health of the lambs. In horses, foals are thought to be at risk if the blood type of the mare does not contain determinants of the A and Q systems present in the stallion. The test to determine the presence of iso-antibodies is usually the haemolytic test, and this can be carried out on serum or pre-colostrum of the mare. These samples should be collected 1–2 weeks before parturition to allow laboratory tests. If haemolysis occurs, the veterinarian should advise the owner to remove the foal from the mare as soon as it is born. Appropriate mating and breeding plans can be used to reduce neonatal erythrolysis to zero.

10.7   LINKAGES BETWEEN MHC ANTIGENS IN DOMESTIC ANIMALS AND DISEASE

Although considerable efforts were expended in looking for linkages between erythrocyte antigens and disease susceptibility or resistance, none have been found for the common diseases of livestock. On the other hand, there is a strong linkage between a chicken lymphocyte antigen and resistance to Marek's disease, and this has spurred on work in mammalian systems.

10.7.1 Marek's Disease in Chickens

The selection of chickens for resistance or susceptibility was carried out by Cole at Cornell in the 1950s and 1960s. Using the response of a sample of progeny as the sole criterion for selection of breeders, a resistant line and a susceptible line of birds with respective susceptibilities of 12.9% and 90.7% were developed after only two generations of selection from a common stock in which the susceptibility was 51.1% (Cole, 1968).

At about the same time, Hansen *et al.* (1967) found a very strong association between susceptibility to the herpesvirus causing Marek's disease and the *B* locus in chickens. Progeny with the B21 antigen had approximately one-half the mortality of progeny with the B19 antigen. The B21 antigen was subsequently found to be present in Cole's resistant line, but, since the same gene was absent in the originally-selected Cornell lines (C and K), it appears that several other genetic alternatives also exist for resistance to the virus.

Removal of the bursa of Fabricius, either surgically or by hormone treatment, does not affect the incidence of the Marek's disease. So the genetic differences in susceptibility to the disease do not appear to result from primary differences in the humoral immune response. However, neonatal thymectomy of genetically-resistant chickens blocks the development of resistance with age. Thymic transplants restore resistance to the resistant strain of birds but not to the susceptible strain.

Other diseases of chickens have been investigated, and several other linkages with the *B* locus have been found. For example, resistance to the transient paralysis syndrome after Marek's virus infection has been linked with B1 and susceptibility with B2. Spontaneous autoimmune thyroiditis in 'obese' strain chickens has been linked with B1. More recent work on Marek's disease itself has suggested that virus strain differences produce different results which depend on the ontogenicity or persistence of the virus in the genetic material of the host. Chickens resistant to the JM-10 strain are completely susceptible to the GA-5 strain.

There are degrees of susceptibility or resistance, with chickens possessing any of the three alleles, *B2*, *B6* or *B21*, exhibiting moderate to strong resistance to Marek's disease, while those possessing a genotypic combination of five other alleles (*B3*, *B5*, *B13*, *B19* and *B27*) experience high levels of susceptibility.

Within strains there are also differences, and chickens homozygous for *B1* (B1/B1) fall into high and low responders to killed *Salmonella pullorum* organisms as measured by agglutination titres in serum after immunisation. Heterozygotes of *B1*, such as B1/B2 or B1/B19, have been found to produce significantly higher titres than the homozygotes (B1/B1) to immunisation with *S. pullorum* organisms. A linkage between the immune reponse to glutamic acid–L-alanine–L-tyrosine (GAT) and the progression of Rous Sarcoma virus (RSV)-induced tumours was found. Birds which were high responders to GAT in the B1/B1 strain were also able to control the progression of the tumour. Conversely, the low-responder B1/B1 birds to GAT were much less able to control the spread of the tumours.

Thus it can be concluded that the *B* locus is closely linked to the immune response of chickens to several antigens and that this locus contains the *Ir* region of the major histocompatibility complex.

Relatively little use has been made of the knowledge of resistant lines to increase resistance to Marek's disease in chickens. This was the result of an effective vaccine against the disease becoming available in the early 1970s. Genetic selection may become more important with newly-recognised highly-oncogenic strains of the virus which are causing vaccine breakdowns. A combination of vaccination and genetically-resistant strains may become important in disease control.

10.7.2   *Trichostrongylus colubriformis* in Sheep

As mentioned in Chapter 8 on immunity to internal parasites, sheep have been bred for resistance or susceptibility to parasites. Dineen and colleagues selectively bred sheep to have a highly-heritable response or lack of it, to vaccination with irradiated *Trichostrongylus colubriformis* larvae and challenge with normal larvae. The OLA type SY 1 is found in high frequency (70%) in high responders and lower frequency (22%) in low responders. The possibility of chance selection of this lymphocyte antigen in the parent flock was excluded when the same association between this antigen and low faecal egg count was found in randomly-selected sheep.

It is interesting that although an effect was found after challenge alone, the most statistically-significant effects were found after vaccination and challenge. If an immune-response gene effect is involved, it seems important to have a strong immune response to demonstrate it. In this case, the immune response is stimulated using the irradiated-larvae vaccine, which leads to the production of higher levels of complement-fixing antibody to parasite antigens in the high responders than in the low responders. Later on, the presence of high levels of antibody denotes a persistent infection and levels are reversed, with the low responders having the higher levels of antibody than the high responders, which have reduced their worm burden by this time.

The genetic linkage between this responsiveness and the *Ir* gene locus of sheep has yet to be confirmed. However, *T. colubriformis* infection of guinea pigs has been found to map in or near the *I* region of the guinea pig MHC. Geczy and

Rothwell (1981) found that the guinea pig *Ia-1,3* gene was associated with susceptibility, while the *Ia-1* gene was associated with resistance. This is a similar experimental system to the sheep, except that the guinea pig is an atypical host. Nevertheless, prospects appear good for finding an association between immune responsiveness to parasites in the sheep and the OLA *Ir* genes.

10.7.3 *Boophilus microplus* in Cattle

As mentioned in Chapter 9 on immunity to external parasites, there are breed differences in resistance to ticks in cattle. The *Bos indicus* breeds acquire a higher degree of resistance than the European cattle to *Boophilus microplus*. However, some of this effect may be due to more efficient grooming and removal of the ticks in the resistant compared with the susceptible cattle.

Nevertheless, within breeds, there is a normal distribution of tick burdens, with some animals apparently being highly resistant and others highly susceptible. There appears to be no bimodal distribution of tick counts as in the faecal egg counts in young lambs infected with *Trichostrongylus colubriformis,* and if immune responsiveness to ticks is involved in the cattle, it is not very obvious.

Work has been published by Stear *et al.* (1982), however, which shows a linkage between tick resistance and the BoLA system. They found a weak but significant correlation between the CA 4 antigen and resistance and between the CA 11 antigen and susceptibility. Again, the connection between these antigens and the BoLA *Ir* genes has yet to be formally established, but the evidence so far suggests that such a connection may also be made in cattle.

If an effective vaccine against ticks can be produced—for example, by directing the immune response against the internal organs of the ticks—it may be possible to vaccinate cattle of known BoLA type. In this case, associations may be more readily found in the presence of an active immune response than by uncontrolled-infestation survey experiments in the field.

10.8 CONCLUSIONS

It is perhaps in the field of internal and external parasite immunity that the detection of *Ir* genes will be important to domestic livestock. Any improvements in the response to vaccines may depend on having a background of selected high responders present in the flock or herd. However, the genes must be already present in high frequency if inbreeding is to be avoided, and the greatest improvements would probably be achieved in the first and second generations of selection. The selective breeding of cattle for hardiness in extensive grazing conditions could well involve basic research on the *Ir* genes and for the first time put such selection on a sound scientific basis.

REFERENCES

Amorena, B. and Stone, W. H. (1980). *Tissue Antigens* **16**, 212–225.

Auer, L., Bell, K. and Coates, S. (1981). *J. Am. Vet. Med. Assoc.* **180**, 729–730.

Bijnen, A. B., Obertop, H., Joling, P. and Westbroek, D. L. (1980). *Transplantation* **30**, 191–195.

Brodsky, F. M. and Parham, P. (1982). *Immunogenetics* **15**, 151–166.

Bull, R. W. (1982). *J. Am. Vet. Med. Assoc.* **181**, 1115–1119.

Calne, R. Y. (1973). Allografting in the pig. *In* 'Immunologic Aspects of Transplantation Surgery' (R. Y. Calne, ed.), pp. 296–316. John Wiley, New York.

Church, W. R., Poulik, M. D. and Reisfeld, R. A. (1982). *J. Immunol. Methods* **52**, 97–104.

Cole, R. K. (1968). *Avian Dis.* **12**, 9–28.

Cullen, P. R., Bunch, C., Brownlie, J. and Morris, P. J. (1982). *Anim. Blood Groups Biochem. Genet.* **13**, 149–159.

Deeg, H. J., Wulff, J. C., De Rose, S., Sale, G. E., Brown, M., Brown, M. A., Springmeyer, S. C., Martin, P. J. and Storb, R. (1982). *Immunogenetics* **16**, 445–457.

Geczy, A. F. and Rothwell, T. L. W. (1981). *Parasitology* **82**, 281–286.

Hansen, M. P., Van Zandt, J. N. and Law, G. R. J. (1967). *Poult. Sci.* **46**, 1268.

Hoffmann, D., Jennings, P. A. and Spradbrow, P. B. (1981). *Aust. Vet. J.* **57**, 159–162.

Klein, J. (1975). 'Biology of the Mouse Histocompatibility-2 Complex'. Springer-Verlag, Berlin and New York.

Lunney, J. K. and Sachs, D. H. (1978). *J. Immunol.* **120**, 607–612.

Millot, P. (1979). *Immunogenetics* **9**, 509–534.

Mottironi, V. D., Perryman, L. E., Pollara, B., Mickey, M. R., Swift, R. and McGrath, P. (1981). *Transplantation* **31**, 290–294.

Oliver, R. A., McCoubrey, C. M., Millar, P., Morgan, A. L. G. and Spooner, R. L. (1981). *Immunogenetics* **13**, 127–132.

Palker, T. J. and Yang, T. T. (1981). *J. Natl. Cancer Inst.* **66**, 779–787.

Pollack, M. S., Mastrota, F., Chin-Louie, J., Mooney, S. and Hayes, A. (1982). *Immunogenetics* **16**, 339–347.

Sachs, D. H., Leight, G., Cone, J., Schwarz, S., Stuart, L. and Rosenberg, S. (1976). *Transplantation* **22**, 559–567.

Saison, R. and Bull, R. W. (1976). Animal blood groups and biochemical polymorphisms. *In* 'Handbook of Laboratory Animal Science' (E. C. Melby and N. H. Altman, eds.), Vol. 3, pp. 463–478. CRC Press, Cleveland, Ohio.

Schierman, L. W. and Nordskog, A. W. (1963). *Nature (London)* **197**, 511–512.

Shinohara, N. and Sachs, D. H. (1982). Interspecies cross-reactions of murine anti Ia allo-antibodies. *In* 'Ia Antigens. Vol. 1: Mice' (S. Ferrone and C. S. David, eds.), pp. 219–240. CRC Press, Boca Raton, Florida.

Spooner, R. L., Leveziel, H., Grosclaude, F., Oliver, R. A. and Vaiman, M. (1978). *J. Immunogenet.* **5**, 335–346.

Stear, M. J., Newman, M. J., Nicholas, F. W., Brown, S. C. and Holroyd, R. G. (1982). *N. S. W. Vet. Proc.* **18**, 36–38.

Stone, W. H. (1967). Immunogenetics of type-specific antigens in animals. *In* 'Advances in Immunogenetics', pp. 173–215. J. P. Lippincott, Philadelphia, Pennsylvania.

Stormont, C., (1975). *Adv. Vet. Sci. Comp. Med.* **19**, 23–45.

Strominger, J. L. (1980). Structure of products of the major histocompatibility complex in man and mouse. *In* 'Immunology 80: Progress in Immunology IV' (M. Fougereau and J. Dausset, eds.), pp. 541–554. Academic Press, New York.

Swift, R. V. and Mottironi, V. D. (1982). *Am. J. Vet. Res.* **43**, 1859–1862.

Theilen, G. H. and Hills, D. (1982). *J. Am. Vet. Med. Assoc.* **181**, 1134–1141.

Vaiman, M., Metzger, J.-J., Renard, C. and Vila, J.-P. (1978). *Immunogenetics* **7**, 231–238.

van Dam, R. H., van Kooten, P. J. S., van der Donk, J. A. and Goudswaard, J. (1981). *Vet. Immunol. Immunopathol.* **2**, 321–330.

Vriesendorp, H. M. (1979). *Adv. Vet. Sci. Comp. Med.* **23**, 229–265.

Yang, T.-J. (1978). *Am. J. Pathol.* **91**, 149–152.

Zinkernagel, R. M. and Doherty, P. C. (1975). *J. Exp. Med.* **141**, 1427–1436.

Appendix
of Methods

ISOLATION OF LYMPHOCYTES FROM BLOOD

The aim of the isolation procedures for blood lymphocytes is to obtain the best recovery possible and at the same time produce a sample which accurately reflects the lymphocyte subpopulations which are present in the original blood sample.

There are two main ways of isolating blood lymphocytes: The first involves the use of a density-gradient mixture such as Ficoll-Paque (Pharmacia, Uppsala, Sweden). The second method involves the selective lysis of erythrocytes in the blood sample, which leaves the leucocytes intact. An example of this method is the glycerol-lysis technique of Binns (1978), which is described herein.

There are advantages and disadvantages to both techniques. The advantage of the Ficoll-Paque method is that it is gentle on the cells and is reasonably rapid. The disadvantage is that it does not always work for blood from domestic animals, such as ruminants, and there appears to be a selective loss of small, dense T-cells. However, if a representative sample of lymphocyte subpopulations is not required for later studies, the Ficoll-Paque method usually works well even in ruminants. Some samples of calf or lamb blood do not separate well on

225

Ficoll-Paque, and for this reason, it may be useful to make the granulocytes more dense than normal by allowing them to ingest carbonyl iron powder before they are placed on the gradient.

The advantage of using carbonyl iron powder is that the cells which ingest the powder can be held back by a strong magnet before the blood is placed on Ficoll-Paque, and this gives a more highly-purified population of lymphocytes than without the carbonyl iron powder treatment. Any carbonyl iron which is not held back, ends up in the red-cell pellet and does not contaminate the lymphocyte sample.

For the lysis techniques, the method of choice appears to be the glycerol lysis of erythrocytes. Other techniques are available which involve the use of distilled water to lyse the erythrocytes followed by rapid restoration of isotonicity with double-strength saline solution, but this method can be detrimental to lymphocyte membranes and can inhibit *in vitro* responses to antigens and mitogens.

The glycerol-lysis technique involves the suspension of the blood for 30 minutes in 5% glycerol–saline, the centrifugation of the blood and removal of most of the glycerol–saline and the rapid suspension of the cell pellet in normal saline. The method depends on the rigidity of the erythrocyte membrane, which is permeable to the glycerol–saline, but in medium of normal saline alone, cannot adjust the osmotic balance rapidly enough to prevent disruption of the membrane and lysis of the erythrocyte. The leucocytes, on the other hand, have membranes which are less rigid than the erythrocytes, and the leucocytes can adjust to the osmotic-pressure change and survive intact but slightly swollen. For this reason, the cells should be allowed to recover their size by incubation for 2 hours in tissue culture medium before being used in cell-sizing experiments or density-gradient centrifugation on gradients of Percoll (Pharmacia, Uppsala, Sweden), for example.

The advantages of this method are the high recovery of lymphocytes ($>90\%$) and the ease with which all species, including the chicken erythrocytes (which are difficult to lyse), have their erythrocytes lysed. It is also much more gentle on the lymphocyte cell membranes than distilled-water lysis, and the assays for lymphocyte membrane markers are usually unaffected by glycerol lysis, compared with the interference found with distilled-water lysis. For the fluorescence-activated cell sorter (FACS) too, there appears to be some advantage in having slightly-swollen cells, which exaggerate size differences between lymphocyte subpopulations.

A disadvantage of the glycerol-lysis technique is the large volume of glycerol–saline required for blood samples greater than 10–20 ml of blood. It is also slower than the Ficoll-Paque technique, in that glycerol lysis requires an equilibration, as well as several centrifugation steps. It does, however, produce a representative sample of cells for lymphocyte subpopulation studies.

Sheep Blood Lymphocyte Preparation
Using Ficoll-Paque

1. Collect blood from the jugular vein of sheep (e.g., 20 ml) using preservative-free heparin (10 IU/ml of blood) or K–EDTA (2 mg/ml of blood) as anticoagulants.

2. Add blood to 0.3 gm of carbonyl iron (Type SF, G. A. F. Corp.) in a Universal bottle, and place on a rotator at 37°C for 45 minutes. The carbonyl iron should be heated before use (in the bottle with the cap off) for 2 hours at 90°C, to break up clumps and sterilise it, and then allowed to cool.

3. Dilute 10 ml of blood containing carbonyl iron with 10 ml of sterile normal saline (SNS), and carefully layer it on top of 15 ml of Ficoll-Paque. Spin the tube at 2000 g for 35 minutes at 4°C in a refrigerated centrifuge. The refrigeration of the sample reduces clumping of the cells during concentration at the plasma–Ficoll-Paque interface.

4. Harvest the white cell layer and the Ficoll-Paque with a pipette, all the way down to the red-cell layer, and transfer to a sterile plastic centrifuge tube. Spin the cells into a pellet at 200 g for 15 minutes after diluting the Ficoll-Paque with saline. The supernate will be cloudy with platelets, which can be discarded if not needed.

5. Lyse contaminating red cells by adding 5 ml of ammonium chloride Tris buffer (ACT) at pH 7.2 at 37°C to the tube for 5 minutes in a water bath. Then fill the tube with SNS and spin into a pellet (200 g for 15 minutes). Discard the supernate and wash once again in the SNS solution.

6. Resuspend the cells in 1 ml of Eagle's minimal essential medium (MEM) or RPMI medium with 100 IU of penicillin and 100 μg of streptomycin per millilitre of medium. Sheep lymphocytes seem particularly susceptible to clumping in a concentrated pellet if serum is added, so add only small amounts (2%) of foetal calf serum (FCS).

7. Count cells in a Coulter Counter or haemocytometer, and adjust the volume to the required cell concentration, such as 10^6 cells/ml.

Pig and Horse Blood Lymphocyte Preparation
Using Ficoll-Paque

Both pig and horse erythrocytes sediment rapidly if left in a tube on the bench, particularly in the presence of added 10% dextran–saline. Therefore, a standard technique is to add dextran–saline (e.g., Dextraven, Fisons) to whole blood in a large tube and allow the red cells to sediment at unit gravity at an angle of 45° in a 37°C water bath.

The supernate contains the leucocytes, which after 30 minutes can be harvested and spun into a pellet to concentrate the cells and platelets. The pellet is then resuspended in a small volume of dextran–saline and separated on Ficoll-Paque, as described for the sheep and cow.

Sheep Blood Lymphocyte Preparation Using Glycerol Lysis

1. Collect blood from the jugular vein of sheep (e.g., 20 ml) with preservative-free heparin (10 IU ml of blood) or K–EDTA (2 mg/ml of blood) used as anticoagulants.

2. Add blood to 0.3 gm of carbonyl iron in a Universal bottle, and place on a rotator at 37°C for 45 minutes. The carbonyl iron should be heated before use (in the bottle with the cap off) for 2 hours at 90°C and then allowed to cool. This reduces the clumps in the carbonyl iron and also sterilises it.

3. Remove the carbonyl iron with a strong magnet placed on the outside of the tube, and pour off approximately equal volumes of blood into two 30-ml centrifuge tubes. Fill each tube with saline. This step is introduced to reduce the number of centrifugations required to wash out the plasma. Since the glycerol-lysis technique depends on osmotic shock, the presence of plasma reduces the osmotic difference between the cells and the medium, and the technique will not work unless very small volumes are used. Spin the blood for 20 minutes at 500 g.

4. Resuspend the cells in five parts of sterile 4% glycerol–saline (v/v) and leave at room temperature for 30 minutes. The glycerol–saline may be sterilised by autoclaving.

5. Spin the cells into a pellet (200 g for 15 minutes) at room temperature. It is important not to spin the cells too hard, or they will be difficult to resuspend. Remove the supernate and add SNS to the pellet with rapid mixing to lyse the red cells. This is a very important step to mix the cells and saline rapidly on a vortex mixer at low speed.

6. Spin the cells into a pellet at 200 g for 15 minutes, and discard the dark-red supernate. Wash once by resuspending the pellet in Hank's balanced salts solution (HBSS), and spin again at 200 g for 15 minutes.

7. Resuspend in 1 ml of Eagle's MEM containing 100 IU of penicillin and 100 μg of streptomycin per millilitre of medium. Pass the tube over the strong magnet again to consolidate the remaining carbonyl iron in a patch on the bottom of the tube, and carefully remove the cell suspension using a Pasteur pipette and transfer to another tube.

8. Count the cells in a Coulter Counter or haemocytometer, and adjust the volume to the required cell concentration (e.g., 10^6 cells/ml).

9. If erythrocyte 'ghosts' and platelets must be removed, the cells are layered over Ficoll-Paque diluted 1:1 with SNS and spun at 500 g for 20 minutes at 4°C. The pellet contains the lymphocytes, but the 'ghosts' and platelets remain at the interface between the Ficoll-Paque and the MEM.

Reference

Binns, R. M. (1978). *J. Immunol. Methods* **21**, 197–210

LYMPHOCYTE MEMBRANE MARKERS

Lymphocyte membrane markers are often the receptors for various components of the immune system such as complement and the Fc pieces of immunoglobulin molecules. There is also a receptor for sheep erythrocytes in the membrane of T-cells, which is useful for some domestic species of animals such as the goat, sheep, pig and cow. These are all available as rosette methods, but in the human they have largely been replaced by fluorescent monoclonal antibodies, which can be measured in the fluorescence-activated cell sorter (FACS).

These methods are, however, not antigen-specific and only reflect broad subpopulations. As long as this limitation is appreciated, the potential of lymphocyte subpopulation measurements can be realistically assessed.

Sheep Erythrocyte (E-) Rosettes with Sheep Lymphocytes

1. Prepare lymphocytes by the glycerol-lysis technique.
2. Resuspend the cells at 10^6 cells/ml in Eagle's MEM containing 2.5% FCS.
3. Prepare sheep erythrocytes from blood, using heparin or EDTA as anticoagulant and washing the erythrocytes five times with SNS. This is done by spinning the cells at 1800 g for 15 minutes into a pellet and then resuspending the cells in SNS each time.
4. Prepare a solution of Ficoll 400 (Pharmacia, Uppsala, Sweden) 24% (w/v) in phosphate-buffered saline (PBS), pH 7.2. Prepare a solution of preservative-free heparin at 200 IU/ml of PBS. Mix the heparin–saline (2 ml) with the Ficoll–saline (2.8 ml), and add 0.1 ml of packed, washed sheep erythrocytes with mixing.
5. Use Dreyer tubes or any small, tapered tubes after cleaning them thoroughly with tissue culture standard detergent (e.g., Decon 90, Decon Laboratories, England). Add to a clean, dry tube one drop of lymphocytes, followed by two drops of sheep erythrocytes in Ficoll–heparin–saline.
6. Spin the tubes at 450 g for 15 minutes at 4°C, and leave overnight at 4°C before reading.
7. The erythrocyte–lymphocyte pellet is resuspended with extreme care by gentle agitation with a stream of fluid slowly sucked up and down through a Pasteur pipette. This is a critical step for the resuspension of the rosettes, and it is important to do this gently. It is also important to do it only just before the rosettes are to be counted under the microscope.

8. It is useful to add three drops of fluorescein diacetate (Sigma Chemical Co.) in saline at 1 : 10,000 (w/v) to each tube and mix this with the rosettes as they are being resuspended.

9. Examine cells on a clean microscope slide under a coverslip using a fluorescence microscope. Living cells show a green fluorescence, and those with five or more erythrocytes attached are counted as rosettes.

Sheep Erythrocyte (E-) Rosettes with Cattle Lymphocytes

The overall technique for E-rosettes with cattle lymphocytes is the same as for sheep lymphocytes except for a difference in Ficoll concentration, which is higher for cattle than for sheep lymphocytes.

A solution of Ficoll 400 is prepared at 24% (w/v) in PBS. Prepare a solution of preservative-free heparin at 200 IU/ml in PBS. Mix the heparin–saline (2 ml) with the Ficoll–saline (4.8 ml), and then discard 1.8 ml. To the remaining 5 ml add 0.1 ml of washed, packed sheep erythrocytes prepared as for sheep lymphocyte E-rosettes.

This produces a rosette-enhancing medium with a higher concentration of Ficoll than for the sheep lymphocytes. The addition of heparin further enhances the percentage of detectable rosettes with both sheep and cattle lymphocytes.

Pig Lymphocytes

The use of dextran–saline was originally described by Binns (1978), as a method for enhancing pig E-rosettes. Ficoll 400 was found to be superior to dextran in promoting E-rosette formation. However, there remained a population of T-cells which could not be induced to form E-rosettes, and these were the thymus-dependent 'null' cells described in Chapter 2 on cellular immunology.

Dog and Cat Lymphocytes

The blood lymphocytes of the dog and cat do not form E-rosettes with sheep erythrocytes, and attempts to enhance rosette formation with Ficoll are not effective. A method using guinea pig erythrocytes has been described, and this appears to be a marker for a subpopulation of T-cells in the dog and cat.

Horse Lymphocytes

Sheep erythrocytes do not form E-rosettes with horse lymphocytes, and there appears to be no generally-available marker for horse T-cells.

Chicken Lymphocytes

Sheep erythrocytes do not form E-rosettes with chicken lymphocytes.

The Detection of Fc Receptors on Lymphocytes
by Rosette Techniques

Membrane receptors for the Fc piece of all the immunoglobulins—IgG, IgM, IgA and IgE—have been detected in human lymphocyte subpopulations. A rosette technique with ox erythrocytes (BRBC) coated with purified immunoglobulin subclasses has been used with IgG and IgM in domestic animals (Fig. A.1). The method involves immunising rabbits with ox erythrocytes and separating the antibody-containing immunoglobulins into IgG and IgM fractions on Sephadex G200 (see section on preparation of immunoglobulins, p. 246. The method relies on the cross-reactivity of the rabbit Fc pieces with the receptors in the membranes of ovine and bovine lymphocytes. There is no reliable way of

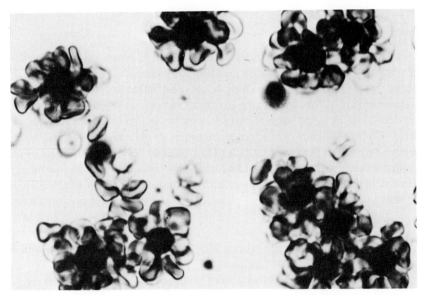

Fig. A.1. The formation of Fc-rosettes between sheep lymphocytes and bovine erythrocytes coated with antibody prepared in rabbits is shown. The rosettes have been fixed with glutaraldehyde and stained with crystal violet, so that the lymphocyte at the centre is darkly stained while the surrounding erythrocytes remain translucent. The erythrocytes are attached in three dimensions around the lymphocyte, so that the plane of focus of the microscope leaves some red cells blurred. The close attachment of the erythrocytes leads to some distortion of the red cells clustered tightly around the lymphocytes. (Reproduced by kind permission of Dr. R. M. Binns ARC, Institute of Animal Physiology, Babraham, Cambridge.)

providing homologous antiserum to ox erythrocytes which can be used in the same way.

Method

1. Sensitise 0.1 ml of packed, washed (five times) BRBC with a subagglutinating concentration of rabbit anti-BRBC (IgG or IgM) for 1 hour at 37°C.
2. Wash and spin the erythrocytes three times at 200 g with SNS at 4°C.
3. Resuspend the erythrocytes in 5 ml of Eagle's MEM containing 100 IU of penicillin and 100 μg of streptomycin per millilitre.
4. Store the sensitised cells at 4°C, and wash again with MEM just before use. Resuspend the erythrocytes in 5 ml of MEM.
5. Proceed with one drop of lymphocytes followed by two drops of sensitised BRBC in Dreyer tubes as for sheep E-rosettes.
6. Spin the tubes at 200 g for 15 minutes at 4°C, and leave overnight in the cold before reading on the fluorescence microscope with added fluorescein diacetate.

Complement Rosettes

This method involves the coating of BRBC with immunoglobulin, followed by the addition of fresh serum which contains complement (C') components. The species from which the fresh serum is obtained influences the percentage of rosettes detected. It has been found that fresh mouse complement, for example, produces a higher percentage of rosettes with bovine lymphocytes than are detected with homologous bovine serum complement (Higgins and Stack, 1978). The reason for this is not clear. It is also important to use serum complement which has been previously absorbed with lymphocytes to remove the low titres of heterophile antibodies directed towards the lymphocytes, which might alter the percentage of rosettes detected.

Method

1. Prepare immunoglobulin-coated BRBC as for Fc-rosettes with 0.1 ml of packed cells.
2. To the pellet of antibody-sensitised erythrocytes add 1 ml of 1:10 mouse serum, and incubate for 1 hour at 37°C.
3. Wash the sensitised erythrocytes five times in SNS, and resuspend the BRBC in 5 ml of Eagle's MEM.
4. Prepare and examine C' rosettes as for Fc-rosettes.

References

Binns, R. M. (1978). *J. Immunol. Methods* **21,** 197–210.
Higgins, D. A. and Stack, M. J. (1978). *J. Immunol. Methods* **20,** 211–224.

Surface Immunoglobulin on B-Cells

Using this assay for cells which have surface immunoglobulin (sIg) in their membranes, the Ig subclass has been shown to be monomeric IgM in all species so far examined. However, anti-IgM is not always necessary for its detection, since cross-reaction between the light chains of IgG and IgM allows the use of polyspecific antisera.

It is recommended that $F(ab')_2$ fragments of antiserum be used to prevent cells labelling with fluorescent immunoglobulin by their Fc receptors. In practise, it is often possible to label sIg using an indirect method with uncleaved fluorescein isothiocyanate (FITC)-labelled anti-immunoglobulin, as long as appropriate controls with FITC-labelled anti-immunoglobulin are made. It appears that labelling cells at 4°C for 15 minutes reduces adsorption of antibody to Fc receptors to a very low level.

Affinity-purified, FITC-labelled anti-immunoglobulin or monoclonal antibodies to immunoglobulin are available for direct labelling of human B-cells. They are also in the form of $F(ab')_2$ fragments, which makes them ideal for the purpose required. Such reagents are not commercially available for the labelling of B-cells in domestic animals, so that the method described here is a compromise between what is ideal and what is practical at this time.

Method

1. Wash lymphocytes five times in HBSS. For critical work it is recommended that the cells be incubated for 2 hours in Eagle's MEM at 37°C in the CO_2 incubator to allow elution or metabolism of the cytophilic antibodies attached to the Fc receptors. Wash the cells once in MEM.

2. Resuspend the cells in MEM at a concentration of 10^6 cells/ml.

3. Add one drop of cells to a small glass tube in an ice-bucket. Tests should be carried out at least in duplicate and preferably in triplicate or quadruplicate for accuracy.

4. Add one drop of rabbit anti-immunoglobulin and leave to react for 15 minutes. It may be necessary to pass the antiserum through a 0.22-μm membrane filter to remove aggregates.

5. Wash the cells twice in ice-cold PBS, and resuspend in one drop of saline.

6. Add one drop of FITC-labelled goat anti-rabbit immunoglobulin to the drop of suspended cells.

7. React for 15 minutes and then wash twice with ice-cold PBS.

8. Transfer the drop of labelled cells to a cleaned microscope slide, attach a coverslip and examine immediately by incident ultraviolet or blue-light excitation on a microscope. The cells may also be resuspended in 0.5 ml of PBS and examined in the FACS.

USE OF THE FLUORESCENCE-ACTIVATED CELL SORTER

The fluorescence-activated cell sorter (FACS) (Fig. A.2) allows the rapid analysis of cells which have been labelled with FITC attached to various membrane probes, such as specific antisera. Because the cells pass through a narrow orifice to cross the path of the laser which excites the fluorescein, the use of the FACS for measuring rosettes is usually not successful. This is because it is difficult to distinguish the clumps of lymphocytes and sheep erythrocytes from the true rosettes. Also it has been found that rosettes, in particular E-rosettes, dissociate into their lymphocyte and sheep erythrocyte components during their passage through the orifice, due to the shearing forces generated there. Attempts have been made to fix the rosettes with glutaraldehyde (Stadler *et al.*, 1980), and these have been successful, except that the cells are killed by the treatment.

In any case, the rosette method coupled with density-gradient centrifugation on Percoll or Ficoll-Paque is a good method for the bulk separation of lymphocyte subpopulations. What the rosette sedimentation method lacks in high purification, it gains in speed of separation. This is because the FACS can take several hours to separate a few million cells of a minor subpopulation due to the sorting time involved even at a rate of 3000 cells/second. This has meant that the

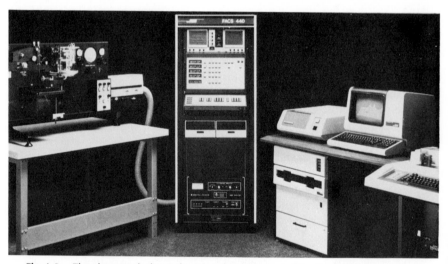

Fig. A.2.   The photograph shows the general arrangement of the Becton-Dickinson fluorescence-activated cell sorter (FACS). The cell separation and analysis is carried out in the apparatus on the left with the argon laser and S-shaped power line attached. In the centre is an analytical module with cathode-ray display, scalers and sorting controls. On the right is the data acquisition and storage module controlled by computer, data storage disk and video display unit for multiparameter analysis. (Reproduced by kind permission of the Becton-Dickinson FACS System, Sunnyvale, California.)

bulk of the work carried out on cell sorters has been analytical, since this takes advantage of the rapid speed with which cell populations can be differentiated by the machine. If sorting is required, it is advisable to concentrate the required cell subpopulation first by a bulk rosette method to reduce the time taken on the FACS.

It is fortunate in the human immunology field that there are commercially-available FITC-coupled monoclonal antibodies for most of the differentiation antigens and some of the MHC antigens of human lymphocytes. These fluorescent probes have largely replaced the rosette methods for differentiation of lymphocyte subpopulations in the human. It has also led to a proliferation of published papers on the distribution of lymphocyte subpopulations in various clinical conditions in humans which has not been paralleled by similar studies in domestic animals.

This is because in the veterinary field, similar types of anti-lymphocyte monoclonal antibodies are not generally available, although there have been some specially produced against ruminant T- and B-cells in several laboratories. These antibodies are not generally available outside the laboratory of origin, so that cell sorters have not been used extensively for analysis of lymphocyte subpopulations in domestic animals. There is published work on the use of a cell sorter for analysis of DNA distribution on biopsy specimens of solid tumours of dogs (Johnson et al., 1981). This involved staining cells with mithramycin to highlight the DNA. So far, no tumour-specific antigens have been detected for dog tumours, although this is the aim of the research.

The important point with flow cytometry is the specificity of the fluorescent staining reaction, and this must be evaluated using a fluorescence microscope before examining the cells in the FACS.

Method

1. Stain cells with required fluorescent label (e.g., for sIg). Check that the cells are properly labelled using the fluorescence microscope.

2. Wash the cells thoroughly (three to five times) in PBS to reduce the non-specific staining, and make up to 2×10^6 cells/ml in PBS.

3. Tune the argon laser in the FACS to the line closest to the optimum excitation wavelength for the fluorochrome (e.g., 488 nm for FITC).

4. Run the cells through the FACS and choose appropriate parameters, such as cell size (scatter or axial light loss) against green or red fluorescence.

5. Enclose by electronic 'gate' the clusters of interest in the cytogram mode or peak of interest in the histogram mode. Store differential counts in notebook or on computer disk.

6. Sort cells of interest into MEM for further microscopic examination or *in vitro* tests.

7. For accurate quantitative data it is necessary to run a normal control and

TABLE A.1

Advantages and Disadvantages of FACS Analysis

FACS	Microscope
Expensive	Cheap
Fast	Slow
Sorting possible	No sorting
Total fluorescence, no cell detail	Cell detail visible
Limitations with double fluorochromes	Discrimination of double fluorochromes
Argon laser limits excitation wavelength for some fluorochromes	Mercury vapour lamp excites most fluorochromes
Cell size measurable	Cell size difficult to measure

use the background-subtraction facility to correct reading on the test sample which follows it.

References

Johnson, T. S., Raju, M. R., Giltinan, R. K. and Gillette, E. L. (1981). *Cancer Res.* **41**, 3005–3009.
Stadler, B. M., Spengler, H. and de Weck, A. L. (1980). *J. Immunol. Methods* **35**, 201–211.

LYMPHOCYTE STIMULATION

A well-established technique for the measurement of lymphocyte responses to antigens and mitogens *in vitro*, lymphocyte stimulation is often used in conjunction with cell sorting or other techniques of lymphocyte subpopulation separation to measure the distribution of responses amongst the various subpopulations.

The technique depends on the incorporation of a DNA precursor, such as [^{3}H]thymidine, into lymphocytes during the period of DNA synthesis associated with transformation of the cells into lymphoblasts. The labelled DNA is then retained by glass-fibre filter disks, which are transferred to the scintillation counter for radioactive counting.

Method

1. Lymphocytes are prepared by Ficoll-Paque or by the glycerol-lysis method.
2. For most species, lymphocytes may be cultured in Eagle's MEM with

bicarbonate or HEPES buffer (Flow Laboratories). However, conditions vary for optimum stimulation in each species of domestic animals. The addition of low concentrations of 2-mercaptoethanol appears to provide a substitute for the lack of accessory cells, such as monocytes, which promote lymphocyte transformation. There is also an optimum concentration of FCS which must be added (10–20%) to ensure survival of the lymphocytes during the culture period. This is used because of its ready availability, but foetal lamb serum for sheep lymphocytes or foetal foal serum for horse lymphocytes may produce better results than foetal calf serum in these species. The important point is to have a serum supplement in the medium, free of immunoglobulins which may contain antibodies to lymphocytes.

3. For ruminants, Eagle's MEM with 2-mercaptoethanol at $5 \times 10^{-5} M$ and 20% FCS appears suitable. The buffer used may be either bicarbonate or HEPES buffer; the bicarbonate buffer is suitable for use in the CO_2 incubator. If the cell cultures must be removed and replaced frequently in the incubator, the HEPES buffer is more effective at maintaining pH than the bicarbonate buffer. All culture media should be prepared using sterile technique.

4. Cells are placed in round-bottom Microtiter trays (Cooke Engineering) with lids. Both trays and lids can be purchased in sterile packs.

5. Dilutions of antigen are prepared so that, for example, four wells contain either no antigen, 1.0 μg, 10 μg or 100 μg of antigen per millilitre of medium. Antigen solutions must be sterilised by 0.22-μm membrane filter before use.

6. Calculate the amount of medium required for each dilution on the basis of 0.2 ml/well at 300,000 lymphocytes per well, multiplied by the number of replicates.

7. Resuspend the lymphocyte pellets in the appropriate antigen concentrations, and dispense 0.2-ml aliquots using an automatic pipettor with sterile tip. Work from the control cells towards the highest antigen concentration without changing the tip.

8. Place the plates, with lids attached, into the 37°C humid incubator with an atmosphere of 5% CO_2 in air.

9. Incubate the cultures for 48 hours with phytohaemagglutinin (PHA), for 72 hours with specific antigen and for 144 hours with mixed-lymphocyte cultures before adding [³H]thymidine for the last 18 hours. The medium above the cells must be changed at 96 hours for the mixed-lymphocyte reactions to restore cell reactivity. This is done by aspirating each well with sterile pipettor and replacing with 0.2 ml of the same medium, without disturbing the cell pellet.

10. [³H]Thymidine (The Radiochemical Centre, Amersham, England) is withdrawn from its vial using a sterile needle and syringe after swabbing the rubber stopper with 70% alcohol. A volume of 0.1 ml is added to 2.5 ml of MEM. This is enough for 100 wells if 0.025 ml is added to each well.

11. Add 0.025 ml of [³H]thymidine to each well at the appropriate time using

a micropipettor with sterile tip, and incubate the cells for a further 18 hours in the CO_2 incubator.

12. Harvest the plates using an automatic sample harvester (e.g. Dynatech, Multiple Cell-Culture Harvester) onto glass-fibre discs.

13. Dry the glass-fibre discs and place them individually into scintillation vials containing scintillation cocktail. Count the vials in a scintillation counter with windows set for tritium and with automatic quench correction.

SEPARATION OF LYMPHOCYTES ON NYLON WOOL

This is a method which has been widely used for the initial separation of blood lymphocytes into B-cell-depleted non-adherent cells and B-cell-enriched adherent cell populations. As mentioned in Chapter 2, the method involves an appreciable loss of cells on the column (14–20%), which are not recoverable. Therefore, it is only used for work in which total recovery of cells is not a critical part of the experiment.

Method

1. Nylon wool (Leukopak, Fenwall Laboratories) is washed 5 times in boiling water and rinsed 10 times in cold distilled water.

2. After drying, the nylon wool is handled with clean forceps, and 0.6-gm amounts are weighed out on a top-loading balance.

3. The 0.6-gm amounts of nylon wool are each packed into 10-ml syringe barrels (Monoject, Becton-Dickinson) fitted with a stopcock and autoclaved in a sterile pack.

4. The columns are equilibrated with MEM containing HEPES buffer and 10% FCS, for 45 minutes at 37°C, prior to loading the lymphocyte suspension.

5. The medium is run out of the column, by opening the stopcock, until the meniscus of the fluid is just above the nylon wool. One hundred million lymphocytes suspended in 2 ml of MEM with 10% FCS, are loaded onto the column by opening and shutting the stopcock to run in the cells and trap them in the interstices of the nylon wool. Fresh medium is added above the nylon wool. The cells are incubated for another 30 minutes at 37°C.

6. The lymphocytes are eluted from the column by 10% FCS in MEM warmed to 37°C and added to the top of the column with the stopcock open. The medium is allowed to flow at approximately 1 ml/minute until the eluate is visibly free of cells. In practice, more than three column-volumes (approximately 30 ml) is needed. These cells are termed the non-adherent fraction and are a population enriched for T-cells and depleted of B-cells.

7. The adherent lymphocytes are then harvested by first inserting a sterile syringe plunger into the barrel and drawing up 10–30 ml of the medium into the

syringe with nylon wool in place, expelling it and repeating the process 20 times before finally expelling the cell suspension into a centrifuge tube. The population of cells so obtained is enriched for B-cells but still contains a significant proportion of T-cells.

8. The adherent and non-adherent populations are transferred to centrifuge tubes, washed twice in MEM and resuspended in 10% FCS in MEM for counting in a haemocytometer or Coulter Counter.

ISOTOPE RELEASE ASSAY

The isotope release assay is for measuring the cytotoxic activity of lymphocytes, macrophages and neutrophils against target cells or microorganisms. The assays usually involve the release of ^{51}Cr from labelled chicken erythrocytes or from ^{51}Cr-labelled tumour cell targets. There is also a direct assay on radiolabelled protozoa, such as *Tritrichomonas fetus* or *Trypanosoma theileri*, which has been used to measure the direct cytotoxic activity of cattle leucocytes.

The most extensively-used assay in the veterinary field has been ^{51}Cr release from chicken erythrocytes. This has been used to measure the activity of neutrophils, macrophages and K-cells in cattle (Grewal et al., 1977). It has even been adapted to measure the activity of leucocytes against chicken erythrocytes coated with protozoan antigens (Duffus et al., 1978).

These assays have demonstrated that the most important effect of leucocytes on protozoan parasites is antibody-dependent. Therefore, a method for measuring antibody-dependent cell-mediated cytotoxicity (ADCC) is described here.

Method

1. Obtain 1–2 ml of chicken blood from the wing vein using a sterile syringe containing heparin anticoagulant to give a final concentration of 10 IU/ml.

2. Wash the chicken red blood cells (CRBC) four times in Eagle's MEM, and remove the buffy coat.

3. Dilute 0.1 ml of washed, packed CRBC to 1.9 ml in Eagle's MEM.

4. Mix 0.1 ml of diluted blood with 0.1 ml of sodium ^{51}Cr (Radiochemical Centre, Amersham, England, Cat. No. CJS IP). A film badge should be worn while handling the isotope to monitor the radiation dose to the operator. Awareness of the hazards of γ-emitting isotopes is vital at all times.

5. Incubate the CRBC with the isotope in an untightened, screw-capped tube for 1 hour at 37°C in a CO_2 incubator. Wash the CRBC four times by centrifugation, and dispose of the washings according to the radiochemical code used in your laboratory. It may be necessary to store the washings in a lead-lined box to allow the ^{51}Cr to decay before final disposal.

6. Dilute the labelled CRBC to a concentration of 2×10^5 CRBC/ml in a

suspension of sheep erythrocytes. This is done to reduce the spontaneous lysis of the CRBC. The sheep erythrocytes are made up as a suspension of 10^7 erythrocytes/ml, after washing four times in MEM. It is essential not to dilute the CRBC until just before use, to reduce spontaneous lysis.

7. For the measurement of K-cell activity, lymphocytes are prepared from blood using Ficoll-Paque. It is not recommended that NH_4Cl–Tris lysis be used, since this reduces the cytotoxic activity of the lymphocytes. It is also not advisable to use carbonyl iron to remove the phagocytic cells, since this may also remove the cytotoxic activity of the cell suspension. An alternative to using carbonyl iron is to pass the cells through a nylon wool column steeped in 100% FCS to remove the phagocytic cells, while retaining K-cell activity.

8. A dose–response curve can be constructed by altering the ratio of lymphocytes to CRBC targets. For example, a ratio of 25 lymphocytes to 1 target CRBC is optimum for mouse spleen cells, but for sheep blood lymphocytes, the ratio is more like 100:1. Therefore, a trial assay should be set up using ratios of 25:1, 50:1 and 100:1 lymphocytes to CRBC in quadruplicate, in a sterile Microtiter plate with round-bottom wells, capacity 0.3 ml/well.

9. The ADCC assay requires antibody to CRBC prepared in rabbits. This is inactivated at 56°C for 30 minutes. The antibody is titrated to this end-point using an agglutination test, and this gives a guide to the dilution required for the ADCC assay.

10. The assay is set up as described in Table A.2. This is repeated for each effector: target cell ratio, so that more than one Microtiter plate may be needed. The lymphocytes are added to the wells first, then antibody and finally the labelled CRBC. It is important to add the CRBC last to reduce the spontaneous lysis. The plates are incubated, with lids on, for 4 hours at 37°C in a CO_2 incubator. Longer incubation times, such as 18 hours, may also be used, as long as the spontaneous release of ^{51}Cr from the CRBC is not excessively high during this period.

11. The released ^{51}Cr is harvested by carefully removing an aliquot (0.15 ml) of the supernate from each well without disturbing the cell pellet. Alternatively, there is a system available for Microtiter plates which uses disposable cylindrical filters which fit snugly inside the wells (Titertek Supernatant Harvester). These soak up the supernates and separate them from the CRBC by means of a glass-fibre disk attached to the end of the filter. Whichever method is used, the supernates are transferred to the γ counter to measure the ^{51}Cr release, with 1-minute counts. Again all radioactive waste must be discarded in the required manner.

12. The calculation of cytotoxicity may be carried out in several ways depending on the baseline taken as spontaneous release. This may be the control with antibody alone or the control with lymphocytes alone. It is sometimes found that the control with lymphocytes alone is less than that with antibody alone.

TABLE A.2

ADCC Assay

Wells (×4)	Lymphocytes (μl)	Antibody (μl)	^{51}Cr-Labelled CRBC (μl)	Saponin (μl)
A	100	50	100	—
B	—	50	100	—
C	100	—	100	—
D	—	—	100	—
E	100	—	100	100

This 'protective effect' is thought to be due to contaminating monocytes which take up the released ^{51}Cr from the supernate, making it unavailable for harvesting.

The accepted formula for calculating the result is as follows:

$$\% \ ^{51}\text{Cr Release} = \frac{A - B \times 100}{E - B}$$

or

$$= \frac{A - C \times 100}{E - C}$$

The letters correspond to the wells in the protocol given in step 10. The final percentage ^{51}Cr released may be used to titrate the antibody to a point where cytotoxicity disappears. There should also be an effect of varying the effector : target cell ratio, with an increase in the higher ratios.

References

Duffus, W. P. H., Butterworth, A. E., Wagner, G. G., Preston, J. M. and Franks, D. (1978). *Infect. Immun.* **22**, 493–501.

Emery, D. L. and Kar, S. K. (1983). *Immunology* **48**, 723–731.

Grewal, A. S., Rouse, B. T. and Babiuk, L. (1977). *Infect. Immun.* **15**, 698–703.

Perlmann, H., Perlmann, P., Pape, G. R. and Hallden, G. (1976). *Scand. J. Immunol., Suppl.* No. 5, 57–68.

Townsend, J. and Duffus, W. P. H. (1982). *Clin. Exp. Immunol.* **48**, 289–299.

INTERLEUKIN II PRODUCTION

The aim of production of the lymphokine, interleukin II (IL II), is to stimulate lymphocytes with phytomitogens or antigens to produce conditioned medium, which can then be used to maintain lymphoblast cell lines. The lymphocyte-stimulating activity is also known as co-stimulator, but the most common term is interleukin II.

The activity is contained in culture supernates, and the evidence so far suggests that the IL II activity is species-specific. The medium used to culture the lymphocytes may contain the usual concentration of 10% FCS, or it may contain a serum substitute, such as polyethylene glycol (PEG) or bovine serum albumin (BSA), as described in the accompanying references. The lack of serum allows further biochemical characterisation of the IL II. The lymphokine appears to have its effects on lymphocytes at short range, and its effect *in vivo* is very likely the recruitment of 'bystander' lymphocytes in the delayed-hypersensitivity skin response to tuberculin.

Method

1. Using clean technique to avoid bacterial contamination, obtain a large volume of blood (500 ml) from a cow or pig using K–EDTA anticoagulant at a final concentration of 2 mg/ml of blood.

2. Concentrate the buffy-coat cells by centrifugation of the blood in large, sterile 250-ml centrifuge bottles using a centrifuge with a swing-out head.

3. Remove the buffy-coat cells by sterile pipette and transfer to a small, sterile narrow-bore centrifuge tube. Spin this at 1000 g for 20 minutes, to concentrate the leucocytes in a narrow band above the red cells. Harvest the leucocytes with a sterile Pasteur pipette and suspend the cells in Eagle's MEM.

4. Prepare culture medium for lymphocytes. This can be Eagle's MEM with bicarbonate buffer and with 0.4% PEG (20,000 MW) and 100 IU of penicillin and 100 μg streptomycin per millilitre of medium. The cells are suspended at 2×10^6 cells/ml of medium, and 200 ml of suspension are cultured in sterilised, flat glass bottles ('medicine flats', 1-litre volume) with a cotton wool plug in the neck. Disposable plastic culture bottles may also be used but are expensive. The cells are best cultured with the bottle flat and a maximum depth of 1 cm medium, which will allow adequate gas exchange in the CO_2 incubator.

5. The cells are cultured for 48 hours with phytomitogens or 96 hours with antigens, and then the supernate is decanted into centrifuge tubes (250ml) and the cells spun into a pellet by centrifugation. The supernate is decanted and concentrated by ultrafiltration, using a filter membrane with 10,000 MW retention limit. It is also advisable to dialyse the concentrated supernate overnight against the final tissue culture medium which is to be used in the interleukin II culture medium. This should be finally sterilised with a 0.45-μm Millipore filter and stored at 4°C until use.

6. Interleukin II activity is assayed using [³H]thymidine uptake by transforming lymphocytes as described previously.

References

Baker, P. E. and Knoblock, K. F. (1982a). *Vet. Immunol. Immunopathol.* **3**, 365–379.
Baker, P. E. and Knoblock, K. F. (1982b). *Vet. Immunol. Immunopathol.* **3**, 381–397.
Gasbarre, L. C., Urban, J. F. and Romanowski, R. D. (1983). *Vet. Immunol. Immunopathol.* **5**, 221–236.
Outteridge, P. M. and Lepper, A. W. D. (1973). *Immunology* **25**, 981–994.

SOURCES OF MACROPHAGES FOR TISSUE CULTURE

The sources of macrophages from the large domestic animals are limited. With laboratory animals, such as the laboratory mouse and rat, there is a normal resident population of macrophages in the peritoneal cavity. This is not so with the larger animals such as the dog and sheep, and migration of macrophages must be elicited by intraperitoneal injection of sterile mineral oil 5 days before harvesting the cells. However, even after oil injection, it is difficult to wash out the elicited macrophages in the sheep, for example, because it is hard to find and tap the pool of cell-laden fluid, using a paracentesis needle. Therefore, alternative sources of macrophages have been explored, and these include the non-lactating mammary gland, the lung and the circulating blood monocytes.

The non-lactating mammary gland contains a population of resident macrophages which may be washed out with Eagle's MEM by perfusing through the streak canal and milking out the cell-laden fluid into a collecting vessel. The method has been used in the mare, cow and ewe with good results, but repeated sampling requires that the cells be elicited by the perfusion of a very small amount of bacterial lipopolysaccharide. This is followed 6 hours later by the migration of large numbers of neutrophils into the mammary cistern. These neutrophils are in high purity (>98%), and they can be harvested by perfusion of MEM followed by milking the gland into a collecting vessel. Five days later, the cells in the milk cistern have changed in character to be predominantly mononuclear cells, with 70% macrophages. These can be harvested in the same way as the neutrophils are harvested.

The lung is also a good source of macrophages, but these may have to be harvested at postmortem by MEM perfusion of isolated lungs with the trachea attached, followed by squeezing out the mucus-laden MEM, which contains the cells, into collecting vessels. The lung macrophages are likely to have bacterial contamination because of the nature of the dusty surroundings of many domestic animals before they are slaughtered.

An alternative method is to anaesthetise the animal and harvest lung macrophages by endobronchial lavage. A method for this has been described for the dog, but for cattle and horses, the procedure is rather arduous and carries some risk to the life of the animal.

Tissue culture of blood monocytes has been described for cattle. However, it is difficult to obtain large numbers in this way, and the blood monocytes do not necessarily mature into macrophages in tissue culture without the stimulus of conditioned media. The blood monocyte has not been used very successfully as a source of macrophages from domestic animals.

References

Mare: Anderson, L. W. and Banks, K. L. (1981). *Am. J. Vet. Res.* **42**, 1956–1958.
Dog: Brown, N. O., Noone, K. E. and Kurzman, I. D. (1982). *Am. J. Vet. Res.* **44**, 335–337.
Ewe: Lee, C. S. and Outteridge, P. M. (1976). *Aust. J. Exp. Biol. Med. Sci.* **54**, 43–55.
Cow: Wardley, R. C., Rouse, B. T. and Babiuk, L. A. (1976). *J. Reticuloendothel. Soc.* **19**, 29–36.

CHEMILUMINESCENCE IN PHAGOCYTOSIS ASSAYS

Chemiluminescence is a useful method for measuring functional differences between neutrophils and macrophages during phagocytosis. It can also be used to measure differences between individual samples of neutrophils which are phagocytosing standard opsonised particles, such as bacteria or yeast cells. The method depends on the amplification of the natural chemiluminescence which occurs when superoxide is released during lysosomal fusion with phagocytic vesicles. The amplification is provided by adding 5-amino-2,3-dihydro-1,4-pthalazine (Luminol) to the cell suspension and measuring the chemiluminescence of the cells in the scintillation counter during phagocytosis of opsonised particles by the cells.

Method

1. One hundred milligrams of Luminol (Eastman Organic Chemicals) are weighed into a screw-cap tube and mixed with 10 ml of heat-inactivated FCS. This is incubated in the 37°C water bath for 1 hour to produce a saturated solution. The undissolved Luminol is removed by centrifugation and the Luminol–FCS solution filtered through a 0.45-µm Millipore membrane filter.

2. One millilitre of bacterial suspension (e.g., *Salmonella typhimurium*, heat-killed, 10^{10} bacteria/ml) is washed four times in MEM, free of phenol red, to remove any preservative added by the manufacturer. For opsonisation, the bacteria are resuspended in 1 ml of homologous serum, containing specific antibodies. If clumping does not occur, the bacterial suspension is left in the serum for the test. If clumping does occur, the opsonised bacteria must be washed in MEM until they form a smooth suspension.

TABLE A.3

Vial Preparation for Phagocytosis Assay

Tube numbers	FCS (ml)	MEM (ml)	Bacterial suspension (ml)	Leucocytes (ml)
1, 2, 3	0.4	3.4	—	0.2
4, 5, 6	0.4	3.4	0.1	0.2

Tube numbers	FCS– Luminol	MEM (ml)	Bacterial suspension (ml)	Leucocytes (ml)
7, 8, 9	0.4	3.4	—	0.2
10, 11, 12	0.4	3.4	0.1	0.2

3. Neutrophils from the blood or another site, such as the mammary gland, are obtained and suspended at 2.5×10^7 cells/ml in MEM without phenol red. This means that 0.2 ml of the suspension contains 5×10^6 cells. In practice, cells such as macrophages are usually obtained in lower concentration than neutrophils and may have to be diluted to 10^7 cells/ml to carry out the required tests in replicate. Blood neutrophils do not have to be purified because the lymphocytes and monocytes contribute little chemiluminescence compared with the neutrophils. A calculation is made to correct each sample for the variations in total neutrophils, so that samples may be compared.

4. Small (5-ml) scintillation vials are washed and sterilised. The tests are carried out in these vials with the volumes of each component as given in Table A.3.

5. Addition of the opsonised particles is carried out last, and the time of addition is carefully noted. The vials are then measured for chemiluminescence in strict order of addition of the particles at precise intervals of 20 minutes. Shorter time intervals are difficult to accommodate because the number of 1-minute counts on each vial soon overlaps the next reading period.

6. Chemiluminescence is measured as counts per minute (CPM) in the scintillation counter, using the same settings as for [³H]thymidine. The results are drawn on a graph as CPM against time after addition of particles.

References

Allen, R. C. and Loose, L. D. (1976). *Biochem. Biophys. Res. Commun.* **69**, 245–252.

Dog: Angle, M. J. and Klesius, P. H. (1983). *Vet. Immunol. Immunopathol.* **4**, 333–344.

Horse: Washburn, S. M., Klesius, P. H. and Ganjam, V. K. (1982). *Am. J. Vet. Res.* **43,** 1147–1151.

Cow: Weber, L., Peterhans, E. and Wyler, R. (1983). *Vet. Immunol. Immunopathol.* **4,** 397–412.

FREEZING LYMPHOCYTES AND MACROPHAGES FOR STORAGE IN LIQUID NITROGEN

1. Make a solution of 40% (v/v) analytical reagent grade dimethyl sulphoxide (DMSO) in MEM. Another solution is made containing 30% FCS in MEM. One part of DMSO–MEM is to be mixed with three parts of FCS–MEM.

2. Suspend the pellet of cells in FCS–MEM at a maximum of 5×10^7 cells/ml, and add the DMSO–MEM drop by drop, cooling the tube on ice.

3. Rapidly transfer the tubes into specially-made plastic screw-cap (2.0–5.0 ml) vials for liquid nitrogen storage (e.g., Nunc, Roskilde, Norway). It is important to cool the cells evenly from the time of adding the DMSO–MEM, without allowing the cells to warm again.

4. Rapidly transfer the vials to a hollow polystyrene plug which fits snugly into the neck of a liquid nitrogen bottle. An example is the Union Carbide Type BF-S plug which fits into the neck of a Linde liquid nitrogen bottle. Push the polystyrene plug containing the vials into the vapour phase of the liquid nitrogen bottle, and leave overnight to freeze the cells.

5. In the morning, the vials are transferred into the liquid phase of the nitrogen for long-term storage.

6. Thawing of the vials after storage should be as rapid as possible up to 37°C in a water bath with shaking by hand.

7. Rapidly transfer portions of the cell suspension from the vials to sterile centrifuge tubes, mixing the cells gently, using a sterile Pasteur pipette, with 2.5 ml of 20% FCS–MEM warmed to 37°C.

8. Spin the cells into a pellet, and repeat the wash in FCS–MEM five times to remove the DMSO. It is important to reduce rapidly the concentration of DMSO around the cells when they are warmed. The cells can then be counted and used in tissue culture.

PREPARATION OF IMMUNOGLOBULINS BY GEL FILTRATION

The fractionation of serum into broad immunoglobulin classes can be carried out using gel filtration on cross-linked dextran gels, such as Sephadex G200 (Pharmacia, Uppsala, Sweden). The principle of the technique is that proteins >800,000 MW are excluded from the gel, and therefore the first fraction to be eluted contains IgM (MW 1,000,000) but not in a chromatographically-pure form. Both α_2-macroglobulin and the serum lipoproteins elute in this fraction, and antisera prepared in rabbits against this fraction will contain antibodies to these other serum proteins as well as IgM.

The advantage of the Sephadex G200 chromatography is that the distribution of antibody activity in serum between IgM and IgG can be measured with minimum denaturation of the protein. The method can also be used to prepare antiserum to bovine red blood cells for use in the Fc-rosette method described earlier.

Method

1. The dry Sephadex gel is weighed out and mixed with the appropriate amount of PBS according to the column size and the manufacturer's instructions.

2. The gel may be left overnight at 4°C on a magnetic stirrer, or, if speed is necessary, the gel may be boiled, although this has some hazards such as caramelisation of the dextran and the possible concentration of salts by evaporation of the buffer.

3. The gel should be de-gassed before pouring into the column. This is because bubbles may form in the column with variations in ambient temperature, and this can distort protein bands during the run. The de-gassing is carried out in a side-arm flask under vacuum, until no more bubbles appear. The boiling technique of swelling the gel automatically de-gasses the gel.

4. The smaller-sized Sephadex spheres or 'fines' should be removed for the best column flow. This is done by allowing the gel to settle at unit gravity for 1 hour and then removing the upper portion of the buffer. The buffer is replaced and the process repeated until the supernate is clear.

5. The column can be packed using an extension tube and with the column outlet open. The open outlet leads to tighter packing than with the outlet closed. With continued use it is advisable to run the column alternately with ascending or descending flow to keep the gel permeable.

6. Modern columns have nylon nets which are in contact with the top and bottom of the gel bed, and this simplifies sample application, which may be accomplished by merely feeding sample in through the peristaltic pump inlet. If a nylon adapter is not used, the sample should be applied very carefully to the top of the column without disturbing the gel. This can be achieved using a small bent glass tube attached to a glass syringe by plastic tubing, so that the stream of serum protein is directed upwards into the PBS above the gel and settles gently onto the gel surface. The narrower the band of serum applied to the gel, the better the separation of the protein peaks.

7. The column should be run as slowly as possible to obtain good separation of the protein peaks. If possible the gel filtration should be carried out at 4°C in

the cold room, to prevent growth in the column of microorganisms, which may cause denaturation and aggregation of the proteins during the run. Columns are best run at 5 to 10 ml/hour for fine separation.

8. The protein peaks are monitored by a flow-through ultraviolet analyser, or individual fractions can be measured in the spectrophotometer at 280 nm.

9. In examining the fractions for antibody activity, it should be remembered that IgM is more efficient in agglutination tests than IgG and that only a small amount of IgM protein will produce high antibody titres.

10. Fractions may be concentrated by vacuum dialysis against saline or using a controlled-pore membrane (e.g., Amicon Corp.). Some loss of protein by adsorption is inevitable whichever method is used. The ascending sides of the first and second peaks offer the best source of partially-purified IgM and IgG immunoglobulins.

Reference

Anonymous. 'Gel Filtration—Theory and Practice'. Available from Pharmacia Fine Chemicals AB, Box 175, S-751 04, Uppsala, 1, Sweden.

SERUM IMMUNOGLOBULIN CONCENTRATIONS

Table A.4 lists the normal serum immunoglobulin concentrations for selected animals.

References

Curtis, J. and Bourne, F. J. (1971). *Biochim. Biophys. Acta* **236**, 319–332.
Jönsson, A. (1973). *Acta Vet. Scand., Suppl.* No. 43, 1–64.
McGuire, T. C. and Crawford, T. B. (1972). *Infect. Immun.* **6**, 610–615.
Penhale, W. J. and Christie, G. (1969). *Res. Vet. Sci.* **10**, 493–501.
Reynolds, H. Y. and Johnson, J. S. (1970). *J. Immunol.* **105**, 698–703.
Watson, D. L. and Lascelles, A. K. (1973). *Aust. J. Exp. Biol. Med. Sci.* **51**, 247–254.
Williams, M. R., Maxwell, D. A. G. and Spooner, R. L. (1975). *Res. Vet. Sci.* **18**, 314–321.

FLUORESCEIN ISOTHIOCYANATE LABELLING OF IMMUNOGLOBULINS

The globulin fraction of serum is obtained by Sephadex G200 gel filtration or by precipitation three times with ammonium sulphate. This method of labelling immunoglobulin with FITC is used routinely in the CSIRO, McMaster Laboratory, by Mr. G. C. Merritt.

TABLE A.4

Normal Serum Immunoglobulin Concentrations

Animal	IgG	IgM	IgA	References
Sows	13.7	1.9	0.93	Jönsson (1973)
Cows	12.9 (3.4–28.5)[a]	2.8 (1.0–7.2)	—	Penhale and Christie (1969)
Bulls	18.5 (13.3–27.0)	3.3 (1.9–5.0)	—	Penhale and Christie (1969)

Animal	IgG$_1$	IgG$_2$	IgM	IgA	References
Porkers	18.31 ± 0.67[b]	12.41 ± 0.48	3.15 ± 0.19	1.44 ± 0.12	Curtis and Bourne (1971)
Sows	24.33 ± 0.94	14.08 ± 0.49	2.92 ± 0.19	2.37 ± 0.20	Curtis and Bourne (1971)
Cows	9.76 ± 2.59	10.91 ± 4.30	2.71 ± 1.22	0.32 ± 0.16	Williams et al. (1975)
Sheep	18.9 ± 1.5	5.8 ± 0.8	1.9 ± 0.2	0.8 ± 0.3	Watson and Lascelles (1973)
Shetland ponies	13.34 (7.2–19.2)	8.21[c] (2.14–15.0)	1.20 (0.82–2.0)	1.53 (0.6–3.5)	McGuire and Crawford (1972)

Animal	IgGa,b	IgGd	IgGc	IgM	IgA	References
Pure-bred dogs	5.12 (2.6–10.2)	3.00 (0.9–6.2)	1.13 (0.6–2.7)	1.56 (0.7–3.0)	0.83 (0.4–2.4)	Reynolds and Johnson (1970)
Mongrel dogs	7.71 (1.2–14.0)	5.62 (1.0–13.0)	1.12 (0.3–3.0)	1.45 (0.8–2.1)	0.79 (0.3–2.4)	Reynolds and Johnson (1970)

Protein (mg/ml)

[a] Mean is given, followed by range in parentheses.
[b] Mean ± SD.
[c] IgG (T).

Method

1. Dialyse the immunoglobulin against 0.1 M PBS, pH 7.6.
2. Estimate the protein concentration of the fraction and dilute in PBS to 5 to 10 mg/ml.
3. Add two volumes of 0.2 M Na_2HPO_4, pH 9.0–9.2.
4. Weigh out sufficient FITC to achieve a ratio of 3 parts of FITC to 100 parts of protein (w/w), and dissolve the FITC in a minimal amount of PBS.
5. Add the FITC to the protein solution with gentle stirring. Allow the reaction to proceed for 60 to 90 minutes at room temperature (approximately 23°C). It seems important not to attempt labelling for a longer period, if the correct fluorescein : protein (F/P) ratio is to be achieved.
6. Remove the unbound FITC by passing the mixture through a Sephadex G25 column in PBS.
7. Collect the ascending side of the globulin peak separately from the descending side.
8. Check both samples for F:P ratio using the formula:

$$\text{F:P Ratio} = \frac{2.87 \times OD_{495\,nm}}{(OD_{280\,nm} - 0.35) \times OD_{495\,nm}}$$

where OD = optical density
9. The optimum F:P ratio for tissue labelling is 1.5:1 and for sIg is 2:1–4:1.
10. The method has the advantage of speed, since the conjugate can be prepared in 1 day. Storage of conjugates is best with pH adjusted to 8.0–8.3.

SERUM AGGLUTINATION TEST

The serum agglutination test for antibodies to *Listeria monocytogenes* is used as an example, because it demonstrates the need to prepare both the antigen and the serum to produce an interpretable result for some bacterial agglutination tests. The *Listeria* agglutination test is used to measure IgG antibodies, indicative of active infection, without the interference from natural IgM antibodies, which can be depolymerised with 2-mercaptoethanol.

The bacteria themselves are briefly treated with trypsin to expose antigens which have been masked by denatured protein during the heat treatment used to kill the organisms.

Listeria Antigen Preparation

1. *L. monocytogenes* organisms are grown in Tryptose broth for 48 hours at 37°C. The organisms are harvested by centrifugation in stainless-steel centrifuge bottles with screw caps or in a hollow-fibre concentrating apparatus.

2. The organisms are washed twice in normal saline, and killed by steaming for 1 hour. The killed cells are then washed twice again with 0.85% saline.

3. The density of the suspension is adjusted so that it allows 50% transmission at 450 nm in the spectrophotometer.

4. Make up trypsin at 1 mg/ml of phosphate buffer (0.066 M, pH 7.3), and add one part of trypsin solution to nine parts of bacterial cells. Incubate for 30 minutes in a water bath at 37°C, shaking the tube every 10 minutes.

5. Wash the bacteria three times with saline and resuspend them at about 1:50, to give a final adjusted optical density of 50% at 450 nm in the spectrophotometer. Formalin is added to 0.25% to preserve the bacteria. The bacteria can also be left undiluted until just before the agglutination test.

Agglutination Test Procedure

1. Each serum sample is tested as both untreated and 2-mercaptoethanol-treated serum.

2. Dilute each serum sample 1:6.25 with 0.85% saline solution.

3. Dilute 2-mercaptoethanol 1:4 with distilled water and add one drop to 1 ml of the diluted serum. Place stoppers on all the treated serum sample tubes and incubate at 37°C for 30 minutes.

4. Carry out doubling dilutions of treated and untreated serum samples in 0.85% saline using 0.5-ml aliquots in glass tubes.

5. Add 0.5 ml of trypsin-treated killed *Listeria* organisms and shake the tubes to mix the contents.

6. Incubate at 50°C for 2 hours, and then leave in the refrigerator for 48 hours before reading. The agglutinated bacteria form a layer over the bottom of the tube, and the unagglutinated bacteria form a button of bacteria visible when viewed from below.

References

Osebold, J. W. and Aalund, O. (1968). *J. Infect. Dis.* **118**, 139–148.
Osebold, J. W., Aalund, O. and Chrisp, C. E. (1965). *J. Bacteriol.* **89**, 84–88.

THE ENZYME-LINKED IMMUNOSORBENT ASSAY

The enzyme-linked immunosorbent assay (ELISA) system has several advantages over other methods for measuring antibodies in serum samples. The test is almost as sensitive as radioimmunoassay methods, but has no radiation hazards. Both IgG and IgM antibodies to specific antigens can be measured, and the assay lends itself to computer-controlled automation.

Method

1. Obtain or prepare specific antisera to the species immunoglobulin to be assayed (e.g., rabbit anti-sheep IgM or IgG).

2. Fractionate the antiserum by ammonium sulphate precipitation or Sephadex G200 filtration to prepare the globulin fraction.

3. Conjugate the rabbit IgG with horse-radish peroxidase (HRP) using the glutaraldehyde or periodate methods (Voller *et al.*, 1979).

4. Before starting the assay, prepare the substrate, which is 4-aminosalicylic acid, recrystallised in the presence of $Na_2S_2O_5$, dissolved at 1 mg/ml in 0.01 M sodium phosphate buffer pH 5.95 and containing 0.1 M EDTA. Store the substrate at $-20°C$,and add H_2O_2 to a final concentration of 2 mM just before use (Ellens and Gielkens, 1980).

5. Coat the wells in flat-bottomed Microtiter plates with the test antigen by adding the antigen to the wells and leaving overnight. The method for each type of antigen—protein or carbohydrate—varies, and the buffer to be used must be determined from the published methods.

6. Wash the wells three times with PBS containing 0.05% polyoxethylene sorbitan monolaurate (Tween 20) to remove the unbound antigen.

7. Carry out serial, doubling dilutions of test serum in glass tubes using PBS containing 0.05% Tween 20 and 0.25% BSA (w/v).

8. Add 0.1 ml of the diluted serum samples serially to the wells of the antigen-coated plates, and leave at room temperature for 1 hour.

9. Wash the plates three times with the PBS containing 0.05% Tween 20, and add 0.1 ml of HRP-conjugated rabbit IgG anti-sheep immunoglobulin reagent and again leave at room temperature for 1 hour. Wash the wells again three times with the PBS containing 0.05% Tween 20, and then wash the whole plate in 0.15 M NaCl solution to remove any contaminating conjugate which may cause 'spotting'.

10. Add 0.1 ml of substrate to each well, and place the plates on the shaker at room temperature for 30 minutes. The plates may be read by eye or by an automatic plate scanner (e.g., Titertek, Multiskan).

11. The controls on each plate should include a standard antiserum and separate wells containing all the reagents except the test serum. The average optical density at 450 nm of the control wells is subtracted from all readings to calculate the titre.

References

Ellens, D. J. and Gielkens, A. L. J. (1980). *J. Immunol. Methods* **37**, 325–332.
Fahey, K. J., McWaters, P. G., Stewart, D. J., Peterson, J. E. and Clark, B. L. (1983). *Aust. Vet. J.* **60**, 111–116.

Voller, A., Bidwell, D. E. and Bartlett, A. (1979). 'The Enzyme-Linked Immunosorbent Assay (ELISA). A Guide with Abstracts of Microplate Applications'. Available from Dynatech Europe, Borough House, Rue de Pre, Guernsey, G.B.

Wardley, R. C. and Crowther, J. R., eds. (1982). 'The ELISA: Enzyme-Linked Immunosorbent Assay in Veterinary Research and Diagnosis', *Curr. Top. Vet. Med. Anim. Sci.* **22**, 319. Martinus Nijhoff, The Hague, for The Commission of the European Communities.

York, J. J., Fahey, K. J. and Bagust, T. J. (1983). *Avian Dis.* **27**, 409–421.

COMPLEMENT FIXATION TEST

A particular complement fixation (CF) test for antibodies to the sheep intestinal parasite *Trichostrongylus colubriformis* is described here. Although the presence of CF antibodies is not indicative of protective immunity in this case, the test does measure humoral antibody levels reliably and without the consumption of large amounts of scarce antigen.

Method

1. Preparations for the CF test may take 1–2 days before the test because of the need to titrate complement, antigen and haemolysin. However, it is well worth the trouble if large numbers of tests are to be carried out, since the interpretation of the results can be made with confidence.

2. Prepare *T. colubriformis* antigen according to the method of Stewart (1950), by disruption of third-stage parasite larvae.

3. Collect sheep red blood cells (SRBC) in Alsever's solution, and store at 4°C for at least 48 hours before use. Wash the SRBC three times in PBS, and resuspend the SRBC in complement fixation test diluent made from CF test diluent tablets (Oxoid Pty. Ltd.).

4. Adjust the concentration of the SRBC to 6% using a spectrophotometer set at 540 nm. The 6% suspension has an OD of 0.45 with SRBC lysed by 0.01% sodium carbonate solution.

5. Prepare pooled guinea pig serum as a source of complement, filter the serum through a 0.45-μm membrane filter and store at −70°C.

6. Sensitise the 6% SRBC suspension by adding an equal volume of titrated rabbit anti-SRBC (haemolysin). This is done by a chequerboard dilution of 0.025-ml volumes of haemolysin against SRBC and complement (both 0.025-ml volumes) in a round-bottom Microtiter plate. The haemolysin should be diluted 1 : 100–1 : 1000 and the complement 1 : 10–1 : 160, at right angles to each other on the plate. The plates are incubated for 1 hour at 37°C with lids attached, then 3% SRBC are added and the plates shaken to mix the components. The plate is incubated at 37°C for another hour and shaken intermittently. The dilution of

haemolysin chosen is that which gives 100% lysis with the highest dilution of complement.

7. The antigen is then tested for anticomplementary activity by another chequerboard dilution on another plate. The dilutions for antigen and for complement are 0, 1:10, 1:20, 1:30, 1:40, 1:60, 1:80 and 1:120. The plates are incubated for 1 hour at 37°C and SRBC added and allowed to react as before. The dilutions of antigen and complement chosen are those which produce 100% lysis.

8. The final dilution of antigen and complement to be used in the test is chosen by titrating some standard sera of known CF titres with dilutions of antigen and complement at about the optimum titres found in the previous assay. Dilutions of antisera are made and several combinations of antigen and complement dilutions are added. The combination of antigen and complement giving a clear end-point at the known titre is selected. This combination varies from run to run and must be tested each time the test is performed.

9. Tests with unknown sera are carried out in Microtiter plates. Each component is added as a 0.025-ml volume with the final total volume being 0.1 ml/well. Doubling dilutions of sera are carried out in 0.025 ml of CFT diluent using microtitration loops. There are automated systems, such as the Titertek Motorised Dispenser, which allow rapid dilution of large numbers of sera. One volume of diluted antigen is added, then one volume of diluted complement and the plate shaken, then incubated at 37°C for 1 hour with cover on. Then one volume of sensitised SRBC is added and the plates covered, shaken and incubated as before.

10. The results are read after the unlysed SRBC have settled into a pellet. The end-point is taken as 50% lysis of the SRBC. A plate-reader which illuminates the plate from below is a useful aid for reading the plates.

References

Stewart, D. F. (1950). *Aust. J. Agric. Res.* **1**, 285–300.
Windon, R. G. and Dineen, J. K. (1981). *Int. J. Parasitol.* **11**, 11–18.

ANTIGENS AND ADJUVANTS

The antigens which have commonly been used for immunological studies in mice and rats include keyhole limpet haemocyanin (KLH) and the chemically-synthesised polypeptides (e.g., poly-L-lysine). These antigens are generally not suitable for extensive studies in the larger animals because of the expense involved. Therefore, basic immunological studies in domestic animals are limited to antigens which are cheap and readily available.

Such antigens include killed bacterial vaccines to which animals have little or no antibody titres. For obvious reasons, SRBC are not used in ruminants, but CRBC are sufficiently antigenic to be used successfully as antigens in these species. Soluble antigens such as ovalbumen, egg lysozyme and BSA have been used successfully in domestic mammals. The formation of haptens between BSA and dinitrophenyl (DNP) salts has proved useful in ruminants, since the DNP–BSA hapten is far more antigenic than BSA alone.

Delayed hypersensitivity can be induced to tuberculin PPD with BCG vaccine, but cattle so sensitised must be classified as tuberculin reactors when they go to slaughter. Dinitrofluorobenzene (DNFB) has been used successfully in pigs to induce delayed hypersensitivity in skin by direct application.

Enhancement of the immune response usually involves the use of precipitated alum adjuvants. Greater stimulation may be achieved with Freund's complete or incomplete adjuvants, but since these are oil-based, the reaction they produce is

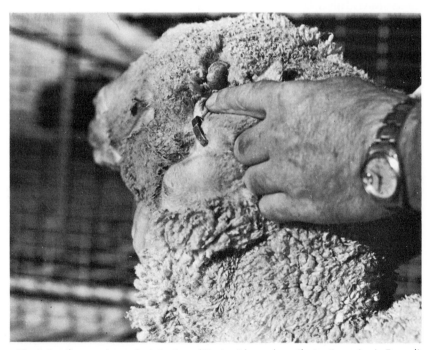

Fig. A.3.   The reaction to the injection of *Bacteroides nodosus* (foot-rot) vaccine in Freund's complete adjuvant is shown beneath the left ear of a sheep. A large subcutaneous abscess has formed which may ultimately break open and discharge into the wool. Although the antibody titres to the vaccine are greatly boosted by the adjuvant, the reaction site is unacceptable for both practical and aesthetic reasons. (Reproduced by kind permission of Dr. D. J. Stewart, CSIRO, Division of Animal Health.)

often unacceptable from an economic, as well as an aesthetic point of view (Fig. A.3). Horses, in particular, react adversely to oily adjuvants, but sheep, cattle and pigs may all react with unsightly granulomas which detract from carcass quality.

The use of the newer synthetic adjuvants such as muramyl dipeptide (MDP) and polyadenylic : polyuridylic acid (poly-A : U) complexes is precluded in large animals because of the expense involved. There remains a great need to develop, for use in domestic animals, cheap, effective adjuvants which present minimal problems with tissue reaction.

Reference

Adjuvants: Osebold, J. W. (1982). *J. Am. Vet. Med. Assoc.* **181,** 983–987.

CROSS-MATCHING OF BLOOD

The cross-matching of blood samples for both dog and cat is carried out by mixing serum and red cells in tubes or on slides, with appropriate controls. Plasma or serum is obtained from both donor and recipient. One method, described for the cat by Auer and Bell, is as follows:

1. Collect blood from donor and recipient using heparin or EDTA anticoagulant. Separate the plasma from the red cells by spinning the blood at 2000 g for 10 minutes or by allowing the samples to stand for at least 30 minutes.

2. Set up four tubes: (a) donor plasma, (b) recipient plasma, (c) a 4% suspension of donor red cells (0.2 ml of red cells plus 4.8 ml of saline), and (d) a 4% suspension of recipient red cells.

3. Set up four slides as follows: slide (1) one drop donor plasma plus one drop donor red cells, slide (2) one drop recipient plasma plus one drop recipient red cells, slide (3) one drop donor plasma plus one drop recipient red cells, and slide (4) one drop recipient plasma plus one drop donor red cells.

4. Rock the slides gently from side to side.

5. Look for agglutination in slides (3) and (4) and compare them with slides (1) and (2), which should be negative controls. Only anti-A will be visible in cats, because anti-B is too weak to be visible by eye. Therefore a group B recipient would probably be positive for slide (4) with a group A donor but be negative for slide (3). If either slide (3) or slide (4) is positive, the donor and recipient are incompatible.

Reference

Auer, L. and Bell, K. (1981). *Anim. Blood. Groups Biochem. Genet.* **12,** 287–297.

THE TWO-STEP MICROCYTOTOXICITY TEST ACCORDING TO TERASAKI

1. Prepare lymphocytes from fresh blood samples using Ficoll-Paque, and resuspend the cells in MEM at 2×10^6 cells/ml.

2. Prepare 60-well Microtest plates (e.g., Nunc, Roskilde, Norway) by filling each well with light mineral oil.

3. Dispense 1 μl of test serum per well using a microsyringe with a repeating dispenser (Hamilton Co., Nevada) as a microdroplet under oil. This is done to prevent evaporation of the serum.

4. Dispense 1 μl of test lymphocyte suspension into each serum droplet so that they mix, and leave the plates at room temperature for 30 minutes.

5. Into each well, dispense 5 μl of mixed serum complement from several young rabbits, which have been screened so that their sera do not contain natural antibodies to sheep lymphocytes. Leave the plates at room temperature for a further 60 minutes.

6. Dispense 5 μl of aqueous eosin Y, which has been filtered before use, into each well.

7. After 2 minutes, dispense 5 μl of neutral, filtered 30–40% formalin, pH 7.2–7.4, into each well.

8. Leave the cells to settle overnight at 4°C before reading the plates.

9. Read the plates on an inverted microscope using phase-contrast optics. The living cells appear small, bright and refractile. The dead cells appear large, dark and non-refractile.

10. A scale of cytotoxicity is set up with five levels of cell killing, where 0 = Not tested or not readable; 1 = Negative (0–10% stained); 2 = Doubtful negative (11–20% stained); 4 = Doubtful positive (21–40% stained); 6 = Positive (41–80% stained); 8 = Strongly positive (81–100% stained).

Glossary

Activation—Usually refers to macrophages with enhanced metabolic activity due to antigenic stimulation

Adjuvant—A substance added to vaccines which boosts antibody production in the recipient

Affinity—The force of attraction between antibody and antigen

Agglutination—The formation of clumps of bacteria or particulate antigens after cross-linking by antibody

Allergy—The altered reaction of the body to a substance as the result of an immune response

Allo-antibodies—Antibodies to tissues of unrelated individuals of the same species

Allogeneic—Genetic dissimilarity between unrelated individuals of the same species

Allograft—A tissue graft between unrelated individuals of the same species; homograft

Allotype—A distinct genetic type recognized in some individuals of a species

Anaphylaxis—A state of acute hypersensitivity induced by parenteral injection or ingestion of antigen and elicited by a second small dose of antigen 1–2 weeks later

Anergy—The lack of expected allergic response to antigen (e.g., in tuberculosis of cattle)

Anti-idiotype—Antibodies to immunoglobulin molecules of a cell clone in an individual of a species

Antibody—An immunoglobulin protein molecule with the capacity to bind with specific antigen as the result of a specific immune response

Antigen—A substance which stimulates production of antibody or sensitized cells during an immune response

Antitoxin—Antibodies which neutralize a harmful toxin

Arthus reaction—Local oedematous reaction which follows the blockage of fine capillaries by antigen–antibody complexes and circulating leucocytes during a Type III hypersensitivity reaction

Autoimmunity—The immune response to self

Autologous—Derived from the same individual

Bence–Jones protein—Immunoglobulin light chains which pass across the glomeruli of the kidney and are found in the urine of individuals with myelomatous tumours

259

Blast cell—A large cell derived from an antigen or mitogen-stimulated lymphocyte and which is synthesizing DNA in preparation for cell division

Capping—The coalescence of patches of lymphocyte membrane proteins cross-linked *in vitro* by fluorescent antibodies

Chemiluminescence—A chemical reaction in phagocytosing leucocytes which results in the production of photons

Chemotaxis—Attraction of leucocytes towards or repulsion from an increasing concentration of chemical substances released during an inflammatory response

Chimaera—An organism consisting of two genetically distinct cell types

E-rosette—A cluster of five or more sheep erythrocytes attached to a T-cell after resuspension of the pellet of lymphocytes and erythrocytes in an *in vitro* test

Endotoxin—A lipopolysaccharide extracted from the cell walls of gram-negative bacteria

Flocculation—Formation of floccules or clumps in suspensions of substances such as antigen-coated bentonite particles, cross-linked by specific antibody

Freemartin—An intersexual female calf with a genetically distinct male twin, both of which share circulating blood cells derived from each other by fused placental circulation *in utero*

Gamma globulin—A serum globulin with antibody activity which moves slowly on electrophoresis

Genetic restriction—The inability of lymphocytes of one histocompatibility type to interact in immune responses with cells of another histocompatibility type

Globulins—Serum proteins of neutral or positive charge during electrophoresis which separates them into α-, β- and γ-regions.

Haemagglutination—Agglutination of erythrocytes caused by cross-linking with specific antibodies or by adsorption of certain viruses

Haplotype—The type of one parent contributed to the offspring as a single set of unpaired chromosomes; also used in reference to MHC antigens contributed by either parent

Hapten—A small non-protein molecule, which must be combined with a larger protein carrier to be antigenic

Heavy chain—A polypeptide chain present in immunoglobulin molecules which differentiates each immunoglobulin class. It has a variable and constant region and is linked to a light chain by disulphide bonds

Heterologous—Derived from a different species

Hinge region—The point of divergence of the two arms of the IgG molecule

Histocompatibility—Usually refers to isoantigens present in the cell membranes of all nucleated cells which are capable of eliciting an immune response leading to graft rejection after tissue transplantation

Homocytotropic—Usually refers to IgE antibody which attaches to mast cells of individuals of the same species but not those of other species

Homologous—Derived from the same species

Hybridoma—A hybrid cell formed by the fusion of a myeloma cell and a specific antibody-forming cell

Hypersensitivity—An altered reaction to an antigen as a result of previous contact with the antigen

Ia antigen—Alloantigen found in the cell membrane of mouse B lymphocytes and which is under the control of the H-2 locus

Idiotype—Refers to individual immunoglobulin molecules which vary in amino-acid sequence as the result of reassortment of the controlling genes

Immunogenic—Refers to a substance capable of inducing an immune response, which is often protective

Immunoglobulin—Serum proteins made up of light and heavy polypeptide chains and divisible into classes, which contain within them antibody activities towards a wide range of antigens

Inoculation—Introduction of an antigen or substance into the body by any route but usually by parenteral means

Interferon—A polypeptide released by virus-infected cells or by transforming lymphocytes which inhibits replication of the virus

Interleukin—A molecule released by a lymphocyte or macrophage which regulates the proliferation of lymphoid cells during the immune response

Iso-antibody—Antibody to antigens of the same species

Isologous—Derived from the same species

Isotype—A genetic type recognized in some individuals of a species

J-chain—Joining polypeptide chain which binds the five monomers of IgM together

K (killer)-cell—Circulating lymphocyte with Fc receptors for IgG and which is cytotoxic for antibody coated target cells

Light chain—A polypeptide chain common to all immunoglobulin classes which has a variable and constant region and is linked to a heavy chain by a disulphide bond

Lymphocyte determined (LD)—Refers to lymphocyte antigens measured by a mixed lymphocyte reaction. It has been replaced by the term class II antigens

Lymphokine—A non-immunoglobulin molecule released by lymphocytes during antigenic or mitogenic stimulation and which in turn has effects on other lymphoid cells in a non-immunological reaction

Microcytotoxicity test—A cytotoxicity test read by microscope and used for detecting antibodies to lymphocyte antigens in MHC typing

Mitogen—Substance which stimulates cell division

Monoclonal—Refers to antibodies produced by a single line of hybridoma cells all directed towards one antigen specificity

Myeloma—Neoplastic proliferation of plasma cells which produce large amounts of immunoglobulin of identical type

Myelopathy—Any disease of the spinal cord or myeloid tissues

Natural-killer (NK) Cells—A subpopulation of T-cells which have no receptors for IgG but which are cytotoxic for virus-infected target cells

Neutralization—A test in which antibody neutralizes the biological effects of a virus or toxin

Null Cells—Cells not recognized by any lymphocyte membrane marker test

Opsonins—Components of serum, such as antibody or complement, which attach to particles and promote their phagocytosis by leucocytes

Paraprotein—Immunoglobulin produced by a myeloma and seen as a sharply defined band on serum electrophoresis

Peyer's Patch—Aggregation of lymphoid cells found in the submucosa of the lower end of the ileum

Phagocytosis—The process of engulfment of particles by cells

Pinocytosis—Selective uptake of fluid into cytoplasmic vesicles by cells

Plasma cell—Antibody-producing cell derived from a B-cell

Polymorphism—The existence of two or more different forms of individuals in the same species

Precipitation—The formation of a visible precipitate between soluble antigen and antibody usually in agar gel or between a serum overlay and antigen in a tube

Properdin—A globulin component of serum which activates complement via the alternative pathway but which is not an immunoglobulin

Prozone—Inhibition of antigen–antibody reactions by high concentrations of serum containing excess or blocking antibodies. The serum may be diluted, and the normal reaction reappears

Purified Protein Derivative (PPD)—A tuberculin derived from heat-killed *Mycobacterium tuberculosis* and capable of eliciting a delayed hypersensitivity response when injected intradermally into animals with tuberculosis

Pyroninophilic—Cells, such as plasma cells, with a high RNA content and which may be stained with Pyronin Y

Reaginic antibody—Immunoglobulin of the IgE or IgG subclass which is characterized by reaction with allergens to elicit an immediate or Type I hypersensitivity

Receptor—A cell membrane component which specifically binds biologically active molecules

Rosette—A cluster of five or more erythrocytes attached to a lymphocyte in an *in vitro* test

Secretory component—A protein bound to IgA which promotes its secretion across epithelial cells of mucous membranes or of liver cells

Self-cure—Type I hypersensitivity reaction to parasite larvae in the small intestine of sheep which promotes expulsion of adult intestinal parasites

Sensitivity—The ability of a test to give a positive result in an individual which has the disease under investigation

Sensitization—Administration of antigen into an individual to provoke a primary response. This may be boosted into a strong secondary immune response by a subsequent injection of antigen

Sero-conversion—A term used to describe the appearance of antibodies to virus in animals not normally exposed to the virus. Used as a measure of spread of virus disease in previously unexposed populations

Serologically determined (SD)—Refers to lymphocyte antigens measured by microcytotoxicity test. It has been replaced by the term class I antigens

Specificity—The ability of a test to give a negative result in an individual which does not have the disease under investigation

Stimulation—Refers to the early contact of macrophages with antigen, which causes these cells to become activated

Thymectomy—Surgical removal of the thymus

Titre—A measure of antibody levels in serum; usually done by doubling dilution to a 50% end point

Tolerance—The failure of an individual to respond to antigenic stimulation with a normal immune response

Toxoid—Chemically inactivated bacterial toxin which can still stimulate production of protective antibodies in the recipient

Variable region—The antigen combining site on an immunoglobulin molecule consisting of a variable part of the heavy chain and a variable part of the light chain

Wasting syndrome—Weight loss and disease susceptibility in mice after neonatal thymectomy

Index

Italic page numbers indicate that the page reference is to a figure, and boldfaced page numbers indicate that the page reference is to a table.

270 Index

Genes (*cont.*)
Class III lymphocyte antigens, 208
generation of diversity, 6, 85
immunoglobulin, 85
J (joining) segment, 85
transplantation antigens, 203
transposition of V region, *86*
μ-chain switch, 50, 86, *87*
V region, 85, *86, 87*
C region, 85, *86, 87*
Genetically-engineered vaccines
Babesia bigemina, 198
Escherichia coli in pigs, 17, 144
Foot-and-Mouth disease, 17, 157
identification of antigens, 18
Genetic resistance
BoLA antigens, 194, 222
B21 in chickens, 153, 220
cattle tick, 191, 193, 222
Marek's disease, 157, 220, 221
OLA antigens, 181–182
transplantation antigens, 205, 219
Trichostrongylus colubriformis, 221, 222
Genetic restriction
domestic species, 153
Lymphochoriomeningitis (LCM) virus, 152, 153, *153,* 205
Theileriosis of cattle, 196
Genetic selection
Boophilus microplus in cattle, 222
cattle, 182, 222
chicken, 220, 221
Cooperia oncophora, 182
guinea pig, 182, 221
Haemonchosis, 180
haemoglobin type, 180, 181
high- and low-responder lambs, 18, 181
Marek's disease of chickens, 220
predictive marker, 18
Salmonella pullorum in chickens, 220
sheep, 18, 180, 181, *181*
Trichinella spiralis in mice, 182
Trichostrongylus colubriformis, 18, 180, 181, 221
Globulin
α, β and γ, 67
β-lactoglobulin in calf urine, 55
β2-microglobulin, 203, *204*
chicken, 210
pig, 212
cow, 213

intestinal absorption of globulin, 54–56, *55*
transmission of γ-globulin across placenta, 53
Goat lymphocyte antigens (GLA), 214
Graft rejection
bone marrow transplant, 212
B-locus in chickens, 209
Canine Venereal Sarcoma, 211
DLA, 210, *211*
foetal lambs, 4, 48, 59
freemartin calves, 59
Grey Collie syndrome, 211
H-2 locus in mice, 205
MHC antigens, 60, 208–214
MLR, 60
production of MHC antisera, 214–216
reciprocal skin grafts, 215
site effect with skin, 60
Grey Collie syndrome
bone marrow transplant as cure, 211

H

[³H]thymidine uptake, *see* Tritiated thymidine uptake
Haemolytic disease
Babesia vaccines, 198, 219
colostral antibodies, 60, 61
dogs, 60
foetal–maternal incompatibility, 61
horses, 217, 219
neonatal isoerythrolysis, 219
pigs, 219
prevention, 60, 217, 219
protozoal diseases, 186
ruminants, 61
Type II hypersensitivity, 186
Heavy chains
antigenic differences between immunoglobulins, 76
canine myeloma sequence, 71
genes, 85, 86
homology between cat, dog and human, 71
molecular weight, 73
structure, *71*
μ-chain switch, 86, *87*
variable regions, *71*
Helper T-cells
collaboration with B-cells, 31